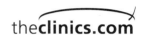

CLINICS IN GERIATRIC MEDICINE

Geriatric Rehabilitation

GUEST EDITOR
Adrian Cristian, MD, FAAPMR

May 2006 • Volume 22 • Number 2

SAUNDERS

An Imprint of Elsevier, Inc.
PHILADELPHIA   LONDON   TORONTO   MONTREAL   SYDNEY   TOKYO

W.B. SAUNDERS COMPANY
A Division of Elsevier Inc.

Elsevier, Inc. • 1600 John F. Kennedy Blvd., Suite 1800 • Philadelphia, PA 19103-2899

http://www.theclinics.com

CLINICS IN GERIATRIC MEDICINE	Volume 22, Number 2
May 2006	ISSN 0749-0690
Editor: Maria Lorusso	ISBN 1-4160-3501-X

Clinics in Geriatric Medicine (ISSN 0749-0690) is published quarterly by W.B. Saunders, 360 Park Avenue South, New York, NY 10010-1710. Months of publication are February, May, August, and November. Business and editorial offices: Elsevier, Inc. 1600 John F. Kennedy Blvd., Suite 1800, Philadelphia, PA 19103-2899. Accounting and circulation offices: 6277 Sea Harbor Drive, Orlando, FL 32887-4800. Periodicals postage paid at New York, NY, and additional mailing offices. Subscription price is $165.00 per year (US individuals), $275.00 per year (US institutions), $215.00 per year (Canadian individuals), $335.00 per year (Canadian institutions), $215.00 per year (foreign individuals), and $335.00 per year (foreign institutions). Foreign air speed delivery is included in all *Clinics* subscription prices. All prices are subject to change without notice. POSTMASTER: Send address changes to *Clinics in Geriatric Medicine* Elsevier Periodicals Customer Service, 6277 Sea Harbor Drive, Orlando, FL 32887-4800. **Customer Service: 1-800-654-2452 (US). From outside of the US, call 1-407-345-4000. E-mail:hhspcs@wbsaunders.com.**

Clinics in Geriatric Medicine is covered in *Index Medicus, EMBASE/Excerpta Medica, Current Contents/Clinical Medicine (CC/CM), and the Cumulative Index to Nursing & Allied Health Literature.*

Printed in the United States of America.

GUEST EDITOR

ADRIAN CRISTIAN, MD, FAAPMR, Chief, Department of Rehabilitation Medicine, James J. Peters Veterans Affairs Medical Center, Bronx; Assistant Professor, Department of Rehabilitation Medicine, Mount Sinai School of Medicine, New York, New York

CONTRIBUTORS

URI ADLER, MD, Director of Stroke Services, Kessler Institute for Rehabilitation, Saddle Brook; Assistant Professor, Department of Physical Medicine and Rehabilitation, University of Medicine and Dentistry, New Jersey Medical School, Newark, New Jersey

ANNE F. AMBROSE, MD, Instructor, Department of Rehabilitation Medicine, Mount Sinai School of Medicine, New York, New York

JULIET ASHLEY, MS, CCC-SLP, Speech-Language Pathologist, James J. Peters Veterans Affairs Medical Center, Bronx, New York

JONATHAN F. BEAN, MD, Assistant Professor, Spaulding Cambridge Outpatient Center, Cambridge, Massachusetts

ADRIAN CRISTIAN, MD, FAAPMR, Chief, Department of Rehabilitation Medicine, James J. Peters Veterans Affairs Medical Center, Bronx; Assistant Professor, Department of Rehabilitation Medicine, Mount Sinai School of Medicine, New York, New York

CATHY M. CRUISE, MD, Clinical Assistant Professor, Department of Rehabilitation Medicine, Rusk Institute of Rehabilitation, New York University School of Medicine, New York; Physiatrist, Veterans Integrated Service Network #3, Northport Veterans Affairs Medical Center, Northport, New York

TEINA DALEY, OTR/L, Chief Occupational Therapist, Clinical Specialist, Department of Rehabilitation Medicine, James J. Peters Veterans Affairs Medical Center, Bronx, New York

MICKEY DUGGAN, MS, CCC-SLP, Senior Speech-Language Pathologist, James J. Peters Veterans Affairs Medical Center, Bronx, New York

STEVEN R. FLANAGAN, MD, Associate Professor, Department of Rehabilitation Medicine, Mount Sinai School of Medicine, New York, New York

MAUREEN FITZPATRICK, OTR, Clinical Specialist, James J. Peters Veterans Affairs Medical Center, Bronx, New York

JASON E. FRANKEL, MD, Instructor and Physiatrist, Department of Physical Medicine and Rehabilitation, New England Sinai Hospital, Stoughton; Tufts New England Medical Center, Boston, Massachusetts

WALTER R. FRONTERA, MD, PhD, Professor and Chairman, Department of Physical Medicine and Rehabilitation, Harvard Medical School/Spaulding Rehabilitation Hospital, Boston, Massachusetts

WAYNE A. GORDON, PhD, Professor, Department of Rehabilitation Medicine, Mount Sinai School of Medicine, New York, New York

EVELYN S. HALEY, PT, Lead Therapist, Spinal Cord Injury Unit, James J. Peters Veterans Affairs Medical Center, Bronx, New York

MARY R. HIBBARD, PhD, Professor, Department of Rehabilitation Medicine, Mount Sinai School of Medicine, New York, New York

JOSEPH M. LANE, MD, Attending Orthopedist, Hospital for Special Surgery, New York; Professor, Department of Orthopedic Surgery, Weill Medical College of Cornell University, New York, New York

MATHEW H.M. LEE, MD, Howard A. Rusk Professor and Chair, Department of Rehabilitation, Rusk Institute of Rehabilitation, New York University School of Medicine, New York, New York

JULIE T. LIN, MD, Assistant Attending Physiatrist, Hospital for Special Surgery, New York; Assistant Professor, Department of Rehabilitation Medicine, Weill Medical College of Cornell University, New York, New York

CYNTHIA MACALUSO, PT, Clinical Specialist, Kessler Institute for Rehabilitation, Saddle Brook, New Jersey

DANIEL E. MACDONALD, DMD, MSD, FAGD, Assistant Clinical Professor, Division of Periodontology, Columbia University College of Dental Medicine, New York; Associate Research Scientist, Columbia University Fu School of Graduate Engineering, New York; Associate Research Scientist, Hospital for Special Surgery, New York, New York; and Director, Spinal Cord Injury Dental Service, James J. Peters VA Medical Center, Bronx, New York

BRITTANY A. MATSUMURA, MD, Clinical Instructor, Department of Rehabilitation Medicine, Mount Sinai School of Medicine, New York, New York

SHAILESH PARIKH, MD, Director, Amputee Rehabilitation, Kessler Institute for Rehabilitation, Saddle Brook; Assistant Professor, Department of Physical Medicine and Rehabilitation, University of Medicine and Dentistry, New Jersey Medical School, Newark, New Jersey

DANIELLE MARIE PERRET, MD, Department of Rehabilitation Medicine, The Mount Sinai Medical Center, New York, New York

BRUCE POMERANZ, MD, Medical Director, Kessler Institute for Rehabilitation, Saddle Brook; Assistant Professor, Department of Physical Medicine and Rehabilitation, University of Medicine and Dentistry, New Jersey Medical School, Newark, New Jersey

SHANA RICHARDS, MPT, Staff Physical Therapist, Department of Rehabilitation Medicine, James J. Peters Veterans Affairs Medical Center, Bronx, New York

BRIAN RIORDAN, MD, Chief Resident, Department of Rehabilitation Medicine, Mount Sinai School of Medicine, New York, New York

JOSEPHINE RIM, MD, Department of Anesthesiology, The State University of New York Health Sciences Center at Brooklyn, Brooklyn, New York

TIMOTHY P. SABOL, PT, DPT, CSCS, Senior Physical Therapist, Spinal Cord Injury Unit, James J. Peters Veterans Affairs Medical Center, Bronx, New York

NICOLE SASSON, MD, Clinical Assistant Professor of Rehabilitation Medicine, Rusk Institute of Rehabilitation, New York University School of Medicine; Chief, Physical Medicine and Rehabilitation Service, Department of Veterans Affairs, New York Harbor Healthcare System, New York, New York

MONIKA V. SHAH, DO, Assistant Professor, Department of Physical Medicine and Rehabilitation; Attending Physician, Traumatic Brain Injury and Stroke Program, The Institute for Rehabilitation and Research; Director, Long-Term Acute Care Brain Injury Program, Kindred Hospital, Baylor College of Medicine, Houston, Texas

NIGEL SHENOY, MD, Resident, Department of Physical Medicine and Rehabilitation, University of Medicine and Dentistry, New Jersey Medical School, Newark, New Jersey

MICHELLE STERN, MD, Assistant Professor, Department of Clinical Rehabilitation Medicine, Columbia University College of Physician and Surgeons, New York, New York

NATALIE SUTCLIFFE, MS, CCC-SLP, Director of Extended Care, James J. Peters Veterans Affairs Medical Center, Bronx, New York

CONTENTS

As the population of older adults increases, so does the number of people aging with a disability. It is more important than ever that clinicians caring for these individuals ask appropriate questions and focus on key areas of the physical examination that are pertinent to the care of this population. This article is meant to provide clinicians with a framework for evaluating the older adult aging with a physical disability in a clinic or hospital setting.

Exercise programs for elderly patients have received much attention recently for their potential role in preventing illness and injury, limiting functional loss and disability, and alleviating the course and symptoms of existing cardiac, pulmonary, and metabolic disorders. The basic components of an exercise training program include strength, endurance, balance, and flexibility. This article reviews the main attributes of each, along with some of the most recent research defining their roles in health care. Where available, it discusses specific recommendations for prescribing exercise modalities. Finally, it presents suggestions for developing integrated exercise programs and enhancing patient compliance.

Rehabilitation of the Older Adult with Stroke 469

Monika V. Shah

Stroke is an increasing public health concern throughout the world as the leading cause of long-term disability. It is well known that there exist differences related to epidemiology, pathophysiology, comorbidity, and functional outcome of stroke patients with advanced age compared with the young. Factors that have been suggested to influence this disparity include age-related complications, availability of resources, lack of aggressive management, and possible diminished capacity for neuroplasticity. This article reviews the current medical and rehabilitative aspects of stroke and the possible disparities related to advanced age.

FORTHCOMING ISSUES

PREVIOUS ISSUES

ELSEVIER
SAUNDERS

Clin Geriatr Med 22 (2006) xiii–xiv

CLINICS IN
GERIATRIC
MEDICINE

Preface

Geriatric Rehabilitation

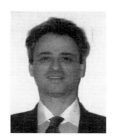

Adrian Cristian, MD, FAAPMR
Guest Editor

Because of advances in health care, Americans are living longer lives. Whereas many individuals have successful and productive later stages in life, a significant number face functional losses secondary to declining health.

The older adult often faces multiple medical problems such as hypertension, diabetes, coronary artery disease, and pain. Superimposed on these diagnoses may be life-altering events such as stroke or amputation. The end results of the combined effects of these conditions are often limited mobility, sedentary lifestyle, increased dependence on others, and a functional decline.

Rehabilitation has a very important role in the care of the older adult living with one or more disabilities. The cornerstone of geriatric rehabilitation is the holistic multidisciplinary approach to the restoration and preservation of function.

This is accomplished through the use of exercises to improve range of motion, strength and endurance; various modalities such as heat, cold, and electrical stimulation for the management of pain; orthotics and prostheses for the improvement of ambulation; adaptive equipment and mobility devices for maximizing function.

The rehabilitation of the older adult is often challenging due to the combination of disease-associated impairments superimposed on normal age-related changes. Cardiac, pulmonary, and weight-bearing precautions have to be monitored during treatment sessions. Progress is often measured in small increments and goals may need prolonged periods of time for completion. A frag-

0749-0690/06/$ – see front matter © 2006 Elsevier Inc. All rights reserved.
doi:10.1016/j.cger.2006.01.001   *geriatric.theclinics.com*

mented social support system, aging caregivers, limited finances, or access to transportation pose additional barriers.

The goal of this issue of the *Clinics in Geriatric Medicine* is to provide geriatricians with practical knowledge that is pertinent to the rehabilitation of the older adult. The first section addresses the basic elements of geriatric rehabilitation-the physiatric assessment of the older adult, the exercise prescription and measurement of outcomes. The second section describes physical, occupational therapy, speech and swallowing disorders, neurogenic bowel and bladder, physical modalities for pain management, mobility devices, prosthetics & orthotics, and balance impairments. The last section focuses on the rehabilitation of impairments often encountered by clinicians—osteoporotic fractures, stroke, and traumatic brain injury. An article on the dental issues facing older adults with physical and cognitive impairments is also included.

Successful aging requires astute, timely, and appropriate observations and interventions on the part of clinicians. It is the hope of this issue to provide some of the knowledge base to help make this possible.

I would like to thank the contributors, who work at various rehabilitation centers around the United States for their contributions as well as to my family and patients for their support and inspiration.

Adrian Cristian, MD, FAAPMR
Department of Rehabilitation Medicine
Room 3D-16
James J. Peters Veterans Affairs Medical Center
130 W. Kingsbridge Road
Bronx, NY 10468, USA
E-mail address: acristianmd@msn.com

CLINICS IN
GERIATRIC
MEDICINE

Clin Geriatr Med 22 (2006) 221–238

The Assessment of the Older Adult with a Physical Disability: A Guide for Clinicians

Adrian Cristian, MD[a,b,*]

[a]Department of Rehabilitation Medicine, Mount Sinai School of Medicine,
One Gustave L. Levy Place, NY 10029, USA
[b]Department of Rehabilitation Medicine, Room 3D-16, 526/117,
James J. Peters Veterans Affairs Medical Center, 130 West Kingsbridge Road, Bronx, NY 10468, USA

According to the United States census conducted in 2000, there are more than 33 million noninstitutionalized Americans older than 65. Of these older Americans, 28.8% reported living with a physical disability and 9.6% reported a self-care disability [1]. According to the National Aging Information Center, 2,192,563 Americans have both a mobility and a self-care limitation. These numbers rise considerably in the 85-plus age group, with 49.8% of people reporting a self-care or a mobility limitation or both [2].

Given these staggering numbers, it is imperative that clinicians caring for this older, frailer population be able to perform a comprehensive medical and psychosocial assessment that adequately addresses its needs and limitations.

The goal of this article is to provide clinicians with descriptions of some of the key elements of the history and physical examination as they pertain to the older adult living with a physical disability.

Disability history

The traditional elements of the medical history include sections on chief complaint, history of present illness, past medical and surgical history, allergies, medications, review of systems, and social history. Many of the issues facing the older adult with a physical disability may be adequately covered in one or more

---

* Department of Rehabilitation Medicine, James J. Peters Veterans Affairs Medical Center, 3D-16, 526/117, 130 West Kingsbridge Road, Bronx, NY 10468.

E-mail address: acristianmd@msn.com

0749-0690/06/$ – see front matter © 2006 Elsevier Inc. All rights reserved.
doi:10.1016/j.cger.2005.12.001

of these sections. However, it is advisable to consider adding a new section to the medical history, entitled "Disability history," because there are certain issues that are common and yet unique to this population. These issues deserve special attention, because they may have a considerable impact on an individual's functionality. This section could be divided into three broad categories: (1) Disability-related symptoms, (2) Mobility and adaptive equipment issues, and (3) Disability-related psychosocial issues.

Disability-related symptoms include impaired communication and swallowing, pain, fatigue, impaired sleep, impaired sexuality, impaired bowel or bladder function, and spasticity. Mobility and adaptive equipment issues include lower limb orthotics, lower limb prosthetics, wheelchairs, ambulation aids (eg, walkers, crutches), and adaptive equipment in the home. Disability-related psychosocial issues include depression, aging caregivers, gaps in care, and limited finances.

In obtaining the disability history, it is important to establish a chronology of the various problems from time of onset of the disability. Key points include when and how the disability started and key moments when there was a change in the person's functionality as a result of the disability. Attempts to limit the disability or improve function should be noted, as well as their level of success. The following sections provide an overview of some of the key elements of the disability history.

Disability-related symptoms

Communication and swallowing

Inability to communicate can lead to social isolation, as well as difficulties in providing information to caregivers about needs or symptoms. Impaired swallowing may lead to poor nutritional intake and aspiration pneumonia. The clinician caring for the older adult with a physical disability should ask both the patient and the primary caregiver about both the intelligibility of speech and the effectiveness of communication. Does the patient use a communication device? If so, how effective is it? Has the patient received speech therapy and, if so, how effective was it? If the patient stopped attending speech therapy, what was the reason for the discontinuation (eg, a recent move to an area with limited access to speech therapy services)?

Some key questions to assess problems with swallowing are, Does the food get "stuck in the throat"? Which food consistencies are most difficult to swallow (eg, meat, thin liquids)? Does the patient cough after ingesting food or water? The caregiver should be asked about a "wet or gurgling" quality to the patient's speech, pocketing of food in the cheeks, or excessive drooling. It is also important to ask about loss of weight or reduced appetite to assess for decreased nutritional intake. Finally, has the patient had a recent swallowing evaluation?

Pain

Pain is common in older adults with physical disabilities and may be multifactorial in origin [3]. Musculoskeletal and neuropathic pains are particularly common. It is therefore important for the clinician to ask questions about the presence of pain. Once one has determined that pain is present, one should ascertain the pain's location, quality, duration, and intensity. It is helpful to determine the intensity of the pain at its worst and at its least, as well as an acceptable level of pain for the patient. Aggravating and alleviating factors provide useful information about activities or movements that may exacerbate or relieve the pain. Particularly relevant is information about the impact of pain on activities of daily living. For example, propelling a wheelchair can cause or worsen shoulder, elbow, and wrist pain. This aggravation in turn may limit the patient's mobility around his or her home or community or make it more difficult to transfer from the wheelchair to another surface.

The patient should also be asked about pertinent tests that were performed to diagnose the origin of the pain (eg, electrodiagnostic and imaging procedures). This question is important to reduce the duplication of tests for a patient who may have limited transportation available. The history of interventions tried offers the clinician an opportunity to assess what has worked and what has not worked in the past. Often the reasons for the failure of an intervention are just as important as the reasons for its success. For example, a patient may have stopped attending physical therapy because of transportation problems or increased pain associated with exercising. Medications may have been discontinued because of side effects such as sedation or increased constipation.

Fatigue

Fatigue is common in adults living with a physical disability such as multiple sclerosis, traumatic brain injury, Parkinson's disease, polio, or cerebral palsy [4–6]. Fatigue can affect activities of daily living and appears to be more common in adults who have mild to moderate disease severity [5,6]. It is associated with anxiety, depression, pain, poor general health, increased functional dependence, and even increased rates of institutionalization and mortality [6].

Several instruments have been described to assess the presence of fatigue in various populations, including the Visual Analogue Scale for Fatigue, the Fatigue Severity Scale [7], and the Fatigue Impact Scale, which measures social, cognitive, and physical aspects of fatigue [8]. If the clinician does not wish to use one of these scales, then some common questions to ask include the following:

Is it predominantly a physical fatigue, a mental fatigue, or both?
What precipitates the fatigue? Is it an activity or perhaps a change
   in temperature?
Which activities of daily living are limited by the fatigue—basic ones, such as
   dressing, bathing, and hygiene, or higher levels of function, such as
   shopping or working?
How has the fatigue affected the patient's hobbies, work, and social relationships? Has the patient cut back on his or her work schedule or limited
   social interactions as a result of the fatigue?

How has the patient modified his or her life to reduce the effect of the fatigue? Has he or she purchased a motorized scooter for community mobility or an air conditioner for the home? How effective have these interventions been?

Falls

Falls are common in the elderly, but the risk for falls is increased in older adults with physical disabilities. The reasons for this increased risk are often multifactorial. Some common examples include weakness in an extremity, impaired sensation, impaired balance, increased use of medications with cognitive side effects, and an ill-fitting prosthesis. Changes in living arrangements or social support system may also lead to increased falls (eg, the patient has to move in with an adult child who works all day and lives in a home that is inappropriate given the patient's disability). It is important for the clinician to ask about falls or "near falls." At what time of day do they occur? How often does the impaired individual fall? Which activity precipitates the fall (eg, walking to the bathroom during the night)? Are there any potential environmental hazards (eg, loose rugs)? Does the person have adaptive equipment in the home to reduce the risk of falling (eg, tub bench, grab bars)?

Sleep

Sleep problems are common in adults with disabilities. Their cause is often multifactorial. Pain, anxiety, and depression have all been linked to impaired sleep [9]. Biering-Sorensen and colleague [10] reported on the results of a sleep questionnaire administered to 408 people living with spinal cord injury. Problems with falling asleep, frequent nightly awakenings, and interrupted sleep due to spasms, pain, paraesthesias, and trouble voiding were all reported. The incidence of sleep apnea syndrome is high in tetraplegics, especially in older men with large necks [11]. Foley and colleagues [12] reported that older adults living with chronic diseases such as obesity, diabetes, lung disease, and stroke have breathing pauses, snoring, and restless legs during sleep. They also have insufficient sleep (<6 hours per night). Depression, heart disease, bodily pain, and memory problems were also associated with more prevalent symptoms of insomnia. Sleep-disordered breathing has been linked to poorer long-term outcomes and increased long-term stroke mortality. Fifty percent of stroke patients have problems with breathing during sleep; 20% to 40% have sleep-wake disorders, insomnia, and excessive daytime sleepiness [13].

In assessing the older adult who has a neurologic impairment such as stroke, it is important to ask about snoring during sleep, difficulty falling asleep, episodes of waking with shortness of breath, daytime prolonged naps, fatigue and sleepiness during the day, the presence of nighttime spasms, frequent nighttime urination, and musculoskeletal pain with movement in bed.

Sexuality

Sexual dysfunction has been reported in adults who have physical disabilities, so clinicians caring for this population should ask about it during clinic visits.

Choi-Kwon and colleagues [14] reported on stroke patients followed 3 months and 2 years after a stroke. Forty-nine percent had decreased libido, 65% had decreased coital frequency, and 20% had decreased erectile function. Emotional incontinence (excessive or inappropriate laughing or crying) was linked to the sexual dysfunction at the 2-year follow-up. Kimura and colleagues [15] reported that 58.6% of men and 44% of women expressed dissatisfaction with sexual function after their stroke. This dissatisfaction was found to be linked to depression, decreased activities of daily living, and left-sided stroke. Similar findings were reported in two Finnish studies performed by Korpelainen and colleagues [16,17]. In one of them, 28% of patients discontinued sexual intercourse at 2 months post-stroke and 14% at 6-month follow-up. Fifty-five percent had impaired nocturnal erections [17]. Spinal cord injured patients have also been reported to have low levels of satisfaction with sexual intercourse. Concerns raised included inability to satisfy the partner, urinary accidents during intercourse, and risks for transmitting or receiving sexually transmitted diseases [18]. Bodenheimer and colleagues [19] reported that, in lower extremity amputees (mean age 57), interest in sexual intercourse was high; however, 63% reported problems with orgasms, and 67% experienced erectile dysfunctions.

Given the high prevalence of sexual dysfunction in adults who have disabilities, it is important for clinicians to ask general questions about this topic, emphasizing potentially treatable conditions. For example, spasticity that interferes with sexual intercourse may lend itself to various pharmacologic interventions. Urinary incontinence may be treated with urinary catheterization before sexual intercourse to empty the bladder. The patient may also be referred for sexual counseling.

Bowel and bladder

Impaired bowel or bladder function is common in adults living with neurologic injuries such as stroke, multiple sclerosis, or traumatic brain injury. Successful bowel and bladder function in individuals who have these conditions is a predictable evacuation at desired times of day or night with no accidents in between.

Appropriate questions about bowel function concern the frequency of bowel movements (eg, daily, every 2 days), their occurrence at predictable times of day, bowel accidents, and changes in bowel habits. The type and effectiveness of previous and current bowel regimens should also be evaluated. For example, if the patient uses stool softeners and mild laxatives, how soon after administration of these agents is there a bowel movement?

Bladder management techniques often involve a combination of catheterizations and medications. Self-catheterization may be more difficult for the older adult because of limited hand function or impaired vision; therefore, questions about decreased hand function or loss of eyesight are appropriate. If these are present, the patient may rely on a family member or an aide to perform the catheterizations; therefore, questions about that individual's technique are important. Frequency of catheterizations or voiding per day, presence of urinary accidents, history of kidney or bladder stones, and urinary tract infections are also important to note.

Spasticity

Spasticity is common after central nervous system injuries such as traumatic brain injury, spinal cord injury, and stroke. It is characterized by increased tone, hyperreflexia, episodic uncontrolled movements, and clonus in the affected limbs. Spasticity may lead to decreased use of a paretic limb, contractures, and skin breakdown.

In evaluating the impact of spasticity on a patient with a neurologic injury, the clinician should inquire about the frequency, duration, and intensity of the spasms, as well as about any inciting or alleviating factors and compensatory techniques used. Painful spasms should be noted, as well as functional impact of the spasms. For example, do the spasms make it difficult to dress an extremity, perform perineal hygiene, or safely transfer from a wheelchair to another surface? Is ambulation impaired by the spasms, placing the patient at greater risk for falling?

Asking patients whether they believe that the spasms need to be treated is helpful, because not all spasms require treatment. The clinician should bear in mind that there are some functional benefits to spasticity. For example, spasticity can make a limb stiff, thereby making it easier for a patient with some preserved motor function in the extremities to transfer from one surface to another. In certain circumstances, it may even make dressing of the lower extremities somewhat easier.

It is also helpful to have a treatment history for the spasticity. What has the patient tried, and how successful was it? Reasons for the discontinuation of a treatment are helpful (eg, the patient did not tolerate the side effects associated with medications).

Mobility and adaptive equipment issues

Lower limb prosthetics

The most common reasons for lower limb amputations in the older adult are complications of diabetes and peripheral vascular disease. Common amputation sites in the lower limb include below the knee (transtibial) and above the knee (transfemoral). The transtibial prosthesis is made up of a suspension, socket, pylon, and foot. The transfemoral prosthesis has similar components but also has a prosthetic knee.

Amputees often have fragile skin and are therefore at a high risk for skin ulcerations, cysts, calluses, blisters, folliculitis, and contact dermatitis. The increased risk is often due to sweat, bacteremia, and high shear forces at the socket and residual limb interface [20].

It is important to ask the older amputee about the fit of the prosthesis. Does it feel too loose or too tight? Does he or she have a difficult time putting it on? Does the residual limb touch the bottom of the socket? The clinician should also ask about recent weight changes, because they can have a significant impact on the fit of the prosthesis. Weight gain may make it more difficult to fit the residual limb in the prosthesis, whereas weight loss or decreased postoperative edema in the residual limb can lead to poor fit.

Often amputees will compensate for a residual limb of reduced size by using more residual limb socks inside the prosthetic socket. Asking about the total number of socks used may be important. Each sock has a certain thickness or ply that is often determined by a number located on the sock itself. The thicker the "ply," the higher the number. If the patient has needed to add residual limb socks that total 13 to 15 ply, then he or she is probably ready for a better fitting socket.

Older amputees should be asked how long they have had the current prosthesis and when the prosthesis was last evaluated by a prosthetist or in a prosthetic clinic. The types of changes made are also useful information (eg, a new socket to accommodate a residual limb of reduced circumference). Patients should be asked how and where they use their prostheses on a daily basis. Is the prosthesis used for short-distance ambulation around the apartment, or is it used for ambulation in the community? Are there any recent changes in their walking distance? Has the amputee limited his or her ambulation because of an ill-fitting prosthesis?

The patient should also be asked about any red marks, skin breaks, drainage, warmth, or other evidence of superficial skin infections. The diabetic amputee is at high risk for amputation in the opposite foot; therefore, similar questions to assess the possibility of infection in that foot are important.

Lower limb amputees have a high risk for falling, especially at times when they may forget that they have an amputated limb—for example, getting up in the middle of the night to go to the bathroom and forgetting to put the prosthesis on. It is important to find out about the circumstances of falls or near falls.

Given the high prevalence of pain in lower limb amputees, it is important to ask the lower limb amputee about pain. Pain may occur in the residual limb or where the amputated limb used to be (phantom pain). Musculoskeletal pain is common in lower limb amputees. Altered gait from an ill-fitting prosthesis may cause increased pain in the low back or other major joints of the lower extremities.

Lower limb orthotics

Several different types of orthotics are worn by older adults with neurologic impairments. Examples of lower limb orthoses include the ankle foot orthosis (AFO) and knee-ankle foot orthosis. It is important to ask questions such as how long the patient has worn the orthosis and why it was prescribed. The name of the vendor may be helpful, as is information about any recent adjustments that have been made.

It is useful to know the age of the brace to determine if it is still appropriate for the patient's neurologic condition. Sometimes an initial brace is not as effective when worn for a long period, because of a deterioration or improvement in the patient's condition. For example, a newly diagnosed stroke patient with a foot drop may be prescribed a solid confining brace soon after the event; however, after several months the patient may have regained significant motor strength and require a less confining brace. It is important to ask how often and when and where the brace is used. Does the patient wear the brace daily for ambulation in the community, or is it only used sporadically during exercise sessions? If it is only used sporadically, the reason should be identified: Is it too painful to wear, or is it too confining and restrictive? Does the patient believe that the brace helps with ambulation? Has the patient had any falls or near falls when walking with the brace, or does he or she experience difficulty putting the brace on or taking it off? Sometimes a brace that is too bulky does not fit in the patient's shoes and as a result is not used frequently. Recent weight gains or losses may lead to an ill-fitting orthosis with resulting pain and skin irritation.

Ambulation aids

Adults who have an impaired gait commonly use walkers, canes, and crutches. They offer a wider base of support and thus added safety during ambulation. It is important to inquire how and where the patient is using the assistive device and whether it is still providing the patient with stability and safety while ambulating. For example, in a progressive neurologic disorder, a cane may initially have been adequate but may currently not be as appropriate as a walker.

Changes in the patient's living arrangements may pose safety challenges. For example, a walker is appropriate for a flat surface but may not be when the patient has moved to a home with many steps to negotiate. It is also helpful to ask the patient about the source of the assistive device. A cane obtained from a family friend or relative may not be appropriate for a patient's condition.

Falls or near falls are a common reason for a patient to obtain an assistive device for ambulation, so questions about falls may yield valuable information about the current effectiveness of these devices.

Wheelchair

Wheelchairs may be a source of problems for patients, and it is a good idea for clinicians to inquire about them during visits. Wheelchairs are typically composed of a back, seat (typically with a cushion), arms, wheels, rims, casters (small wheels in the front), brakes, leg-rests, and footrests. The wheelchair user should be asked about several issues, but the most important ones are related to use, fit, and safety.

One should find out how the patient is using the wheelchair and whether there are any limitations on its use. Is the patient using it primarily in a small, confined space or for outdoor long-distance travel on various terrains? Is the wheelchair used as the primary source of mobility on a daily basis or used infrequently as back-up? The patient should also be asked about limitations of the current wheelchair—what does the patient wish it to do that it cannot? Difficulty with transporting the wheelchair in automobiles may also limit the mobility of the patient and should be assessed. This factor can be especially problematic for the aging spouse, who may need to lift the wheelchair in and out of the vehicle.

Because the older wheelchair user may spend a considerable amount of time in the wheelchair, proper fit is important to minimize the risk of skin breakdown and maximize comfort. Weight changes may affect proper fit. Weight gain may make it difficult for a patient to fit in a wheelchair (especially during inclement weather when additional clothing is worn). Weight loss may be associated with reduced skin padding over bony prominences, which in turn can lead to skin breakdown. The age and type of cushion, as well as a history of skin breakdown over the sacrum, ischial tuberosities, and greater trochanters, can provide useful information about adequate pressure relief. Patients who have inadequate pressure relief may also complain of persistent low back and buttock pain.

Safety-related questions include inquiries about the effectiveness of the brakes—are they easy to use and effective in stopping the wheelchair? If the patient has had a stroke and has limited use of an arm, he or she may benefit from an extended wheelchair brake. Questions about the safety of transfers from the wheelchair to other surfaces, such as a bed or regular chair, may help determine whether this important function is performed appropriately for the existing wheelchair. The age of the wheelchair and its repair history shed light on its overall structural integrity.

A frequent manual wheelchair user is at risk for repetitive musculoskeletal injuries, especially in the shoulders, elbows, and wrists. Pain in these areas may subsequently have an impact on the patient's mobility and activities of daily living. Active patients with motorized wheelchairs may have mechanical problems with the motor and electrical system of their wheelchair, including stalls or difficulty in starting the engine.

Finally, it is helpful to know where the patient obtained the wheelchair. Was it prescribed through a wheelchair clinic at a rehabilitation hospital or rehabilitation department, obtained from a surgical supply store or vendor, or obtained from a friend or family member? A wheelchair borrowed from a friend does not guarantee a good fit.

Home adaptive equipment

Older adults with disabilities have limitations in performing activities of daily living. They often need increased assistance from caregivers as well as from modified equipment [21,22]. Sorensen and colleagues [23] reported that stroke survivors are dependent on assistive devices and environmental modifications even several years following the stroke. Bingham and colleague [24] surveyed 500 adults living with multiple sclerosis and spinal cord injury and noted that half of them had indicated a need for assistive equipment in the previous 12 months.

It is helpful for the clinician to get a clear sense of how the disabled person accomplishes these tasks and how much assistance he or she requires to do so. Questions about dressing, hygiene, bathing, bowel and bladder care, feeding, transfers, food shopping, and banking can yield valuable information about gaps in the patient's care.

It is also important to ask patients about activities they find particularly meaningful but are having difficulty performing (eg, hobbies, travel). What is difficult about the activities, and what do they think that they need to perform them?

An abundance of devices are intended to lessen the functional burdens faced by older adults with disabilities. Unfortunately, not all of them may be appropriate for the patient's use. The clinician should inquire about how the patients have compensated for their deficits in activities of daily life. What kind of equipment have they obtained, and when and where did they obtain it? For example, an individual with a lower extremity amputation may have received a commode from a friend but not have been trained in how safely to transfer on and off it, and as a result may be at increased risk for falling. Or a family member may have given a heating pad to a stroke patient for shoulder and arm pain, not realizing that sensory deficits can lead to burns.

The age of the adaptive equipment is also important. An older device may no longer function well and may place the patient at risk in its use. For example, loose grab bars in the shower may place the patient at risk for falling. Both the patient and the primary caregiver should be asked about any problems associated with adaptive equipment.

Disability-related psychosocial issues

Depression

Depression is reported to be common in adults living with disabilities. Among stroke survivors, 24% to 33% experience it [4,25], and among spinal cord injury survivors there is a 24% to 57% prevalence [26]. Comparable numbers have been reported for amputees [27,28]. Mild depression has been reported in 40% of PD patients, and moderate to severe depression in 16.7% of patients [28]. Depression in PD may be accompanied by anxiety, apathy, and cognitive impairment [28,29].

Hence it is important for the clinician to inquire about the presence of depression from the patient as well as from the primary caregiver.

Aging caregivers

Older adults who have physical disabilities increasingly rely on spouses and family members for day-to-day care. These individuals are asked to assume great responsibility for the activities of daily life and transportation. Additionally, they often bear the sole responsibility for administering complex medication regimens to their loved ones and perform assessments of their effectiveness. They often come to these tasks with limited education or training yet are asked to be the primary link between the patient and his or her community and medical providers.

Often these caregivers are older and have medical needs and impairments of their own that may affect the care of an even frailer spouse. Therefore, it is important for the clinician caring for an older adult with a physical disability to spend time discussing the concerns of the primary caregiver.

The caregiver can also provide valuable information about the functionality of the patient in the community and shed light on potential problem areas, both medical and social. It is not uncommon for the caregiver to give a more realistic account of the patient's condition than does the patient. Inquiries about caregivers' roles in patients' care should include the number of hours they are with patients on a daily basis and the amount of assistance they provide for activities of daily living (bathing, hygiene, dressing, feeding, shopping, cooking, cleaning, and banking are some common examples). If they accompany patients around the community and to physician visits, it is helpful to detail how this is accomplished (eg, public transportation, cabs, private car).

The clinician should ask what sorts of difficulties the caregiver has observed in the care of the patient. Does it take a long time to dress the patient or put on a prosthesis or a brace? Is it difficult to maneuver the current wheelchair or to place it in the trunk of a car? The caregiver may also be asked questions about the presence of pressure ulcers in areas that the patient may not be able to visualize or about side effects of medications, such as drowsiness, dizziness, or changes in mental status. Are there other family members nearby who can offer assistance? Is there a reliable back-up provider in case the caregiver is ill or has to keep a doctor's appointment?

Questions about the general health of the caregiver are also relevant. For example, an overweight, aging spouse with advanced osteoarthritis of the hips and back may have difficulties with patient transfer and pushing a wheelchair. Does the caregiver get enough exercise? How has the caregiving affected his or her hobbies, professional career, or friendships? Has the caregiver sought medical or psychiatric care for any problems? Anticipated changes in the caregiver's role should also be explored. For example, an upcoming surgery and hospitalization for the spouse will have a direct impact on the care of the patient, perhaps even requiring a temporary nursing home stay.

Is the caregiver experiencing feelings of stress, anxiety, or depression? Evidence suggests that caregivers are at risk for depression and increased mortality as a result of providing care. The prevalence of depression among caregivers of stroke survivors ranges from 34% to 52% [30]. Schulz and colleague [31] reported a 63% higher mortality among older caregivers than non-caregivers.

Areas identified as particularly difficult and time consuming for the caregiver include managing finances, providing emotional support, transporting the patient, managing behaviors, administering medications, carrying out household chores, such as cleaning, and finding adequate care while he or she is away [32,33]. Caregivers often find themselves unexpectedly in the caregiver role and do not believe they have adequate knowledge about the patient's medical condition (eg, bowel and bladder care) or skills to be effective caregivers [34]. This can be a source of stress. They report feelings of a "heavy responsibility" and constant worries about their loved ones [35]. Scholte op Reimer and colleagues [36] reported that 6 months after discharge for a stroke was the time of the highest unmet needs. Pierce and colleagues [37] also described the lack of a formal and informal support system and the impact of the disability on the couple's interpersonal relationship. Similar concerns have been reported for caregivers of amputees and patients who have Parkinson's disease [38] and spinal cord injury [39]. Thompson and colleague [40] reported on 109 helpers for amputees and found that they assessed their health as poor, with feelings of anxiety, depression, interrupted sleep, and need for continuous vigilance. Financial pressures associated with decreased income and inability to leave the home for extended periods were also of concern. Martinez-Martin and colleagues [41] reported that in PD, the patient's functional state and disease severity were predictors of the caregiver's psychosocial burden.

Gaps in care

The clinician should inquire about gaps in the care of the patient or times of day when the caregiver feels particularly stressed and cannot provide adequate care. Red flags should be raised in the clinician's mind when he or she encounters an isolated caregiver caring for a disruptive, cognitively impaired patient. Inquiries should also be made about tasks that the caregiver is having a particularly difficult time carrying out. For example, a complex medication schedule may be simplified or the patient may be referred to a social worker for assistance in obtaining a home health aide to help with dressing and bathing. Caregivers should be encouraged to seek professional help for their own medical and emotional needs.

Limited finances

The older adult living with a disability faces the daunting task of dealing with increased medical and social needs while living on a fixed or declining source of income. As a result, the patient's choices of equipment, home modifications, living arrangements, and medical treatments may be significantly limited. The clinician caring for the older adult who has a physical disability should ask questions about the impact of these constraints on the patient's well-being. Can the patient afford currently prescribed medications? If not, perhaps less expensive medication regimens may be prescribed. Is it difficult for the patient to afford transportation for thrice-weekly outpatient physical therapy? If so, perhaps home therapy or fewer sessions followed by a home exercise program may be helpful. The clinician should ask the patient and the caregiver openly how limited finances have affected the patient's well-being. Is the patient not filling all of his or her prescriptions? Is the patient isolated because he or she cannot get out of a wheelchair-inaccessible building? Have the patient and spouse stopped socializing with family and friends? Although many of these problems do not have easy solutions, a referral to a social worker may be warranted. It is important for the clinician to understand that the most sophisticated and elaborate treatment plan may fail because of financial factors. Therefore, one should know about these limitations early on and find ways to minimize their impact on the patient.

Physical examination

The physical examination of the older adult with a physical disability combines elements of the traditional physical examination with an additional emphasis on key systems that are particularly stressed by long-standing disability. These include the nervous system, musculoskeletal system, and skin. In addition, mobility devices that are in constant contact with the patient should be evaluated. These include the lower limb brace, lower limb prosthesis, and wheelchair.

Nervous system

Cognition

The patient's level of alertness and ability to follow instructions on a consistent basis should be evaluated. The Mini–Mental Status examination may be a useful screen that is easily administered in the clinic setting or at the bedside. The Geriatric Depression Screen may be helpful in identifying the patient with underlying depression.

Cranial nerves

Vision, hearing, and swallowing should be checked for possible correctible impairments (eg, ear wax, need for a stronger prescription of eyeglasses).

Motor/Sensory

The strength of the muscles of the upper and lower limbs should be evaluated. Decreased strength can place the individual at increased risk for loss of functionality, contractures, and accidents. Sensation should also be evaluated, especially in areas where a brace or prosthesis comes in contact with the skin.

Balance

Balance should be evaluated initially with the ambulatory patient in a static standing position and subsequently, if deemed safe, challenged by a slight perturbation to assess for dynamic stability. In the ambulatory patient, ambulation with a current assistive device can yield additional information.

In the nonambulatory patient, trunk stability and balance may be assessed with the patient either sitting in a wheelchair or on the side of a mat. Information thus obtained may be of value in deciding on the type of trunk support needed for a wheelchair.

Wheelchair evaluation

A brief evaluation of the wheelchair and the person in it should be an integral part of the clinical visit. Evaluation of the wheelchair begins with an overview for any obvious signs of wear and tear. Does the wheelchair appear sturdy? Are there any rips in the back of the seat or the cushion material? Are there any parts missing (eg, leg rests, seat belt)? As mentioned earlier, the cushion and seat back are integral parts of the wheelchair. If they are not in good condition, the patient is at high risk for skin breakdown, typically in the sacral area.

The wheelchair cushion should provide adequate pressure relief. If an air cushion is used, it should be adequately inflated. If it is flat when pressed, this may be due to inadequate inflation or an air leak; in this case, the cushion is not providing adequate pressure relief. Do the tires appear to be adequately inflated? Check the brakes of the wheelchair. Do they open and close well? Does the wheelchair still move when the brakes are locked? In the motorized wheelchair, does the joystick operate well? Does the wheelchair start and stop appropriately? Once in motion, does the motorized wheelchair stop suddenly or lose power?

Next, observe the patient in the wheelchair. Does he or she appear to be slipping out of the wheelchair or leaning too much to one side? Does the wheelchair appear too small for the patient? Typically, one should be able to fit two or three fingers between the arms of the wheelchair and the patient. The uppermost part of the back of the wheelchair should be at the same level as the inferior border of the scapula. The patient's hips and knees should be at right angles to the chair seat. It is also important to evaluate the patient's trunk control while seated in the wheelchair. Poor trunk control is demonstrated by slouching of the patient either to the front or sides.

Because wheelchair users are at risk for skin breakdown, it is imperative that a thorough skin check be performed on a regular basis, especially in older patients with insensate skin, incontinence, and bony prominences. Areas at highest risk include the sacrum, ischial tuberosities, and greater trochanters. However, patients with spasticity and contractures in the lower limbs are also at higher risk for skin breakdowns in areas such as the heels and around the fibular heads.

Once the physical assessment is complete, it is helpful to watch the patient transfer from the wheelchair to a mat or bed if he or she has intact upper body strength. This observation provides the clinician with valuable information about this critical functional aspect of wheelchair use.

Musculoskeletal system

Because of the high prevalence of musculoskeletal pain in adults who have physical disabilities, it is important to perform a thorough physical examination of this vital system, including examination of the spine and upper and lower limbs. Areas to focus on include range of motion limitations around key joints, presence of contractures, and tender points in muscles and over bony prominences.

The examination of the upper extremities is a key component of the physical assessment of the older adult who spends most of the day in a wheelchair, especially a manual one. A considerable degree of wear and tear to the arms develops from the chronic propulsion of a wheelchair. It is common to find rotator cuff tears, shoulder impingement syndrome, bicipital tendonitis, lateral epicondylitis, wrist sprains, and carpal tunnel syndrome in wheelchair users.

Orthosis

The main reasons for wearing an orthosis are to support or protect a weak extremity or assist weakened muscles around a joint in performing their function. In a patient wearing an orthotic device, the clinician should evaluate the brace's structural integrity, fit, and functional benefit. The orthosis should first be checked for evidence of abnormal wear and tear, such as irregular surfaces that could be a source of skin irritation, straps that are worn out or dirty, and deformities of the material. Next, the relevant body part should be checked for any potential problem areas for orthotic fit, such as edema, contractures, and spasticity. Once these steps are completed, the brace should be fitted to the body part in question. Areas where the brace appears to be irritating the skin surface should be noted. The patient should then be asked to move around with the brace on. For a lower extremity brace, it is important to evaluate the gait of the patient with and without the brace. The purpose of the lower extremity AFO is to assist in clearance of the foot during the swing phase of the gait cycle. If this is not adequately accomplished with the brace on, then the brace may not be effective in assisting the patient during ambulation and may predispose the patient to falls. Evaluation of the skin before and after use of the orthosis is important to document any areas of erythema or skin breakdown. Areas with bony prominences (eg, medial and lateral malleoli, the plantar aspects of the feet and the fibular head) should be inspected carefully.

Prosthesis

The evaluation of the prosthesis is comparable to that of the orthosis. The structural integrity, fit, and function of the prosthesis are key components of the assessment. The prosthesis should be evaluated for any abnormal wear and tear, such as tears in a suspension sleeve or irregular surfaces for the socket that may be a source of irritation for the skin. Typically, the patient wears one or more socks or a silicone liner between the socket and the residual limb (stump) to protect it. However, the socks or gel liner may also be worn or torn. Small tears in the silicone liner may cause cuts in the skin. These are typically identified when examining the inside of the liner, especially at its distal end or at the crease lines. Some patients may have thigh straps to provide more stability, which may also show signs of wear and tear with aging. After evaluating the prosthesis, one should examine the residual limb. Important observations include the presence of a hip or knee contracture, weakness of key muscle groups such as the hip flexors and quadriceps, and any evidence of skin irritation, breakdown, or blisters. The bony residual limb with little distal or circumferential soft tissue padding and tightly adherent overlying skin is especially at risk for skin breakdown.

After evaluating the residual limb and the prosthesis, one should ask the patient to put on the prosthesis. This provides valuable information about the patient's ability to apply the prosthesis safely. In addition, areas of potential problems may be quickly identified. For example, the patient may apply the socks inappropriately, or weakness in the hands may make it difficult for the patient to advance the residual limb inside the socket. Inadequate fit of the residual limb in the socket due to changes in circumference is also notable (eg, fluctuating edema in a dialysis patient). Once the prosthesis is on, the patient should be asked to walk, preferably in a wide open space such as a hallway, with the pant leg on the amputated side raised. This measure makes it easier to evaluate the gait of the patient. It is helpful to look at each joint on the affected side as it goes through the gait cycle. What is happening at the hip, knee, and foot? Does the patient appear to be "sinking" into the prosthesis with each step, or, alternatively, does the patient report that the distal end of the residual limb is hitting the bottom of the socket? This problem may be due to a socket that is too big for the residual limb. Does the patient have difficulty clearing the ground with the prosthetic foot during ambulation or actually trip over the prosthetic foot? During ambulation, additional information may be obtained about the patient's balance, the effectiveness of assistive devices such walkers or canes, and the ability to rise from a seated position and sit back down.

After ambulation, the prosthesis should be removed and the skin checked for any areas of erythema over bony prominences, such as the tibia or medial and lateral aspects of the knee. Areas of erythema over the patellar tendon or muscles such as the anterior tibialis are to be expected. Vision, grip strength, and upper extremity strength should also be evaluated as part of the clinical assessment of the older amputee. Before the conclusion of the visit, the clinician should check the foot on the nonamputated side for any evidence of skin breakdown, especially on the plantar aspect of the foot and in between the toes.

Functional assessment—transfers, gait

In the nonambulatory patient, it is important to assess the ability to transfer in and out of the wheelchair from one surface to another. The degree of assistance required for transfer should be noted. Can the patient do it independently, or is the assistance of another person required? If the transfer is independent, is the patient safe, or does another person need to be nearby? If assistance is required, then the degree of assistance should be noted—minimal, moderate, or total.

Transfers should also be assessed for the ambulatory patient. Typically, this may be accomplished in a coordinated effort with the gait evaluation. The patient is asked to stand from a seated position and then walk for 20 ft, stop, turn, walk back, and sit back down in the chair. If the patient uses an assistive device, such as a walker or a cane, he or she should use this device. The patient's balance, fluidity of movement, and safety should be evaluated. If the clinician does not believe that the patient is safe, then an alternative assistive device may be tried to see if the patient is safer. (For instance, if the patient is not safe with a cane, a walker may be tried.) The clinician should focus on the major joints during ambulation. For example, does the knee appear to buckle or "snap back"? Is there a "foot-drop" with an audible foot slap when the patient walks? This finding may indicate a weakness of the anterior tibialis muscle that helps to elevate the foot during ambulation. Shoe examination may also yield valuable information about problems during gait. Scuff marks on the shoes may indicate a mild foot-drop, whereas wear patterns on the bottom of the shoes may provide evidence of pes-planus.

Summary

Because more and more older adults are living with significant physical impairments, it is important for clinicians to be able adequately to assess their needs. The purpose of this article is to serve as a guide for geriatricians on the key components of the history and physical examination of the older adult with a physical disability.

References

[1] Census 2000 data on aging. Available at: http://www.aoa.dhhs.gov.

[2] National Aging Information Center. Older persons with mobility and self-care limitations: 1990. Available at: http://www.aoa.dhhs.gov.

[3] Cristian A, Thomas J, Nisenbaum M, et al. Practical considerations in the assessment and treatment of pain in adults with physical disabilities. Phys Med Rehabil Clin N Am 2005; 16:57–90.

[4] Choi-Kwon S, Han SW, Kwon SV, et al. Post-stroke fatigue: characteristics and related factors. Cerebrovasc Dis 2005;19(2):84–90.

[5] DeGroot MH, Phillips SJ, Eskes GA. Fatigue associated with stroke and other neurologic conditions: implications for stroke rehabilitation. Arch Phys Med Rehabil 2003;84(11):1714–20.

[6] Jahnsen R, Villien L, Stanghelle JK, et al. Fatigue in adults with cerebral palsy in Norway compared to the general population. Dev Med Child Neurol 2003;45(5):296–303.

[7] Krupp LB, LaRocca NG, Muir-Nash J, et al. The Fatigue Severity Scale: application to patients with multiple sclerosis and systemic lupus erythematosis. Arch Neurol 1989;46:1121–3.

[8] Fisk JD, Ritvo PG, Ross L, et al. Measuring the functional impact of fatigue: initial validation of the Fatigue Impact Scale. Clin Infect Dis 1994;18:S79–83.

[9] Norrbrink Budh C, Hultling C, Ludenberg T. Quality of sleep in individuals with spinal cord injury—a comparison between patients with and without pain. Spinal Cord 2005;43(2):85–95.

[10] Biering-Sorensen F, Biering-Sorensen M. Sleep disturbances in spinal cord injury: an epidemiological questionnaire. Spinal Cord 2001;39(10):505–13.

[11] Stockhammer E, Tobon A, Michel F, et al. Characteristics of sleep apnea syndrome in tetraplegic patients. Spinal Cord 2002;40(6):286–94.

[12] Foley D, Ancoli-Israel S, Britz P, et al. Sleep disturbances and chronic disease in older adults: results of the 2003 National Sleep Foundation Sleep in America Survey. J Psychosom Res 2004;56(5):497–502.

[13] Bassetti CL. Sleep and stroke. Semin Neurol 2005;25:19–32.

[14] Choi-Kwon S, Kim JS. Post-stroke emotional incontinence and decreased sexual activity. Cerebrovasc Dis 2002;13(1):31–7.

[15] Kimura M, Murata Y, Shimoda K, et al. Sexual dysfunction following stroke. Compr Psychiatry 2001;42(3):217–22.

[16] Korpelainen JT, Nieminen P, Myllyla W. Sexual functioning among stroke patients and their spouses. Stroke 1999;30:715–9.

[17] Korpelainen JT, Kauhanen MI, Kemola H, et al. Sexual dysfunction in stroke patients. Acta Neurol Scand 1998;98(6):400–5.

[18] White MJ, Rintala DH, Hart KA, et al. Sexual activities, concerns, and interests of men with spinal cord injury. Am J Phys Med Rehabil 1992;71(4):225–31.

[19] Bodenheimer C, Kerrigan AJ, Garber SL, et al. Sexuality in persons with lower extremity amputations. Disabil Rehabil 2000;22(9):409–15.

[20] Dudek NL, Marks MB, Marshall SC, et al. Dermatologic conditions associated with use of a lower extremity prosthesis. Arch Phys Med Rehabil 2005;86:659–63.

[21] Thompson L. Functional changes in persons aging with spinal cord injury. Assist Technol 1999;11(2):123–9.

[22] Gerhart KA, Bergstrom E, Charlifue SW, et al. Long-term SCI-functional changes over time. Arch Phys Med Rehabil 1993;74(10):1030–4.

[23] Sorensen HV, Lendal S, Schultz-Larsen K, et al. Stroke rehabilitation: assistive technology devices and environmental modifications following primary rehabilitation in hospital—a therapeutic perspective. Assist Technol 2003;15(1):39–48.

[24] Bingham SC, Beatty PW. Rates of access to assistive equipment and medical rehabilitation services among people with disabilities. Disabil Rehabil 2003;25(9):487–90.

[25] Hackett ML, Yaga C, Parag V, et al. Frequency of depression after stroke. Stroke 2005;36: 1330–40.

[26] Consever A, Uzun O, Yildiz C, et al. Depression in men with traumatic lower part amputation: a comparison to men with surgical lower part amputation. Mil Med 2003;168(2):106–9.

[27] Kashani JH, Frank RG, Kashani SR, et al. Depression among amputees. J Clin Psychiatry 1983;44(7):256–8.

[28] Rojo A, Aguilar M, Garolera MT, et al. Depression in Parkinson's disease—clinical correlates and outcomes. Parkinsonism Relat Disord 2003;10(1):23–8.

[29] Schrag A. Psychiatric aspects of Parkinson's disease—an update. J Neurol 2004;7:795–804.

[30] Han B, Haley WE. Family caregiving for patients with stroke. Review and analysis. Stroke 1999;30:1478–85.

[31] Schulz R, Beach SR. Caregiving as a risk factor for mortality: the Caregiver Health Effects Study. JAMA 1999;282:2215–9.

[32] Bakas T, Austin JK, Jessup SL, et al. Time and difficulty of tasks provided by family caregivers of stroke survivors. J Neurosci Nurs 2004;36(2):95–106.

[33] Bakas T, Austin JK, Okonkwo KF, et al. Needs, concerns, strategies and advice of stroke caregivers in the first 6 months after discharge. J Neurosci Nurs 2002;34(5):242–51.

[34] Weppner DM, Brownscheidle CM. Healthcare needs of women with disabilities. Prim Care Update Ob Gyns 1998;5(4):210.

[35] Scholte op Reimer WJ, deHaan RJ, Rijnders PT, et al. The burden of caregiving in partners of long-term stroke survivors. Stroke 1998;29:1605–11.

[36] Scholte op Reimer WJ, deHaan RJ, Rijnders PT, et al. Unmet care demands as perceived by stroke patients: deficits in health care? Qual Health Care 1999;8:30–5.

[37] Pierce LL, Steiner V, Govoni AL, et al. Caregivers dealing with stroke pull together and feel connected. J Neurosci Nurs 2004;36(1):32–9.

[38] Thommessen B, Aarsland D, Braekhus A, et al. Psychological burden on spouses of the elderly with stroke, dementia and Parkinson's disease. Int J Geriatr Psychiatry 2002;17(1):78–84.

[39] Weitzencamp DA, Gerhart KA, Charlifue SW, et al. Spouses of spinal cord injury survivors: the added impact of caregiving. Arch Phys Med Rehabil 1997;78(8):822–7.

[40] Thompson DM, Haran D. Living with an amputation: the helper. Soc Sci Med 1985;20(4): 319–23.

[41] Martinez-Martin P, Benito-Leon J, Alonso F, et al. Quality of life of caregivers in Parkinson's disease. Qual Life Res 2005;14(2):463–72.

CLINICS IN
GERIATRIC
MEDICINE

ELSEVIER
SAUNDERS

Clin Geriatr Med 22 (2006) 239–256

Exercise in the Elderly: Research and Clinical Practice

Jason E. Frankel, MD[a,b], Jonathan F. Bean, MD[c,d],
Walter R. Frontera, MD, PhD[c,*]

[a]New England Sinai Hospital and Rehabilitation Center, Department of Physical Medicine and
Rehabilitation, 150 York Street, Stoughton, MA 02072, USA
[b]Department of Physical Medicine and Rehabilitation, Tufts New England Medical Center,
750 Washington Street, Box 400, Boston, MA 02111, USA
[c]Department of Physical Medicine and Rehabilitation,
Harvard Medical School/Spaulding Rehabilitation Hospital, 125 Nashua Street,
Boston, MA 02114, USA
[d]Spaulding Cambridge Outpatient Center, Box 9, 1575 Cambridge Street,
Cambridge, MA 02138, USA

A surge of recent inquiries into the preventive health benefits of exercise in elderly patients has been generated by the growing percentage of seniors in the population. Some data are preliminary, but many important conclusions can be drawn that may positively affect the care and functional capacity of elderly patients.

Exercise programs generally consist of four major components: strength, endurance, balance, and flexibility. This article outlines the normal physiology of each component, the natural effects of aging and the effects of medical comorbidities on each, research into the primary effects of exercise in elderly patients, and specific prescription recommendations.

Except where otherwise indicated, the research cited in this article pertains specifically to older adults. Although many studies are prospective in design and allow the reader to draw at least some generalizable conclusions, much of this work is still preliminary in nature. Further studies with larger patient cohorts are needed, and the recommendations contained herein reflect this need. A summary of the recommendations to follow is found in Table 1.

* Corresponding author. 125 Nashua Street, Boston, MA 02114.
E-mail address: wfrontera@partners.org (W.R. Frontera).

0749-0690/06/$ – see front matter © 2006 Elsevier Inc. All rights reserved.
doi:10.1016/j.cger.2005.12.002   *geriatric.theclinics.com*

FRANKEL et al

Table 1
Summary of exercise recommendations for older adult patients

Mode	Benefits	Prescription	Precautions
Strength	Improve daily function Reduce disability Reduce blood pressure Reduce arthritis pain Increase aerobic capacity in congestive heart failure	Moderate-to-high-intensity strength training 2–3×/wk May start with low-intensity PRT in deconditioned or poorly compliant patients May add task-specific exercise to improve function	Monitor vital signs in patients with known coronary artery disease, pulmonary dysfunction. Monitor patients with neurologic insults for fatigue. Begin with reduced weight bearing in patients with unstable knee OA.
Endurance	Reduce blood pressure Improve lipid profiles Lower cardiac mortality Improve insulin sensitivity Improve symptoms of pulmonary disease and reduce associated disability Reduce CVA-associated weakness and improve energy expenditure Reduce pain and improve function in OA and rheumatoid arthritis	5–6 METs or more for 30 min 5×/wk Heart rate 60%–70% of projected max or Borg Scale of Perceived Exertion level 11–13	Monitor SpO_2 in patients with pulmonary disease and use supplemental oxygen where needed. Monitor vital signs in patients with cardiac and pulmonary impairment. Patients with vascular claudication exercise to just below the point of pain. Monitor patients with neurologic deficits for fatigue and schedule exercise and rest accordingly.
Balance	Fall risk reduction Improved quadriceps strength Improved functionality	Tai Chi, or weighted vest exercises, or high-velocity ankle exercises 3–4×/wk in combination with other modes	Control pain where needed. Prescribe appropriate assistive devices adjunctively. Consider DEXA scan where appropriate; supplement Vitamin D and Calcium.
Flexibility	Not well studied	4–5 repetitions, held for 30 s apiece, incorporating both static and dynamic exercises Combine routinely with other modes.	No clear contraindications Begin with gentle, supervised stretching where healing orthopedic injuries are present.

Abbreviations: CVA, cerebrovascular accident; DEXA, dual emission x-ray absorptiometry; METS, metabolic equivalents; OA, osteoarthritis; PRT, progressive resistance training; SpO_2, saturation by pulse oximetry.

General considerations

Because of a number of societal and medical factors, securing seniors' long-term compliance with exercise regimens can be most challenging. Transportation difficulties, financial constraints, and insurance payer limitations may all contribute [1]. A study by King and colleagues [2] in 2002 best illustrates this phenomenon. Eighty subjects were enrolled in an intense, supervised, multidisciplinary exercise program at a therapy center. They exercised in this setting thrice weekly for 6 months, weekly for the next 6 months, and then with a home exercise program twice weekly for another 6 months. Various functional tasks were monitored, such as chair rise, 6-minute walk, signing one's name, tandem stance, and others. Progress was compared with a control group of 75 patients who received only home exercise instructions. For the first 12 months, the center-based exercise program showed clear advantages over the home-based program in improving function. However, the transition to home-based exercise for months 13 to 18 saw a quick reversal of these functional advantages. Based on this finding, the authors conclude that some long-term center-based supervision may be necessary to secure compliance with an exercise regimen in older persons.

These data support the notion that supervised or group settings may be preferable for elders, with regard to both safety and compliance. Finding a "workout buddy" for regular exercise sessions may be helpful. Inexpensive community options, such as Tai Chi or more traditional aerobics, may exist for elders who do not have friends nearby with whom to exercise. Researchers have also noted strength gains with the use of Tai Chi group exercise programs, which have the added benefit of providing social activity [3].

Strength

Strength is defined as the instantaneous maximal force generated by a muscle or group of synergistic muscles at a given velocity of movement. *Power* describes the product of the force generated and the velocity of movement. Both of these aspects are physiologically dependent on both the number and diameter of myofibrils within muscle cells, on the fiber type, and on the coordination of the neurologic elements that control the contraction of skeletal muscle.

Physiology and the effects of aging on strength

Advanced age is associated with decreasing strength, and declines in the physiologic properties of muscle mentioned earlier are contributing factors [4–7]. Declining muscle mass and poor overall function in seniors relate significantly to inactivity. Mobility and the ability to perform activities of daily living and instrumental activities of daily living decline accordingly. More specific health problems have also been noted in the presence of poor strength. Quadriceps muscle weakness predisposes to osteoarthritis (OA) of the knee [8]. Decreased body and muscle mass is a risk factor for osteoporotic fractures after falls [9–12].

Benefits of strength training

The process by which muscle tissue is strengthened and trained has been studied for many years. The first systematic clinical research was undertaken by T.L. Delorme in the 1940s [13]. *DeLorme's Axiom* states that training using high repetitions of low-weight tasks will produce improvements in endurance, whereas fewer repetitions of high-weight exercise will lead to increases in strength. The axiom further states that these effects are mutually exclusive, so that exercise geared toward one sort of training will not bring about improvements in the other. More recent research confirms the first two ideas but finds the third assertion incorrect, indicating that strength training is best understood as a continuum between pure endurance training and pure strength training [14,15].

Many patients and physicians believe strength training occurs in a health club or gymnasium-based program, but in fact this need not be the case. Progressive resistance training (PRT) consists of moving the major joints repeatedly through the full range of motion several times weekly, with or without some form of resistance. For patients who are severely deconditioned from extended bed rest or other relative immobilization, PRT can be initiated using only gravity as resistance. However, even frail elders have tolerated high-intensity PRT in studies [5]. An advantage of PRT is that exercise can easily be completed at home, in bed or in a seated position. Conventional weights are often added to the routine to reach a moderate- or high-intensity goal. Weighted vests worn during gait-focused exercise have also been shown to improve strength, power, and physical performance in a pilot study [16].

PRT has been extensively studied, especially in patients at risk for adverse cardiac events such as myocardial infarction (MI) and congestive heart failure (CHF). Research suggests that it is a safe yet efficient training stimulus for these patients [5,17–22]. Moreover, benefits are seen in patients who already have symptomatic cardiovascular disease. Women who have disabilities secondary to known coronary artery disease (CAD) may experience improvements in various aspects of daily physical function [23], and older patients who have CHF can increase strength, endurance, and submaximal aerobic capacity using PRT [24]. Finally, for older patients with borderline high blood pressures, strength training may normalize blood pressure [25].

In addition to its cardiovascular benefits, strength training can decrease disability and is associated with a lower risk for falls in patients with hip fractures [26–29]. Studies using home-based programs demonstrated such benefits. PRT, especially in combination with balance and walking exercises, leads to increased body mass and bone density and appears otherwise to modify the risk for falls [5,30–32]. Patients who have knee OA report reduced pain and increased independence in functional tasks after specific quadriceps-strengthening exercises [33].

Some data also exist regarding the role of strength training in patients with disability secondary to a stroke. In a study by Rimmer and colleagues [34], 12 weeks of exercise, including strength training, were undertaken by African American stroke survivors. At the end of the study, improvements in oxygen consumption (VO_2) and strength were noted. Whether such gains could amount to a reduction in stroke-related disability was not specified. Another study by Oullette and colleagues [35] randomly assigned stroke patients to either high-intensity PRT or stretching routines and noted gains in both unaffected and hemiparetic leg strength. Improvements were seen in self-reported function.

Exercise prescription

In younger patients, abruptly starting vigorous exercise carries a slight risk of malignant cardiac arrhythmia or MI with sudden death. The American College of Sports Medicine recommends exercise stress testing for all men over 40 and women over 50 years of age before beginning any strenuous exercise program [5,23,36,37]. Whether this is advisable for older adults is not clear. Some data indicate that only approximately 26% of patients older than 75 years were able to reach projected maximum heart rate during treadmill testing, and the relevance and financial feasibility of pharmacologic stress testing have not been clearly established [38]. Although there is most likely an initial increase in cardiac mortality for older adults following the start of vigorous cardiac exercise, its effects are quite possibly offset by the resulting improvements in cardiovascular function.

Although specific, scientifically based algorithms for pre-exercise screening have not been delineated, Box 1 itemizes conditions that warrant further diagnosis and treatment before beginning exercise. They include but are not limited to undiagnosed murmurs, bruits, resting tachycardia or bradycardia, enlarged aorta, undiagnosed hernia, and delirium. These all warrant further evaluation, and blood pressure above 200/110 should be treated before initiating exercise. Despite these necessary precautions, the prescribing physician must not lose sight of the benefits of strength training for elderly patients described earlier. When the initial prescription is low intensity, increases are introduced slowly and progress monitored closely.

For severely deconditioned elders and those who have established cardiac risks, PRT or another low-intensity program may be prescribed as little as twice weekly, with the use of only body weight as resistance. Patients should perform 10 to 15 repetitions per set in each of the major upper and lower extremity muscle groups and three sets per session for each muscle group. Frequency should then be increased to three to four times weekly, and then light resistance such as soup cans or wrist weights may be added. Once this goal has been achieved, transition to a supervised, center-based, moderate-to-high-intensity physical therapy program two to three times per week is desirable. Alternatively, a less frequent but higher-intensity PRT program performed at a therapy gym can lead to substantial improvements in strength and neuromuscular performance. This finding

---

Box 1. Contraindications to participation in an exercise program

- Unstable angina or severe left main coronary disease
- End-stage congestive heart failure
- Severe valvular heart disease
- Malignant or unstable arrythmias
- Elevated resting blood pressure (ie, systolic >200 mm Hg, diastolic >110 mm Hg)
- Large or expanding aortic aneurysm
- Known cerebral aneurysm or recent intracranial bleed
- Uncontrolled or end-stage systemic disease
- Acute retinal hemorrhage or recent ophthalmologic surgery
- Acute or unstable musculoskeletal injury
- Severe dementia or behavioral disturbance

From Bean JF, Vora A, Frontera WR. Benefits of exercise for community-dwelling older adults. Arch Phys Med Rehabil 2004; 85(Suppl 3):S33; with permission.

---

appears to be true for even a once-weekly program. Where compliance or transportation to the therapy setting is at issue, this may be the most effective starting point [39]. Ultimately, the patient should be able to perform all exercise without supervision.

Although PRT is known to improve strength, the major controversy regarding it is whether it is the most effective means of improving muscle power and mobility skills. Declining muscle power is well documented in older adults and has also been more strongly associated with declines in functional performance than declines in strength. High-velocity training has been shown to improve power [40], and comparison between this and PRT alone is in the earliest stages. Another option to improve function may be to add task-specific exercises to PRT. These exercises simulate daily functional tasks to the greatest extent possible and are associated with functional gains [5].

Some further precautions are advised. In patients who have known severe cardiovascular or pulmonary disease, initial supervision by a physical therapist or nurse may be warranted, using blood pressure, pulse, and saturation by pulse oximetry (SpO_2) monitoring. Patients who have knee pain from severe OA may benefit from strength training, but weight-bearing exercises may worsen symptoms where knee malalignment and ligamentous laxity are evident [41]. Non–weight-bearing exercises or water-based programs may be a better initial prescription for these patients [42]. Patients with impairments such as cerebrovascular accident or multiple sclerosis, which affect muscles and motor neurons, may experience easier fatigue in these distributions. Strengthening is still beneficial to these patients but may need to be introduced and advanced more slowly.

The ultimate goal of any exercise program is transition to ensure compliance and adherence. One means of accomplishing this goal is to offer varied, low-cost programs in environments that are close to individuals' homes. Many physical therapy centers offer membership at a low rate for use at their gyms; senior centers have exercise classes, and community gym memberships may offer discounts to elders. Researchers have also noted strength gains using Tai Chi group exercise programs, which have the added benefit of providing social activity [3].

Endurance

Endurance is the ability to maintain a given level of exercise over time or to perform a given task repeatedly without fatigue that prevents further such activity. This factor is rooted in numerous physiologic parameters: air exchange in the lungs, heart function, blood circulation and patency of blood vessels, and the biochemical characteristics of individual muscle cells. Diseases or conditions such as coronary or peripheral vascular disease, restrictive or obstructive pulmonary disease, general deconditioning, and malnutrition may therefore adversely affect endurance.

Several terms are used to monitor endurance. *VO2 peak* represents the peak amount of oxygen that may be transported to the active muscles during exercise and is used extensively to chart progress in cardiac and pulmonary rehabilitation. Exercise intensity and caloric expenditure in general may be defined in terms of metabolic equivalents, or *METs*, where one MET is equivalent to the oxygen uptake of a person at rest or approximately 3.5 mL per minute. Subsequent METs represent multiples of this basal rate. Housework, such as vacuuming or mopping, uses approximately two to four METs; moderate exercise such as jogging uses five to six METs. Exercise over six METs is considered high intensity.

Elderly patients develop poor endurance as a result of many factors. Aging itself is associated with declining skeletal muscle mass and capillary blood flow, poor nutritional intake, and impaired oxygen uptake [43]. In addition to these factors, several common disease processes in elderly patients are shown to affect endurance. Approximately 11% of patients older than 70 have chronic obstructive pulmonary disease, which further decreases oxygen exchange in the lungs [44]. In addition to being a common cause of poor endurance, cardiovascular disease (including CHF and CAD) is the second most common ailment and the leading cause of death in older people [45]. General deconditioning from inactivity is common in older adults and contributes to poor endurance [46]; it may predispose to diabetes mellitus. With its associated neuropathies, pain syndromes, and attendant risk for cardiac disease, diabetes is both a risk factor for further inactivity and poor endurance and the sixth leading cause of death in adults 65 and older [47].

Benefits of endurance training

The benefits of endurance exercise in elderly patients have been studied, although some data are generalized from non–age-group specific studies. (In this article, the terms endurance and aerobic exercise are used interchangeably.) For patients at risk for cardiovascular disease, such as those who have hypertension and elevated lipid profiles, aerobic exercise has been associated with average decreases of 11 mm Hg in systolic blood pressure and 8 mm Hg in diastolic blood pressure [5,48,49]; in one study it was associated with both lowered total cholesterol and lowered low density lipoprotein levels. Cardiac mortality has been shown to be lowered by 31% [50]. In a study by Kavanagh and colleagues [51], patients with a recent history of cardiac illness who were enrolled in an aerobic exercise program increased their average VO_2 peak and improved their prognosis.

For patients who have diabetes, endurance exercise can have beneficial effects. Studies have shown improvements in insulin sensitivity as measured by glucose uptake after aerobic exercise training, both in experimental animals [52] and in humans [53]. Diabetic patients also show improved lipid profiles, blood pressure, and energy expenditure with endurance exercise programs [54–56].

Pulmonary disease is common in elderly patients, but data focusing on the effects of exercise in elders with respiratory problems are lacking. A great deal of data exists for the younger population of patients who have lung disease and shows that endurance exercise can improve both objective measures of lung function and perceived symptoms [5,57–59]. Endurance exercise may also reduce disability in patients who have lung disease. One randomized, controlled study showed that 18 months of aerobic exercise in patients aged 65 to 69 resulted in progressive improvements in functional tasks, including a 6% improvement in 6-minute walk tests, an 11% faster stair climbing speed, and reduced self-reported disability [60]. Further studies are required to evaluate the effects of exercise in older adults with pulmonary disease.

Where elders with specific disabilities are concerned, research again focuses mostly on stroke. Cycle ergometry modified for hemiparetic stroke patients, used thrice weekly for 30 minutes, produced improvements in workload, VO_2 maximum, exercise time, and systolic blood pressure [61]. Treadmill exercise in chronic stroke patients can also produce reductions in energy expenditure and cardiovascular demands during walking at a given exercise intensity [62]. For elders who have gait difficulty secondary to OA or rheumatoid arthritis, aerobic exercise can reduce pain and increase function [42,63].

Exercise prescription

Moderate-to-high-intensity aerobic exercise (five to six METs or more) for 30 minutes is a desirable goal for any patient but is obviously not a practical or safe starting point for deconditioned elders [64]. Any male patient older than 40 years and any female patient older than 50 to be enrolled in an endurance training program should first undergo a thorough medical examination, including a resting EKG and an exercise test [5,23,30,31]. (See previously discussed prescription information regarding strength training for specific contraindications and conditions requiring further evaluation and treatment.)

The starting point for this mode of exercise depends largely on baseline conditioning, transportation resources, and compliance. For a deconditioned older adult or one who will be more able to comply with a home-based program, low-intensity exercise may be the safest place to start. At this intensity, the patient should complete four to five sessions per week. The goal should be the prescription of exercises that maintain heart rate at an elevated level of 60% to 70% of the maximum age-predicted rate or perceived exertion of 11 to 13 on the Borg scale throughout the duration of exercise [65]. Aerobic exercises such as treadmill or street walking, bicycling, swimming, dancing, and the like are appropriate. These may be started twice weekly for 20 to 30 minutes but increased as rapidly as tolerated to approximately 30 minutes of moderate-intensity aerobic exercise on most if not all days of the week. Patients should be instructed to increase the duration of exercise before increasing intensity.

For patients who have pulmonary disease, it is commonly accepted practice to use supplemental oxygen where necessary to keep SpO_2 at greater than 88%. These patients, as well as others with known cardiac or vascular impairments, should be monitored for vital signs in a therapy gym by qualified staff, at least initially. Some conditions require special monitoring. Where vascular claudication is present, patients are usually instructed to exercise to just before the point of pain and try to maintain this level of intensity. Patients with impaired autonomic nervous systems, such as those with diabetic neuropathy, may be asked to employ alternative means of monitoring intensity, such as the Borg Scale of Perceived Effort. Another option is the "talk test," in which the patient's ability to engage in conversation during exercise is monitored and maintained [66,67].

Patients who have neurotrauma, stroke, multiple sclerosis, or late effects of poliomyelitis commonly experience physical and psychic fatigue at predictable points in the day and may fatigue more easily in affected muscle groups. However, the physiatric community has known for many years that endurance exercise introduced gradually and concurrently with energy conservation techniques throughout the day may alleviate these symptoms. Patients are generally encouraged to schedule more strenuous activity and therapies for earlier in the day, when energy is usually more abundant, and to make liberal use of naps in the afternoon and rest breaks throughout the day to replenish energy.

Balance

The topic of balance and its relationship to falls in the elderly is covered in great detail elsewhere in this issue. Balance is a complex trait and relies on the collective integrity of multiple peripheral and central nervous system components. These include Golgi organs, Ruffini corpuscles, muscle spindles, large myelinated proprioceptive nerve fibers, the posterior spinal cord columns, the medial lemniscus and cerebellum, and the vestibular and visual systems. Together these may be thought of as a "postural control system," with multiple redundant systems being employed to keep the body upright [68].

Effects of aging on balance

Deterioration in one or more aspects of the postural control system may occur naturally with age. Consequently, falls are the leading cause of accidental death in older persons [68]. When activity declines greatly with a lengthy hospital stay or other period of extreme immobility, general deconditioning may adversely affect balance [37]. Additionally, vascular disease, diabetes, excessive alcohol use, medications, and nutritional deficiencies may cause damage to peripheral nerves carrying proprioceptive information. Finally, Parkinson's disease and other common neurologic disorders have been shown adversely to affect balance [23].

Benefits of balance training

Most research on balance training addresses effects on falls and osteoporosis, for which weight-bearing exercise, including balance components such as weight shifting or postural sway, is often prescribed. Tai Chi is a form of exercise training that shows positive effects on balance [69,70]. One study suggests that Tai Chi participants were 27% less likely to fall than control counterparts [71], and other studies have shown improvement in fall risk assessment scores such as those on the Berg scale [72,73]. Training with weighted vests also benefits balance and is associated with reduction in fall risk indices [74]. Balance exercises for adults with specific disabilities have received limited research attention. For adults who have diabetic peripheral neuropathy, a brief course of high-velocity standing ankle exercises improved balance scores [75].

Exercise prescription

The superiority of one form of balance exercise over another has yet to be determined, so prescriptions must be made using common sense. First, the use of an assistive device such as a cane or walker concurrently with exercise should be considered when specific impairments increase fall risk. Pain control should also be provided by the most effective, least sedating means possible. The physician may wish to screen patients with recent falls or fractures, low body mass index, decreased safety awareness due to dementia, poor vision or hearing, reduced proprioception due to neuropathy, or balance deficits secondary to parkinsonism for low bone density using dual emission x-ray absorptiometry scan before initiating a balance exercise regimen. Appropriate disease-specific pharmacologic treatment may then be prescribed, such as Vitamin D, calcium, or bisphosphonates. Some data suggest that Vitamin D repletion may have an independent effect on falls and balance [76,77]. If exercise is chosen as a means of enhancing bone density, more strenuous, weight-bearing forms of exercise offer the greatest protective effect against bone loss. Moderate-to-high-intensity aerobic exercise and strenuous PRT are shown to have the greatest benefit in comprehensive literature reviews [5]. Patients and therapists should be counseled that improvements in bone density are generally seen over the course of a year or more. Importantly, these forms of exercise also improve body mass and decrease risk for falls.

When balance exercises are prescribed, aspects such as postural sway, weight shifting, strength, and speed work should be emphasized. These may initially be taught and monitored by a qualified therapist, but the patient should ultimately be able to continue independently. Another option for balance is Tai Chi exercise. Most insurance payers will not reimburse the patient for classes, but Tai Chi may have additional cost-effect advantages. It is often supervised by a highly trained instructor, which may enhance safety. It is also a sociable activity, which may improve long-term compliance. Such classes, however, may be deferred until after low-intensity exercise and pharmacologic treatment when osteoporosis is present.

Balance exercise may easily be incorporated into strength or endurance routines three or four times weekly. The American College of Sports Medicine recommends that a balance exercise program include both static and dynamic balance components [57]. The former include wide-base stance, narrow-base stance, and single-leg stance held for 30 or more seconds with eyes closed. The latter generally consist of walking exercises with various bases of support, beginning with normal gait and progressively narrowing the base to heel-to-toe gait. For both of these components, intensity may be varied by initially using an aid such as a raised bar or countertop, then withdrawing the aid. Although adults who have disabilities resulting from stroke, multiple sclerosis, neurotrauma, or amputation may require assistance and supervision from others when starting balance exercise, the prescribing practitioner should bear in mind the special importance for these patients of achieving independence in this modality.

Flexibility

Flexibility describes the range of motion (ROM) around a joint or joints in the body. The extensibility and intactness of many structures contribute to flexibility, including joint articular surfaces and capsules, loose connective tissue about muscles, joints and tendons, and the physical characteristics of muscles and tendons themselves.

The American College of Sports Medicine specifies two forms of flexibility exercise [57]. In dynamic stretching, the joint is moved through its full range repetitively. Static stretching involves moving the joint to end range and holding it there for some time. An additional form of flexibility training, *proprioceptive neuromuscular facilitation* (PNF), was developed shortly after the Second World

War to rehabilitate patients who had developed spasticity and contractures from injuries sustained in battle. This technique involves moving the affected joint diagonally through multiple planes just to the point of a spastic response, which is when the muscle spindle organs in the muscle group, being stretched, begin to trigger the hyperactive reflex that causes spasticity in that muscle group. The muscle group is then contracted at 50% to 100% intensity for 6 to 8 seconds, which inhibits the reflex and allows the joint to be moved beyond this point [78]. With time, substantial gains in ROM can be achieved.

Effects of aging on flexibility

The aging process results in decreased collagen synthesis in skin, ligaments, tendons, and underlying tissues, which may lead to slower healing and adaptation to changing movement patterns. Blood flow through these tissues and through muscle also decreases, further inhibiting these processes. Prolonged bed rest or common neurologic impairments in the elderly population that weaken muscles or cause spasticity lead to contracture by several mechanisms [37]. First, joint capsules and surrounding loose connective tissue form collagen cross links that may lead in time to irreversible contracture. Tendons and muscles, when maintained in a single position for extended periods, also become structurally altered and can shorten permanently. It is not known whether the relative inactivity characteristic of many elderly patients can produce similar permanent changes in ROM with time.

Fractures that displace tendons or rupture of tendons themselves enhances the risk for contracture, because tendon repair will produce disorganized collagen fibers unless tension is applied through the tendon in the post-repair period. Overlying conditions in elderly patients, such as inflammatory or noninflammatory arthritis, trauma, central nervous system insult, or pain, may foster contracture and impair function.

Benefits of flexibility training

Of all exercise modes, flexibility is the least studied in elderly patients. Investigators have generally performed studies of flexibility while concurrently studying other modes of exercise. For instance, the aforementioned study by Rimmer and colleagues [29] examined a group of predominantly African American stroke survivors, using an exercise regimen that included discrete components of strength, endurance, and flexibility training. Improvements were seen in hamstring and low back flexibility. Another group studied the specific effects of strength and cardiovascular training on flexibility [79]. Strength training both alone and in combination with aerobic training produced the greatest effects on flexibility around the elbow, knee, shoulder, and hip. In both these examples, it is not clear what functional advantage flexibility gains may have conferred.

Exercise prescription

No clear precautions against or contraindications to flexibility exercise exist, although gentle stretching should be used at first to avoid injury. Stretching should ideally be performed daily. A general prescription recommended for other age groups is four to five repetitions of approximately 30 seconds each for the most important joints and muscle groups [57]. Flexibility training may be incorporated into strength or endurance training or performed independently of other exercises. The routine should include both dynamic and static components. Prescribing physicians should also recommend techniques such as PNF in the presence of specific disabilities such as spasticity, resulting from disorders such as stroke or multiple sclerosis. Flexibility exercises are low intensity and can be performed sitting or lying down. They may be an especially useful warm-up for patients with impairments in endurance and balance.

Summary

This article incorporates some of the latest available data on the benefits of exercise in the elderly. The authors' methods are sound and frequently innovative. Even so, research methods in this field are not yet as sophisticated as in areas such as stroke and neurotrauma. Most studies use only local samples, often drawn by convenience. The Western world would no doubt benefit from a more unified and balanced approach to exercise research in this rapidly growing patient population. Interfacility databases, similar to those for brain and spinal cord injury, could be used to create study populations that are more indicative of the population of elders as a whole, permitting the drawing of stronger conclusions. Furthermore, few studies focus on disabled elders. Because the incidence of stroke, cardiac dysfunction, and related impairments is high in these patients, wider study of this population would be beneficial.

Although this article focuses on individual types of exercise and their contributions to patient health, any exercise program for a senior will incorporate aspects of them all. The program must be tailored to the individual needs of the patient, based on physical examination and laboratory and diagnostic data. (See case study in Box 2.)

The American College of Sports Medicine, while acknowledging that severely deconditioned older adults may prefer to begin with a low-intensity program such as twice weekly PRT, advises that frequency and intensity be increased to achieve an overall moderate-to-heavy-intensity goal. This principle holds especially true for endurance exercise, which is the best demonstrated by research to have a positive impact on health [57].

The community physician will undoubtedly encounter questions about whether exercise is safe for a deconditioned elder. Taking into account the aforementioned data, most physiatrists would advocate that the question be recast as one of whether an elder is safe remaining sedentary. A comprehensive over-

---

Box 2. Case study

An 82-year-old white female is hospitalized for a femoral neck fracture after tripping over her cat at home. She undergoes urgent hip hemiarthroplasty and makes an uneventful recovery, save for acute pain. You are called 3 days into her hospital course to consult for pain control and discharge recommendations. The patient was widowed 10 years ago and lives alone in a high-rise apartment building with ground-level entry and elevator. She does not smoke or drink. She rarely goes out, except to the grocery store across the street. She has a few friends in her building, with whom she visits a couple of times a week, but no family nearby. She reads avidly and does crossword puzzles. Her past medical history is significant for anxiety, for which she takes Ativan as needed. She also underwent closed reduction and casting for a Colles' fracture of the wrist 7 years ago.

- What are the possible deficits that put this patient at risk for her fracture? Include observations about premorbid physical conditioning as well as underlying medical conditions.
- What further work-up may be indicated?
- Develop an exercise plan for this woman. What is the best short-term plan while she heals from her surgery? What long-term physical fitness goals do you advise?

---

view of secondary prevention cardiovascular rehabilitation programs by Lisa Womack, MEd, found that a major contributing factor to poor patient compliance is "lack of physician endorsement" [80]. Accordingly, the physician should always emphasize to elders not only the specific recommended exercise program but also the benefits to be expected from it.

References

[1] Worsowicz GM, Stewart DG, Phillips EM, et al. Social and economic implications of aging. Arch Phys Med Rehabil 2004;85(Suppl 3):S3–6.

[2] King MB, Whipple RH, Gruman CA, et al. The performance enhancement project: improving physical performance in older persons. Arch Phys Med Rehabil 2002;83:1060–9.

[3] Wu G, Zhao F, Zhou X, et al. Improvement of isokinetic knee extensor strength and reduction of postural sway in the elderly from long-term Tai Chi exercise. Arch Phys Med Rehabil 2002;83(10):1364–9.

[4] Aniansson A, Gustafsson E. Physical training in elderly men. Clin Physiol 1981;1:87–98.

[5] Bean JF, Vora A, Frontera WR. Benefits of exercise for community-dwelling older adults. Arch Phys Med Rehabil 2004;85(Suppl 3):S31–42.

[6] Frontera WR, Meredith CN, O'Reilly KP, et al. Strength conditioning in older men: skeletal muscle hypertrophy and improved function. J Appl Physiol 1998;64:1038–44.

[7] Metter EJ, Conwit R, Tobin J, et al. Age-associated loss of power and strength in the upper extremities in women and men. J Gerontol A Biol Sci Med Sci 1997;52:B267–76.

[8] Loeser Jr RF. Aging and the etiopathogenesis and treatment of osteoarthritis. Rheum Dis Clin North Am 2000;26:547–67.

[9] Dargent-Molina P, Favier F, Grandjean H, et al. Fall-related factors and risk of hip fracture: the EPIDOS prospective study. Lancet 1996;348:145–9 [Published erratum in: Lancet 1996; 348:416.].

[10] Greenspan SL, Myers ER, Maitland LA, et al. Fall severity and bone mineral density as risk factors for hip fracture in ambulatory elderly. JAMA 1994;271:128–33.

[11] Kanis JA. Diagnosis of osteoporosis and assessment of fracture risk. Lancet 2002;359:1929–36.

[12] Phillips EM, Bodenheimer CF, Roig RL, et al. Physical medicine and rehabilitation interventions for common age-related disorders and geriatric syndromes. Arch Phys Med Rehabil 2004; 85(Suppl 3):S18–22.

[13] Delorme TL. Restoration of muscle power by heavy resistance exercises. J Bone Joint Surg Am 1945;27:645–67.

[14] de Lateur BJ, Lehmann JF, Fordyce WE. A test of the DeLorme Axiom. Arch Phys Med Rehabil 1968;49:245–8.

[15] de Lateur BJ. Therapeutic exercise. In: Braddom RL, Buschbacher RM, Dumitru D, et al, editors. Physical medicine and rehabilitation. 2nd edition. Philadelphia: WB Saunders; 2000. p. 392–412.

[16] Bean JF, Herman S, Kiely DK, et al. Increased velocity exercise specific to task (InVEST) training: a pilot study exploring effects on leg power, balance, and mobility in community-dwelling older women. J Am Geriatr Soc 2004;52:799–804.

[17] Fiatarone MA, O'Niell EF, Ryan ND, et al. Exercise training and nutritional supplementation for physical frailty in very elderly people. N Engl J Med 1994;330:1769–75.

[18] Fiatarone-Singh MA. The exercise prescription. In: Fiatarone-Singh MA, editor. Exercise, nutrition and the older woman: wellness for women over 50. Boca Raton (FL): CRC Pr; 2000. p. 37–104.

[19] Gordon NF, Kohl 3rd HW, Pollock ML, et al. Cardiovascular safety of maximal strength testing in healthy adults. Am J Cardiol 1995;76:851–3.

[20] McCartney N, Hicks AL, Martin J, et al. Long-term resistance training in the elderly: effects on dynamic strength, exercise capacity, muscle and bone. J Gerontol A Biol Sci Med Sci 1995; 50:B97–104.

[21] McCartney N. Acute responses to resistance training and safety. Med Sci Sports Exerc 1999; 31:31–7.

[22] Singh MA. Exercise comes of age: rationale and recommendations for a geriatric exercise prescription. J Gerontol A Biol Sci Med Sci 2002;57:M262–82.

[23] Borchu M, Savage P, Lee M, et al. Effects of resistance training on physical function in older disabled women with coronary heart disease. J Appl Physiol 2002;92:672–8.

[24] Pu CT, Nelson ME. Aging, function and exercise. In: Frontera W, editor. Exercise in rehabilitation medicine. 3rd edition. Champaign (IL): Human Kinetics; 1999. p. 391–424.

[25] Martel GF, Hurlbut DE, Lott ME, et al. Strength training normalizes resting blood pressure in 65 to 73-year-old men and women with high normal blood pressure. J Am Geriatr Soc 1999;47:1215–21.

[26] Cifu DX, Burnett D, McGowan JP. Rehabilitation after hip fracture. In: Grabois M, Garrison SJ, Lehmkuhl D, editors. Physical medicine and rehabilitation: the complete approach. Malden (MA): Blackwell Science; 2000. p. 1534–50.

[27] Mitchell SL, Stott DJ, Martin BJ, et al. Randomized controlled trial of quadriceps training after proximal femoral fracture. Clin Rehabil 2001;15:282–90.

[28] Roig RL, Worsowicz GM, Stewart DG, et al. Physical medicine and rehabilitation interventions for common disabling disorders. Arch Phys Med Rehabil 2004;85(Suppl 3):S12–7.

[29] Sherrington C, Lord SR. Home exercises to improve strength and walking velocity after hip fracture: a randomized controlled trial. Arch Phys Med Rehabil 1997;78:208–12.

[30] Buchner DM, Cress ME, de Lateur BJ, et al. The effect of strength and endurance training on gait, balance, fall risk, and health services use in community-living older adults. J Gerontol A Biol Sci Med Sci 1997;52:M218–24.

[31] Campell AJ, Robertson MC, Gardner MM, et al. Falls prevention over 2 years: a randomized controlled trial in women 80 years and older. Age Ageing 1999;28:513–8.

[32] Nelson ME, Fiatarone MA, Morganti CM, et al. Effects of high-intensity strength training on multiple risk factors for osteoporotic fractures: a randomized controlled trial. JAMA 1994; 272:1909–14.

[33] Nicholas JJ. Rehabilitation of patients with rheumatological disorders. In: Braddom RL, Buschbacher RM, Dumitru D, editors. Physical medicine and rehabilitation. 2nd edition. Philadelphia: WB Saunders; 2000. p. 743–61.

[34] Rimmer JH, Riley B, Creviston T, et al. Exercise training in a predominantly African-American group of stroke survivors. Med Sci Sports Exerc 2000;32:1990–6.

[35] Oullette MM, LeBrasseur NK, Bean JF, et al. High-intensity resistance training improves muscle strength, self-reported function, and disability in long-term stroke survivors. Stroke 2004; 35(6):1404–9.

[36] Seto CK. Preparticipation cardiovascular screening. Clin Sports Med 2003;22:23–35.

[37] American College of Sports Medicine Position Stand. Exercise and physical activity for older adults. Med Sci Sports Exerc 1998;30:992–1008.

[38] Gill TM, DiPietro L, Krumholz HM. Role of exercise stress testing and safety monitoring for older persons starting an exercise program. JAMA 2000;284(3):342–9.

[39] Taaffe D, Duret C, Wheeler S, et al. Once-weekly resistance exercise improves muscle strength and neuromuscular performance in older adults. J Am Geriatr Soc 1999;47(10):1208–14.

[40] Fielding R, LeBrasseur N, Cuoco A, et al. High-velocity resistance training increases skeletal muscle peak power in older women. J Am Geriatr Soc 2002;50(4):655–62.

[41] Sharma L, Dunlop DD, Cahue S, et al. Quadriceps strength and osteoarthritis progression in malaligned and lax knees. Ann Intern Med 2003;138:613–9.

[42] Minor MA, Hewett JE, Webel RR, et al. Efficacy of physical conditioning exercises in patients with rheumatoid arthritis and osteoarthritis. Arthritis Rheum 1989;32(11):1396–405.

[43] Chandler J, Studenski S. Exercise. In: Duthie E, Katz P, editors. Practice of geriatrics. Philadephia: WB Saunders; 1998. p. 131–44.

[44] Alba AS. Concepts in pulmonary rehabilitation. In: Braddom RL, Buschbacher RM, Dumitru D, et al, editors. Physical medicine and rehabilitation. 2nd edition. Philadelphia: WB Saunders; 2000. p. 687–701.

[45] Kramorow E, Lenttzer H, Rooks R, et al. Health and aging chartbook. Health, United States, 1999. Hyattsville (MD): National Center for Health Statistics; 1999.

[46] Buschbacher RM, Porter CD. Deconditioning, reconditioning and the benefits of exercise. In: Braddom RL, Buschbacher RM, Dumitru D, et al, editors. Physical medicine and rehabilitation. 2nd edition. Philadelphia: WB Saunders; 2000. p. 702–76.

[47] Desai MM, Zhang P, Hennessy CH. Surveillance for morbidity and mortality among older adults—United States, 1995–1996. MMWR CDC Surveill Summ 1999;48:7–25 [Published erratum in: MMWR CDC Surveill Summ 2000;49:14,23.].

[48] Kelley GA, Kelley KS. Progressive resistance exercise and reducing blood pressure: a meta-analysis of randomized controlled trials. Hypertension 2000;35:838–43.

[49] Kokkinos PF, Narayan P, Papademetriou V. Exercise as hypertension therapy. Cardiol Clin 2001;19:507–16.

[50] Jolliffe JA, Rees K, Taylor RS, et al. Exercise-based rehabilitation for coronary heart disease. Cochrane Database Syst Rev 2001;1:CD001800.

[51] Kavanagh T, Mertens DJ, Hamm LF, et al. Prediction of long-term prognosis in 12,169 men referred for cardiac rehabilitation. Circulation 2002;106:666–71.

[52] Ivy JL. Muscle insulin resistance amended with exercise training: role of GLUT4 expression. Med Sci Sports Exerc 2004;36(7):1207–11.

[53] Hamdy O, Goodyear LJ, Horton ES. Diet and exercise in type 2 diabetes mellitus. Endocrinol Metab Clin North Am 2001;30:883–907.

[54] Hu FB, Stampfer MJ, Solomon CG, et al. The impact of diabetes mellitus on mortality from all causes and coronary heart disease in women: 20 years of follow-up. Arch Intern Med 2001;161: 1717–23.

[55] Hu FB, Stampfer MJ, Solomon C, et al. Physical activity and risk for cardiovascular events in diabetic women. Ann Intern Med 2001;134:96–105.

[56] Horton ES. Diabetes mellitus. In: Frontera WR, editor. Exercise in rehabilitation medicine. 3rd edition. Champaign (IL): Human Kinetics; 1999. p. 211–25.

[57] Casaburi R, Patessio A, Ioli F, et al. Reductions in exercise lactic acidosis and ventilation as a result of exercise training in patients with obstructive lung disease. Am Rev Respir Dis 1991;143:9–18.

[58] Celli B. Respiratory disease. In: Frontera WR, editor. Exercise in rehabilitation medicine. 3rd edition. Champaign (IL): Human Kinetics; 1999. p. 193–210.

[59] Levine S, Johnson B, Nguyen T, et al. Exercise retraining. In: Cherniack NS, Altose MD, Homma I, editors. Rehabilitation of the patient with respiratory disease. New York: McGraw Hill; 1999. p. 417–30.

[60] Berry MJ, Rejeski WJ, Adair NE, et al. A randomized, controlled trial comparing long-term and short-term exercise in patients with chronic obstructive pulmonary disease. J Cardiopulm Rehabil 2003;23:60–8.

[61] Potempa K, Lopez M, Braun LT, et al. Physiological outcomes of aerobic exercise training in hemiparetic stroke patients. Stroke 1995;26:101–5.

[62] Macko RF, DeZouza CA, Tretter LD, et al. Treadmill aerobic exercise training reduces the energy expenditure and cardiovascular demands of hemiparetic gait in chronic stroke patients: a preliminary report. Stroke 1997;28:326–30.

[63] Ettinger Jr WH, Burns R, Messier SP, et al. A randomized trial comparing aerobic exercise and resistance exercise with a health education program in older adults with knee osteoarthritis. The Fitness Arthritis and Seniors Trial (FAST). JAMA 1997;277:25–31.

[64] US Department of Health and Human Services. Physical activity and health: a report of the Surgeon General. Atlanta (GA): Centers for Disease Control and Prevention, National Center for Chronic Disease Prevention and Health Promotion; 1996.

[65] Borg G. Perceived exertion as an indicator of somatic stress. Scand J Rehab Med 1970;2:92–8.

[66] Moldover JR, Bartels MN. Cardiac rehabilitation. In: Braddom RL, Buschbacher RM, Dumitru D, et al, editors. Physical medicine and rehabilitation. 2nd edition. Philadelphia: WB Saunders; 2000. p. 665–86.

[67] Cress ME, Buchner DM, Prohaska T, et al. Physical activity programs and behavior counseling in older adult populations. Med Sci Sports Exerc 2004;36(11):1997–2003.

[68] Studenski S, Wolter L. Instability and falls. In: Duthie E, Katz P, editors. Practice of geriatrics. Philadephia: WB Saunders; 1998. p. 199–206.

[69] Wolf SL, Barnhart HX, Kutner NG, et al. Reducing frailty and falls in older persons: an investigation of Tai Chi and computerized balance training. Atlanta FICSIT Group. Frailty and Injuries: Cooperative Studies of Intervention Techniques. J Am Geriatr Soc 1996;44:489–97.

[70] Wolf SL, Coogler C, Xu T. Exploring the basis for Tai Chi Chuan as a therapeutic exercise approach. Arch Phys Med Rehabil 1997;78:886–92.

[71] Li F, Harmer P, Fisher KJ, et al. Tai Chi: improving functional balance and predicting subsequent falls in older persons. Med Sci Sports Exerc 2004;36(12):2046–52.

[72] Tsang WWN, Hui-Chan CWY. Effects of Tai Chi on joint proprioception and stability limits in elderly subjects. Med Sci Sports Exerc 2003;35(12):1962–71.

[73] Tsang WWN, Hui-Chan CWY. Comparison of muscle torque, balance, and confidence in older Tai Chi and healthy adults. Med Sci Sports Exerc 2005;37(2):280–9.

[74] Shaw JM, Snow CM. Weighted vest exercise improves indices of fall risk in older women. J Gerontol A Biol Sci Med Sci 1998;53:M53–8.

[75] Richardson JK, Sandman D, Vela S. A focused exercise regimen improves clinical measures of balance in patients with peripheral neuropathy. Arch Phys Med Rehabil 2001;82:205–9.

[76] Bischoff HA, Stahelin HB, Dick W, et al. Effects of vitamin D and calcium supplementation on falls: a randomized controlled trial. J Bone Miner Res 2003;18(2):343–51.

[77] Bischoff HA, Stahelin HB, Tyndall A, et al. Relationship between muscle strength and vitamin D metabolites: are there therapeutic possibilities in the elderly? J Rheumatol 2001;59(Suppl 1): 39–41.

[78] Anderson R, Burke ER. Stretching. In: DeLee JC, Drez D, editors. Orthopaedic sports medicine: principles and practice. 2nd edition. Philadelphia: WB Saunders; 1985. p. 383–4.

[79] Fatouros IG, Taxildaris K, Tokmakidis SP, et al. The effects of strength training, cardiovascular training and their combination on flexibility of inactive older adults. Int J Sports Med 2002; 23(2):112–9.

[80] Womack L. Cardiac rehabilitation secondary prevention programs. Clin Sports Med 2003;22: 135–60.

CLINICS IN
GERIATRIC
MEDICINE

Clin Geriatr Med 22 (2006) 257–267

Rehabilitation Outcomes in the Older Adult

Cathy M. Cruise, MD[a,b,*], Nicole Sasson, MD[a,c],
Mathew H.M. Lee, MD[a]

[a]Rusk Institute of Rehabilitation, New York University School of Medicine, Suite 600,
400 East 34th Street, New York, NY 10016, USA
[b]Physical Medicine and Rehabilitation Service/117, Veterans Integrated Service Network #3,
Northport Veterans Affairs Medical Center, 79 Middleville Road, Northport, NY 11768, USA
[c]Physical Medicine and Rehabilitation Service/117, Department of Veterans Affairs,
New York Harbor Healthcare System, 423 East 23rd Street, New York, NY 10010, USA

There are numerous studies supporting the use of rehabilitative interventions in the older adult. Given the many fiscal challenges in health care today, it is of utmost importance that patient care dollars be placed toward rehabilitation that results in fruitful outcomes.

Rehabilitation of the older adult encompasses two populations: the elderly who become disabled and the disabled who become elderly. It is common knowledge that the size of the population over the age of 65 years is increasing rapidly. Americans aged 65 years and older numbered 35.9 million in 2003, an increase of 3.1 million or 9.5% since 1993. By the year 2030 the older population is expected to double to 71.5 million. Individuals over the age of 85 comprise the fastest growing segment of this population and the group that requires the greatest amount of help because of disability. The 85-plus population is expected to increase from 4.7 million in 2003 to 9.6 million in 2030 [1]. These factors, combined with economic challenges within society make it essential that rehabilitative health care be put to good use. Decisions as to what type of rehabilitation practices to use in the older adult should be based on objective outcome measures.

* Corresponding author. Rusk Institute of Rehabilitation, New York University School of Medicine, Suite 600, 400 East 34th Street, New York, NY 10016.
  E-mail address: cmcruise@optonline.net (C.M. Cruise).

Outcome measures

There are a variety of outcomes measures that can be used to determine rehabilitation potential and progress in the elderly. These can be most easily grouped
into individual and programmatic measures.

Setting goals

Goals for rehabilitation in the elderly must be set by the rehabilitation team in
conjunction with the patient and caregiver. Goals should be as realistic as possible, and be aimed at improving function and independence. Individual patient
goals may be successfully viewed in terms of the theoretically achievable goal
score. The theoretically achievable goal is the ultimate attainment in rehabilitation that a disabled person can reach under the most ideal conditions: physical,
intellectual, mental, physiologic, social, economic, and environmental. Although
the theoretically achievable goal score is greatly influenced by age, it can vary
within the same age group, depending on the individual. The theoretically
achievable goal score sharply increases in early life, reaches a maximum at approximately 20 to 35 years of age, and then gradually declines as age advances
(Fig. 1) [2].

Individual measures

The functional independence measure (FIM) is perhaps one of the most
widely used standard tools for collecting data about patients' functional performance on entry into and discharge from an acute inpatient rehabilitation setting.
A recent retrospective review provides evidence for the validity of using FIM
items to derive four domains of functional independence (mobility, activities of
daily living, sphincter management, and executive function) in patients receiving

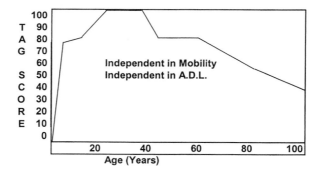

Fig. 1. Theoretically Achievable Goal (TAG) score according to age. Score sharply increases in early
life, reaches maximum at approximately 20 to 35 years of age, and gradually declines as age advances. (*From* Lee M, Itoh M. Geriatric rehabilitation management. In: Goodgold J, editor. Rehabilitation medicine. St. Louis: CV Mosby; 1988. p. 396; with permission.)

rehabilitation in skilled nursing facilities [3]. Taking the FIM a step further, the Functional Status and Outcomes Database has been developed within the Veterans Health Administration. This database allows FIM scores to be tracked for all veterans receiving rehabilitation for new-onset stroke, amputation, and traumatic brain injury. FIM scores are collected on initial evaluation by rehabilitation providers and then followed until the veteran completes his or her rehabilitation course. This expands the data collection window from the inpatient rehabilitation course to the full spectrum of rehabilitation care, potentially ending in home or outpatient therapy [4]. Functional independence staging has been introduced by Steinman and coworkers [5] to address limitations experienced in applying continuous aggregate FIM scores in clinical practice.

Quality, patient satisfaction, and lifestyle measures may also be used to determine individual outcomes in the elderly. Further, the number of hospital and nursing home admissions, emergency room visits, and unscheduled clinic visits represent important metrics that are often followed. Cost is important to consider, although very difficult to calculate accurately given the complexity and inclusiveness of the rehabilitation process.

Program evaluation outcomes

Programmatic outcomes measures and accreditation processes allow one to assess the effectiveness of interdisciplinary processes. The mission of CARF, the Rehabilitation Accreditation Commission, is to promote the quality, value, and optimal outcomes of services through accreditation that centers on enhancing the lives of the persons served. More than 38,000 programs are CARF accredited within the United States, Canada, and Europe. The variety of programs accredited includes comprehensive medical rehabilitation, employment and community services, child and youth services, behavioral health, and aging services. Within medical rehabilitation, there is specific accreditation for traumatic brain injury, spinal cord injury, pain management, and other programs [6]. The Joint Commission on Accreditation of Health Care Organizations is the nation's leading standards-setting and accrediting body in health care, focused on improving the quality and safety of care provided by health care organizations. Accreditation is a distinction given to an organization when its performance meets or exceeds the Joint Commission's standards and quality expectations [7].

Benefit of rehabilitation in the elderly

Specific rehabilitative interventions have been found to be very effective in the elderly, and can be demonstrated through numerous studies. Progressive resistive muscle strength training has been found to be beneficial in hospitalized frail elderly. Sullivan and coworkers [8] noted that a 10-week program of lower limb progressive resistive strength training resulted in improved sit-to-stand maneuver times, one repetition maximum, and improved maximum safe gait speeds. Morey and coworkers [9] demonstrated in a prospective longitudinal study of 69 patients over the age of 64 years given 90 minutes of exercise three times per week at 70% of maximal capacity including stationary cycling, stretching, weight training, and walking that the exercise group increased metabolic equivalents, treadmill time, hip flexibility, and abdominal strength and decreased submaximal and resting heart rates with no major complications. Additionally, weight training has been shown to improve walking endurance in healthy elderly persons [10].

Specialized evaluation of the older adult has been found to result in improved rehabilitative outcomes. In a controlled trial of inpatient and outpatient geriatric evaluation and management published by Cohen and coworkers [11], frail patients 65 years of age or older who were hospitalized at 11 Veterans Affairs Medical Centers were evaluated. After their condition had been stabilized, patients were randomly assigned to receive either care in an inpatient geriatric unit or usual inpatient care in the hospital followed by either care at an outpatient geriatric clinic or usual outpatient care. The interventions involved teams that provided geriatric assessment and management according to Veterans Affairs standards and published guidelines. The primary outcomes were survival and health-related quality of life measured with the Short Form-36 1 year after randomization. Secondary outcomes were the ability to perform activities of daily living, physical performance, use of health services, and costs. It was concluded that although the care provided in inpatient geriatric units and outpatient geriatric clinics had no significant effects on survival, there were significant reductions in functional decline with inpatient geriatric evaluation and management and improvements in mental health with outpatient geriatric evaluation and management, with no increase in costs.

Specific rehabilitative conditions

Stroke

Adults over the age of 55 years have a lifetime risk for stroke of greater than one in six [12]. Many have underlying diabetes, hypertension, and cardiovascular disease. Additionally, cognitive deficits may result from stroke, which may influence rehabilitation outcomes. The choice of setting for rehabilitation for the stroke patient is an important one. In a study by Kramer and coworkers [13], outcomes and costs after hip fracture and stroke were compared. It was noted that there were enhanced outcomes for elderly patients with stroke treated in rehabilitation hospitals but not for patients with hip fracture. Subacute nursing homes were found to be more effective than traditional nursing homes in returning patients with stroke to the community, despite comparable functional outcomes. Comparison of subacute with acute rehabilitation by Keith and coworkers [14] showed that acute rehabilitation involved twice as much cost and twice as many treatment hours but resulted in greater functional gains and no difference in discharge disposition. The cost per successful discharge was greater than twice as much for acute rehabilitation. Clearly, this study highlights the importance of carefully examining the costs and benefits of acute versus subacute rehabilitation.

The proper selection of patients to receive rehabilitation for stroke in a nursing home setting is essential. A recent retrospective cohort study by Murray and coworkers [15] examined the effects of stroke rehabilitation in the nursing home on community discharge rates and functional status among patients stratified by propensity to receive rehabilitation, using a propensity score based on clinical and social characteristics, including 108 patient descriptors in the Minimal Data Set recorded at the time of nursing home admission. It was noted that, with respect to community discharge, patients who were less likely to receive rehabilitation therapy seemed to receive greater benefit from the rehabilitation services than those who were more likely to receive rehabilitation. This finding raises concerns about current selection practices for rehabilitation services. Research is needed to identify the patients most likely to benefit, especially in the present fiscally constrained reimbursement environment.

Traumatic brain injury

Older adults are at increased risk of traumatic brain injury, usually sustained through a fall or a motor vehicle accident. These individuals often tend to have worse functional outcomes and greater disability [16–18]. The impact of age on health problems related to traumatic brain injury was recently examined using a survey instrument. It was noted that individuals with traumatic brain injury reported significantly more overall health problems than those without traumatic brain injury. Younger subjects with traumatic brain injury reported more problems than their nondisabled aged-matched peers with their patterns of sleep and with their metabolic-endocrine, neurologic, and musculoskeletal systems. Older people with traumatic brain injury were also more likely than nondisabled, age-matched peers to report problems with their metabolic-endocrine and neurologic systems. Younger people with traumatic brain injury were more likely than older people with traumatic brain injury to report difficulty falling asleep [19].

The ultimate goal of a traumatic brain injury rehabilitation program is to return the individual to his or her premorbid functional status, which is dependent on several factors including the ability to perform functional tasks, presence of behavioral or cognitive dysfunction, level of family support, and amount of financial resources. Traumatic brain injury patients discharged from acute medical and rehabilitation hospitals often require continuing rehabilitation services. These may be provided through home services, outpatient rehabilitation clinics, residential care programs, day treatment centers, and skilled nursing facilities. In all cases a great deal of community support is essential [20].

Telephone counseling shows promise as a low cost, widely available rehabilitation intervention for traumatic brain injury. Scheduled telephone counseling

262   CRUISE et al

and education results in improved overall outcome, particularly for functional status and quality of well-being, when compared with usual outpatient care [21].

Spinal cord injury

Patients surviving late-life spinal cord injuries are more likely to have incomplete injuries, perhaps because of a higher mortality rate with high-level complete injury. Conditions found to be more prevalent in the older population with spinal cord injury include carpal tunnel syndrome, chronic obstructive pulmonary disease, myocardial infarction, diabetes, kidney stones, pressure ulcers, and hypertension [22]. In addition to increased numbers of elderly surviving spinal cord injury, the number of years of survival with spinal cord injury is increasing. Duration of spinal cord injuries has been associated with decreased financial security and an increase in symptoms and illnesses [23]. The ultimate goal of the rehabilitation process is to integrate the individual with spinal cord injuries into the community. The level of participation in family, vocational, avocational, and civic activities is influenced by the severity of impairment and presence of secondary conditions and the magnitude of financial resources, level of family support, and scope of psychologic adjustment. Educational and professional achievement before acquiring spinal cord injuries also influences community reintegration [24]. A recent retrospective review examined what effect the injury-to-rehabilitation interval has on the outcome of spinal cord injury rehabilitation. Early rehabilitation seemed to be a relevant prognostic factor of functional outcome. Rehabilitation intervention in patients with spinal cord injuries should begin as soon as possible in a specialized setting because delay may adversely affect functional recovery [25]. The role of the caretaker in the rehabilitation of patients with spinal cord injury is extremely important. The caretaker should be included in all rehabilitation plans and with goal setting.

Amputation

There is an increased incidence of amputation in the elderly likely caused in part by the increased prevalence of vascular insufficiency and diabetes mellitus in this population. Amputees of older age are more likely to present problems in rehabilitation because of a decrease in cardiopulmonary capacity, poor neuromuscular coordination, visual impairment, weakened musculature, or limitations in range of joint movement that impose restrictions on the intensity of preprosthetic and prosthetic training programs. The goals for rehabilitation of geriatric amputees should be realistic. Generally, the most common needs are the restoration to premorbid levels of activities of daily living and recreation. When prosthesis is selected, safety must be emphasized. To enable amputees to become as functional and as independent as possible, one should not hesitate to provide a wheelchair if needed [8]. This is particularly true if the patient must negotiate long distances to perform his or her activities of daily living or instrumental activities of daily living independently.

Post–hip fracture

Optimal outcomes after a hip fracture may only be achieved when the cause of the hip fracture is addressed. Risk factors noted potentially to lead to hip fractures include lower limb dysfunction, neurologic conditions, barbiturate use, and visual impairment [26]. The recommended components of clinical assessment and management of older persons living in the community who are at risk for falls include circumstances of previous falls, medication use, vision, postural blood pressure, balance and gait, targeted neurologic examination, targeted musculoskeletal examination, targeted cardiovascular examination, and home hazard evaluation after hospital discharge [27]. In a prospective study examining falls, injuries caused by falls, and risk of admission to a nursing home it was noted that falls are a strong predictor of placement in a skilled nursing facility [28].

Early mobilization after hip fracture is important to prevent pneumonia, deep venous thrombosis, pulmonary embolus, and urinary tract infection and to decrease the amount of deconditioning and decrease the incidence of decubitus ulcers. The choice of setting for rehabilitation is very important. Recently FIM instrument motor outcomes were compared between hip fracture survivors undergoing rehabilitation in inpatient rehabilitation facilities and skilled nursing facilities. It was concluded that the patients admitted to an inpatient rehabilitation facility had superior 12-week functional outcomes, as measured by the FIM motor score, compared with those treated in a skilled nursing facility. The improved outcomes occurred during a significantly shorter rehabilitation length of stay and remained even when statistically controlling for baseline differences between groups. The data suggest that hip fracture survivors should not be excluded from receiving inpatient rehabilitation services [29].

Post–joint replacement

Rehabilitation after joint replacement surgery should be a delicate balance of rest and activity. Individuals must avoid overuse of joints yet at the same time prevent deconditioning. Treatment should combine psychologic, pharmacologic, and physical measures. Munin and coworkers [30] prospectively studied factors predicting successful discharge of 162 patients who underwent elective hip or knee arthroplasty from a rehabilitation unit with the primary outcome measure of discharge to home or to a rehabilitation unit. Patients discharged to an inpatient rehabilitation unit tended to live alone; were significantly older (average age 74 versus 65); and had increased comorbid conditions. Patients discharged to inpatient rehabilitation had higher pain levels. For patients who lived alone, the inability to attain a supervision level with sit-to-stand transfers after three physical therapy sessions predicted 76% of discharges to inpatient rehabilitation. Interestingly, the surgeon, type of prosthesis, surgical sequence, and weight-bearing status were not predictive of discharge destination.

The choice of setting for rehabilitation in the older adult

The rehabilitation team must often decide if an individual will benefit most from rehabilitation therapies provided on an inpatient unit, as an outpatient, or in the home setting. Gill and coworkers [31] studied 188 patients over the age of 75 who underwent a 6-month intervention program that included physical therapy and focused primarily on improving underlying impairments in physical abilities including balance, muscular strength, ability to transfer from one position to another, and mobility versus an educational program (control group). It was concluded that a home-based program targeting underlying impairments in physical abilities can reduce the progression of functional decline among physically frail, elderly persons who live at home. Another question often posed is if better rehabilitation outcomes are achieved by an interdisciplinary rehabilitation unit compared with usual hospital care. In a prospective study published by Landefeld and coworkers [32], 327 patients were randomly assigned to an interdisciplinary program stressing function and rehabilitation where programs for preventing disability were reviewed daily, whereas 324 patients were randomly assigned to receive usual care elsewhere in the hospital. Change in activities of daily living score between admission and discharge was used as the main outcome measure. It was noted that at the time of discharge, patients in the intervention group had significantly more restoration and preservation of function. Additionally, fewer patients in the intervention group were discharged to long-term care facilities. The study concluded that attention to preservation and restoration of functional status should be part of every care plan. The relationship between therapy intensity including physical therapy, occupational therapy, and speech and language therapy provided in a skilled nursing facility setting and patients' outcomes as measured by length of stay and stage of functional independence as measured by the FIM instrument were recently reviewed by Jette and coworkers [33]. Higher therapy intensity was associated with better outcomes as they relate to length of stay and functional improvement for patients who have stroke, orthopedic conditions, and cardiovascular and pulmonary conditions and are receiving rehabilitation in a skilled nursing facility setting.

Rehabilitation in the community

Functional decline in physically frail, elderly persons is associated with substantial morbidity. In a recent study by Gill and coworkers [31], 188 persons 75 years of age or older who were physically frail and living at home were randomly assigned to undergo a 6-month home-based intervention program that included physical therapy and focused primarily on improving underlying impairments in physical abilities, including balance, muscle strength, ability to transfer from one position to another, and mobility, or to undergo an educational program as a control. The primary outcome was the change between baseline and 3, 7, and 12 months in the score on a disability scale based on eight activities of daily living: (1) walking, (2) bathing, (3) upper body dressing, (4) lower body dressing, (5) transferring from a chair, (6) using the toilet, (7) eating, and (8) grooming. Participants in the intervention group were found to have less functional decline over time, according to their disability scores, than participants in the control group. The benefit of the intervention was observed among participants with moderate frailty but not severe frailty. The frequency of admission to a nursing home did not differ significantly between the intervention group and the control group. The authors concluded that a home-based program targeting underlying impairments in physical abilities can reduce the progression of functional decline among physically frail, elderly persons who live at home. Because it is often difficult for elderly persons to find an appropriate setting for exercise, easy to implement programs are often most effective. Walking has been shown to be extremely beneficial and is often very appealing to the older adult because it is inexpensive and can be done almost anywhere. Additionally, walking has been shown to have a positive effect on cardiovascular events in women. In a recent study reported by Manson and coworkers [34], the risk of cardiovascular events was lowest among women with high levels of energy expenditure from both walking and vigorous exercise, but for women with no history of vigorous exercise, high weekly levels of walking were associated with significant reductions in cardiovascular events. The optimal intensity of exercise is best determined after an exercise stress test, particularly in patients with a history of or risk factors for cardiovascular disease.

New directions

Telemedicine is increasingly being used to deliver rehabilitative care to older adults both in the clinic setting and at home. Health-related outcomes during a 1-year period were compared for two groups of frail elders, one that received care coordination by distance monitoring (home telehealth) and one that received no intervention. Subjects in both groups had primary diagnoses of hypertension, diabetes, respiratory disease, or heart disease. The groups were similar in age, race, marital status, and independence in instrumental activities of daily living at baseline. Over 1 year the intervention group showed significant improvement in instrumental activity of daily living scores, FIM motor scores, and FIM cognitive scores. This evidence supports the use of a specific home telehealth strategy for care coordination to improve functional independence in noninstitutionalized veterans with chronic disease [35]. Telehealth is increasingly being used to deliver rehabilitative services to elderly individuals in remote areas where specialist expertise is rare. Communication by telemonitors allows older adults to receive specialist consultation without unnecessary travel, often enabling the individuals to receive orthotic and prosthetic equipment that otherwise could not be prescribed.

Future directions

The complexity of the health care system is increasing rapidly and economic challenges are becoming more severe. This is particularly true when decisions regarding services to be provided to the elderly are involved. Older adults are surviving stroke, traumatic brain injury, spinal cord injury, amputation, and falls, resulting in fracture in greater numbers. Life expectancy in general, and particularly post these traumatic events, is increasing. It is known that specific rehabilitative interventions can be very successful, yet more detail is needed regarding exactly which interventions for which conditions provide the most cost-effective results. In addition to function, clinicians must increasingly look toward quality of life and patient satisfaction measures to assess outcomes. Of growing interest is the provision of telehealth services to the elderly and their ability to result in effective rehabilitative outcomes.

References

[1] Administration on Aging Statistics. A profile of older Americans: 2004. Available at: www.aoa.dhhs.gov/prof/statistics/profile/2004. Accessed July 11, 2005.
[2] Lee M, Itoh M. Geriatric rehabilitation management. In: Goodgold J, editor. Rehabilitation medicine. St. Louis: CV Mosby; 1988. p. 393–406.
[3] Jetted DU, Warren RL, Writable C. Functional independence domains in patients receiving rehabilitation in skilled nursing facilities: evaluation of psychometric properties. Arch Phys Med Rehabil 2005;86:1089–94.
[4] Physical Medicine and Rehabilitation. Department of Veterans Affairs. Functional status and outcomes database. Available at: vaww1.va.gov/health/rehab/FSOD.htm. Accessed July 11, 2005.
[5] Steinman MG, Ross RN, Fielder R, et al. Staging functional independence: validity and applications. Arch Phys Med Rehabil 2003;84:38–45.
[6] The Rehabilitation Commission. The Commission on Accreditation of Rehabilitation Facilities, 2003. Available at: www.carf.org. Accessed June 27, 2005.
[7] The Joint Commission on Accreditation of Healthcare Organizations. Quality check. Who is the Joint Commission? What is Accreditation? Available at: www.jcaho.org. Accessed June 27, 2005.
[8] Sullivan DH, Wall PT, Bariola JR, et al. Progressive resistance muscle strength training of hospitalized frail elderly. Am J Phys Med Rehabil 2001;80:503–8.
[9] Morey MC, Cowper PA, Feussner JR, et al. Evaluation of a supervised exercise program in a geriatric population. J Am Geriatr Soc 1989;37:348–54.
[10] Ades P, Ballor DL, Ashikaga T, et al. Weight training improves walking endurance in healthy elderly persons. Ann Intern Med 1996;124:568–72.
[11] Cohen HJ, Feussner JR, Weinberger M, et al. A controlled trial of inpatient and outpatient geriatric evaluation and management. N Engl J Med 2002;346:905–12.
[12] Heart disease and stroke statistics–2005 update. American Heart Association. Available at: www.americanheart.org/downloadable/heart. Accessed July 11, 2005.
[13] Kramer AM, Steiner JF, Schlenker RE, et al. Outcomes and costs after hip fracture and stroke: a comparison of rehabilitation settings. JAMA 1997;227:396–404.
[14] Keith RA, Wilson DB, Gutierrez P. Acute and subacute rehabilitation for stroke: a comparison. Arch Phys Med Rehabil 1995;76:495–500.
[15] Murray PK, Dawson NV, Thomas CL, et al. Are we selecting the right patients for stroke rehabilitation in nursing homes? Arch Phys Med Rehabil 2005;86:876–80.

[16] Howard MA, Gross AS, Dacey RG, et al. Acute subdural hematomas: an age-dependent clinical entity. J Neurosurg 1989;71:858–63.

[17] Pennings JL, Bachulis BL, Simons CT, et al. Survival after severe brain injury in the aged. Arch Surg 1993;128:787–94.

[18] Teasdale G, Skene A, Parker L, et al. Age and outcome of severe head injury. Acta Neurochir Suppl (Wien) 1979;28:140–3.

[19] Breed ST, Flanagan SR, Watson K. The relationship between age and the self-report of health symptoms in persons with traumatic brain injury. Arch Phys Med Rehabil 2004;85:S61–7.

[20] Scherer T. Community reintegration. In: Woo BH, Nesathurai S, editors. The rehabilitation of people with traumatic brain injury. Malden, MA: Blackwell Science; 2000. p. 1110–3.

[21] Bell KR, Temkin NR, Esselman PC, et al. The effect of a scheduled telephone intervention on outcome after moderate to severe traumatic brain injury: a randomized trial. Arch Phys Med Rehabil 2005;86:851–6.

[22] McGlinchey-Berroth R, Morrow L, Alquist M, et al. Late-life spinal cord injury and aging with a long term injury: characteristics of two emerging populations. J Spinal Cord Med 1995; 18(3):183–93.

[23] Pentland W, McColl MA, Rosenthal C. The effect of aging and duration of disability on long term health outcomes following spinal cord injury. Paraplegia 1995;33:367–73.

[24] Meyers AR. Community reintegration. In: Woo BH, Nesathurai S, editors. The rehabilitation of people with spinal cord injury. Malden, MA: Blackwell Science; 2000. p. 13–6.

[25] Scivoletto G, Morganti B, Molinari M. Early v. delayed inpatient spinal cord injury rehabilitation: an Italian study. Arch Phys Med Rehabil 2005;86:512–6.

[26] Grisso JA, Kelsey JL, Strom BL, et al. Risk factors for falls as a cause of hip fracture in women. N Engl J Med 1991;324:1326–30.

[27] Tinetti ME. Preventing falls in elderly persons. N Engl J Med 2003;348:42–9.

[28] Tinetti ME, William CS. Falls, injuries due to falls and risk of admission to a nursing home. N Engl J Med 1997;337:1279–84.

[29] Munin MC, Seligman K, Dew MA, et al. Effect of rehabilitation site on functional recovery after hip fracture. Arch Phys Med Rehabil 2005;86:367–72.

[30] Munin MC, Kwoh CK, Glynn N, et al. Predicting discharge outcome after elective hip and knee arthroplasty. Am J Phys Med Rehabil 1995;74:294–301.

[31] Gill TM, Baker DI, Gottschalk M, et al. A program to prevent functional decline in physically frail elderly persons living at home. N Engl J Med 2002;347:1068–74.

[32] Landefeld CS, Palmer RM, Kresevic DM, et al. A randomized trial of care in a hospital medical unit especially designed to improve the functional outcomes of acutely ill older patients. N Engl J Med 1995;332:1338–44.

[33] Jette DU, Warren RL, Wirtalla C. The relation between therapy intensity and outcomes of rehabilitation in skilled nursing facilities. Arch Phys Med Rehabil 2005;86:373–9.

[34] Manson JE, Greenland P, LaCroix AZ, et al. Walking compared with vigorous exercise for prevention of cardiovascular events in women. N Engl J Med 2002;347:716–25.

[35] Chumbler NR, Mann WC, Wu S, et al. The Association of home-telehealth use and care coordination with improvement of functional and cognitive functioning in frail elderly men. Telemed J E Health 2004;10:129–37.

ELSEVIER
SAUNDERS

CLINICS IN
GERIATRIC
MEDICINE

Clin Geriatr Med 22 (2006) 269–279

The Role of the Physical Therapist in the Care of the Older Adult

Shana Richards, MPT*, Adrian Cristian, MD

*Department of Rehabilitation Medicine, Room 3D-16,
James J. Peters Veterans Affairs Medical Center, 130 West Kingsbridge Road, Bronx, NY 10468, USA*

Physical therapy is a profession that incorporates theory and clinical applications to provide the highest level of care and to achieve maximum physical functional outcome. A physical therapist is a state-licensed professional who may practice in hospitals, schools, short-term or long-term rehabilitation facilities, and outpatient and sports settings, as well as in the home. These professionals serve all age groups, from infants to the elderly. With the increase in the number of older adults in our society, the need for physical therapists to practice in rehabilitation settings with a large elderly population is on the rise.

Older adults often have many different medical ailments, such as hypertension, diabetes, heart disease, and arthritis. Superimposed on these diseases may be catastrophic conditions, such as stroke or amputation. The combination of all these conditions may lead to physical disability, frailty, and loss of function. The physical therapist (PT) plays a vital role in improving or restoring current physical function and preventing worsening of the patient's physical condition and loss of functionality.

Physical therapy consultation

In some states, such as New York, a therapist cannot initiate care of a patient unless a consult is received from a physician or health care provider. Following receipt of the consult, physical therapy begins. The initial meeting between the therapist and the patient is known as the "initial evaluation." Five elements

---

* Corresponding author.
E-mail address: shana.richards@med.va.gov (S. Richards).

are part of this session: examination, evaluation, diagnosis, prognosis, and in-tervention [1]. The initial evaluation starts with a detailed examination of the patient. It entails gathering a complete history related to the patient's condition, performing appropriate systems review, and carrying out test and measures.

History

A detailed review of the patient's medical history should include the chief complaint, history of present illness, medications, pertinent review of systems, prior functional status and activity level, living arrangements, social support system, and work history. The information is collected from chart review, from the team, and by interviewing the patient. The data collected provide the PT with a global picture of the older adult's current disability level, his or her existing social support system, and the impact of his or her medical conditions on physical status.

Precautions

It is important for the referring physician to provide the treating therapist with as much information as possible about restrictions on and precautions for treatment by means of the medical chart or consultation request. This measure ensures that the treatment sessions will be conducted with minimal risk to patients. Key precautions include presence of deep venous thrombosis, risk for falls, hypoglycemic risk (ie, uncontrolled diabetes), severe cardiopulmonary diseases, severe anemia, and limitations on weight bearing or range of motion.

An acute deep venous thrombosis in a lower extremity can theoretically dis-lodge during active movement of the limb, so it is advisable that weight-bearing activity on that leg be limited once it has been identified. The duration of this restriction should be clearly communicated to the treating therapist.

In orthopedic cases, information about the weight-bearing status of the joint is required. The weight-bearing status is documented as full, partial, toe-touch, or non–weight bearing (Table 1) [2]. Knowing the precautions enables the therapist safely to treat the patient and helps to prevent any future complications.

Any other orthopedic precautions should be clearly communicated to the therapist, including restrictions on range of motion. For example, following a hip replacement, typically there is no hip flexion past 90°, no hip adduction, and no internal rotation of the involved extremity. The therapist adheres to this guideline to reduce the risk for hip dislocation.

Cardiovascular disease has been mentioned as a cause of disability in older adults [3]. Because exercise is a primary intervention in physical therapy, the heart will work harder during therapy sessions. This condition can pose an increased risk in a patient with limited cardiac function due to congestive heart failure or myocardial infarction. Cardiac precautions can reduce that risk. Typical cardiac precautions impose an upper and lower limit to heart rate and blood pressure during treatments. Target heart rate may be calculated using various formulae (eg, $[(220 - \text{age}) \times 50\% - 60\%]$) or from stress test results. If these are

Table 1
Descriptions of weight-bearing status

Weight-bearing status	Description
Toe-touch weight bearing (TTWB)	The toes of the involved extremity can rest on the floor but should not bear weight.
Partial weight bearing (PWB)	Limited amount of weight is allowed on the involved extremity. The physician determines the amount of weight.
Full weight bearing (FWB) or weight bearing as tolerated (WBAT)	Full weight is allowed on the involved extremity. or The patient determines the amount of weight to place on the involved extremity based on tolerance.
Non–weight bearing (NWB)	The involved extremity should not touch the ground.

From Duesterhaus Minor MA, Duesterhaus Minor S. Patient care skills. Stamford (CT): Appleton & Lange; 1999. p. 298; with permission.

not available, a safe range that may be used is 20 beats above resting heart rate. However, given the effect of cardiac medication (eg, beta blockers) on blood pressure and heart rate, checking the blood pressure and heart rate may not accurately indicate the patient's response to exercise.

The Rate of Perceived Exertion (RPE) scale may be used to measure the patient's perception of the level of difficulty of the exercise or task. It allows the patient to rate the level of difficulty on a scale ranging from "very, very light" to "very, very hard." A numerical scale (6–20) accompanies these descriptors [4]. An example of a safe exercise range is 11 to 12 on the RPE scale.

Some weight-training exercises may lead to marked elevation of blood pressure; hence blood pressure recordings should be clearly stated for systolic and diastolic readings. Ideally, hypertension should be adequately treated before inception of a therapy program.

Patients who have significant pulmonary disorders such as emphysema may have additional precautions imposed for acceptable breathing rates during exercise sessions. Pulse oximetry may also be indicated to maintain oxygenation levels within a specified range.

Restrictions on use of equipment commonly encountered in the physical therapy treatment areas should also be clearly indicated. For example, blood pressure readings should not be taken in a dialysis patient over the access site.

Another precaution is awareness of the presence, location, and severity of pressure ulcers. Sacral ulcers may be worsened during transfer training by the potential shearing forces generated.

Review of systems

It is important for the PT to perform a pertinent review of systems, with special emphasis on the cardiopulmonary, musculoskeletal, neuromuscular, and integumentary systems. Like the interview process, reviewing these systems provides the therapist with an understanding of the patient's current health and its effect on physical functioning. The therapist is also able to use these data to predict the elder's expected functional outcome.

Data collected also helps to identify specific precautions to be used later, during treatments. For example, cardiac conditions such as congestive heart failure or myocardial infarction necessitate specific precautions during treatment sessions to establish ranges for blood pressure and heart rate that are safe for the patient. A recent hip replacement may necessitate specific ranges of motion for the affected joint to reduce the risk of hip dislocation.

The PT also evaluates for the presence of pain, because this may have an impact on the patient's progress during treatments. Pertinent information about the pain includes location, duration, radiation, quality, intensity, aggravating or alleviating factors, and previous treatments.

Another factor to assess is the older adult's ability to learn, because learning is an important part of the physical therapy program. Impaired ability to learn can have a negative impact on the therapy program. The older adult is asked which medium of instruction is best suited for him or her—visual, auditory, or written.

Physical examination—test and measures

The physical examination is a detailed process that provides the therapist with information regarding the impairments, functional limitation, and disability of the patient. It begins with an assessment of the patient's level of alertness and cognitive function. Impaired mental abilities due to delirium or dementia can have a direct impact on the therapy program. Ideally, these abilities need to be optimized before the start of rehabilitation.

Vital signs also provide valuable information about the patient's current medical status. Febrile episode, hypotension, marked hypertension, bradycardia, tachycardia, and tachypnea may all be absolute or relative contraindications to therapy, depending on their severity.

A pertinent physical examination focuses primarily on the neuromusculoskeletal and integumentary systems. Key components in the evaluation of the nervous system include sensation, proprioception, and balance. Key components of the musculoskeletal system include joint range of motion, joint integrity, muscle strength, muscle flexibility, and tender points. Dermatologic evaluation focuses on the skin's integrity and preventive measures to reduce the risk of skin breakdown. A vital component of the skin examination is identifying pressure ulcers over bony prominences, such as the sacrum, ischial tuberosities, greater trochanters, and heel. Assessment of the skin is especially important in patients who have moderate to severe functional limitation and in those who wear a prosthesis or orthosis. Frequent evaluation of the prosthesis or orthosis is also recommended, especially where it comes into contact with the patient's skin.

Part of the physical examination is an evaluation of the patient's functional mobility. This includes an assessment of the patient's ability to transfer on and off different surfaces (eg, bed, chair, and floor), ascend and descend stairs and curbs, ambulate on different types of terrain, and propel a wheelchair. The amount of assistance provided by the therapist during the evaluation is also recorded on a scale from minimum to maximum assistance. When no assistance is necessary, but supervision is required, the type of supervision needed is noted as close or distant. Ambulation distance or wheelchair propulsion is also measured and recorded.

Goal setting and treatment program

Once impairments and functional limitations have been identified, goals are set and a therapy program is designed. This program may last for several weeks to months and occur at various frequencies, depending on the setting. It is not uncommon for an outpatient program to occur three times per week and an inpatient program to occur three to six times per week. The duration and the setting of the program are usually determined through a collaborative effort by the PT and referring physician. Factors that are taken into consideration in this decision-making process include the patient's physical limitations, disease process, cognitive status, and motivation level.

Goal setting

Goal setting is a collaborative effort between the patient and the treating therapist. The goals are specific, measurable, achievable, result bounded, and time specific. The length of time necessary to accomplish the goals is also taken into account. It is common to have several short-term and long-term goals for a treatment program.

For example, a patient with hemiparesis following a stroke may have unilateral muscle weakness, gait disorder, impaired balance, limited stamina for ambulation, and difficulty with transfers. Appropriate goals may be developed for each of these areas for a specified time frame. The goals are reviewed at regular intervals and modified as necessary. If goals are not met, original goals may be modified or the time frame to accomplish them extended. Once goals have been met, new goals may be set or the patient may be discharged from the program.

Treatment

The treatment program may be rendered in a variety of settings. Some common sites include the bedside on an acute medical or surgical ward, an inpatient rehabilitation unit, an outpatient physical therapy clinic, and the patient's home. During the initial treatment session, the patient is provided with an equipment orientation and education about exercises to be performed, appropriate clothing to wear (loose, comfortable clothing, sneakers), and exercise precautions based on his or her medical condition.

The cornerstone of the treatment session is exercise. One or more types of exercise may be incorporated into the treatment program. Exercises to improve range of motion and flexibility, strength, and endurance are typically used. Each exercise session consists of a warm-up, exercise period, and cool-down. The warm-up and cool-down sessions may consist of gentle stretches or a low-intensity exercise. The equipment used during the exercise session depends on the type of exercises to be performed. Strengthening exercises may be performed with dumbbells, rubber bands, or sophisticated weight machines. Endurance exercises may be performed on treadmills, stationary bicycles, and elliptical trainers. Exercises are often performed for a set number of minutes, when cardiovascular endurance is being emphasized, or for a specified number of sets and repetitions, when muscle strengthening or enhanced muscle endurance is recommended. Exercises are discussed in greater detail elsewhere in this issue. The patient is also instructed in a home exercise program that is typically performed on a daily basis.

Modalities also tend to be used during treatment sessions, often for pain conditions of the musculoskeletal system. They are discussed in greater detail elsewhere in this issue.

Gait training

Because a common reason for referral to physical therapy is gait abnormalities, the remainder of this article is devoted to an overview of the role of therapy in gait training and a brief discussion of various assistive devices to make ambulation safer.

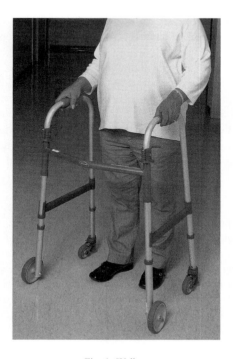

Fig. 1. Walker.

Gait abnormalities are often due to muscle weakness, impaired neurologic function, impaired balance, or skeletal abnormalities. Often the causes are multifactorial, and the treatment program reflects this reality. A typical treatment program often consists of muscle strengthening exercises, balance training exercises, and gait training with appropriate assistive devices. Braces and prostheses are also useful to maximize the individual's ability to ambulate.

Key muscle groups to be strengthened include the hip extensors, hip flexors, quadriceps, and anterior tibialis. Reducible contractures often occur in muscles that cross two joints, such as the hamstrings and gastronemius. This problem may be addressed through a stretching program. Balance training exercises on an increasingly narrow base of support may also be used to improve gait. The goal of gait training is to provide locomotion in the safest possible manner with the most stable assistive device that the individual requires. Initially a patient may require the assistance of two therapists to ambulate the length of a parallel bar. However, with gait training and encouragement, the individual may progress to a walker, crutch, cane, or no assistive device. This is often a gradual process in the older adult. Progress is measured in small increments. Gait training is performed in a variety of settings and over various terrains, including flat surfaces in a medical or nursing home facility, stairs, outdoor sidewalks, and even the patient's home. Not all patients advance to the point where they do not re-

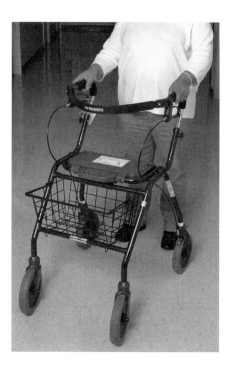

Fig. 2. Rollator.

quire assistive devices, but a primary goal of a gait-training program is to identify the safest way for the patient to ambulate. If the patient is not deemed safe to ambulate, the PT may recommend a wheelchair or powered mobility device. These are discussed elsewhere in the text.

Assistive devices for ambulation

The most common forms of assistive equipment used to aid in locomotion are walkers, crutches, and canes. The device most suitable for the patient is determined based on structural deformity, presence of disease such as arthritis, injury, muscle weaknesses, joint range of motion, and decreased balance [2]. Cognition and coordination play a role in this decision-making process as well.

All assistive devices must be height appropriate for the patient and, in the case of walkers, width appropriate. The devices come in different sizes: tall, regular, and junior. They are used primarily to aid in locomotion such as negotiating ramps, curbs, and stairs and walking. When one is teaching an individual to negotiate stairs, the preferred and safest devices to consider are crutches and canes. Walkers may be unsafe and cumbersome and present a safety risk in elders.

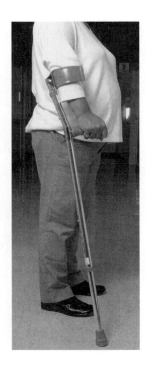

Fig. 3. Crutches.

Walker

Walkers provide the greatest stability of all walking aids. They are characterized by their four legs and thus provide the patient with a wider base of support. They are most often prescribed for older adults. Walkers are beneficial to individuals with poor balance and coordination, generalized weakness, debilitating conditions, and weight-bearing restrictions on one or both lower extremities. Wheeled walkers are more often used than standard walkers, although standard walkers provide more stability. The four-wheeled walker is easier to maneuver in the community than the two-wheeled one and is usually preferred (Fig. 1).

Rollator

The rollator is a form of four-wheeled walker. It has a different shape from the typical rolling walker and a more modern appearance. It has a basket that may be used for carrying small objects and a seat that will allow the older adult to sit and rest (Fig. 2). Two brakes may be activated to stop it from moving. The pressure-activated brake allows the individual to control the speed of movement. The push-to-lock brake stops the rollator from any type of movement. This brake should be activated before the patient sits on or stands up from the seat. The disadvantage of this type of walker is that it is less stable than the others.

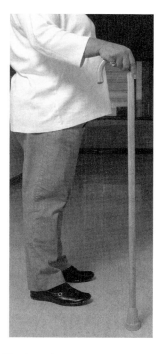

Fig. 4. Straight or single-point cane.

Crutches

Crutches come in pairs, but it is up to the therapist's discretion whether the patient uses a single crutch or both crutches. A pair of crutches provides more stability and balance than a single crutch. Crutches are more stable than canes. The two types of crutches are axillary crutches and lofstrand or forearm crutches (Fig. 3). They are recommended for individuals who have pain or weakness in one or both lower extremities, who may need additional trunk support, or who have weight-bearing restrictions. Forearm crutches are easier to maneuver and lighter than axillary crutches and so are generally preferred by patients. Axillary crutches provide more support than lofstrands.

Canes

Canes are distinguished from other devices by the handle and the various types of base. The base gives the cane its name. A single-point cane is called a straight cane (Fig. 4) and is the most frequently used cane. Quad canes have four points and are narrow or wide based (Fig. 5). Canes provide the least stability of all walking aids. They are issued to individuals who are able to ambulate but require minimal physical support and balance, or who may have minimal weakness or pain in the lower extremity.

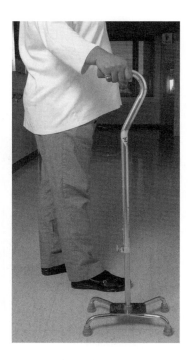

Fig. 5. Quad cane.

Summary

PTs play an important role in the care of older adults with physical disabilities. Proper patient selection, a thorough medical, social, and functional history, and a physical examination emphasizing the neuromusculoskeletal system are the cornerstones of the evaluation process. Treatment is individualized and goal driven, with appropriate precautions being followed. Gait training is an integral part of the treatment process for many older adults with disabilities, and various assistive devices may be used to ensure safe mobility.

References

[1] American Physical Therapy Association. A description of patient client management. In: Revised guide to physical therapy practice. Alexandria (VA): 1999. p. 1–5.
[2] Duesterhaus Minor MA, Duesterhaus Minor S. Patient care skills. Stamford (CT): Appleton & Lange; 1999. p. 298.
[3] Guccione AA. Implications of an aging population for rehabilitation: demography, mortality, and morbidity in the elderly. In: Geriatric physical therapy. 2nd edition. St. Louis (MO): CV Mosby; 2000. p. 11.
[4] Borg GA. Psychophysical bases of perceived exertion. Med Sci Sports Exerc 1982;14(5):377–81.

ELSEVIER
SAUNDERS

CLINICS IN
GERIATRIC
MEDICINE

Clin Geriatr Med 22 (2006) 281–290

The Role of Occupational Therapy in the Care of the Older Adult

Teina Daley, OTR/L*, Adrian Cristian, MD,
Maureen Fitzpatrick, OTR

James J. Peters Veterans Affairs Medical Center, 130 West Kingsbridge Road, Bronx, NY 10468, USA

Occupational therapy (OT) is skilled treatment that helps individuals achieve independence in all areas of their lives [1]. An OT is a board-certified licensed professional who may practice in a wide variety of settings for the geriatric population, including hospitals, nursing homes, skilled nursing facilities, and homes. Treatment involves providing people with the skills necessary for independent and satisfying lives. Services typically include

- Customized treatment programs to improve the client's ability to perform daily activities
- Comprehensive home and job-site evaluations with adaptation recommendations
- Performance skills assessments and treatment
- Adaptive equipment recommendations and usage training
- Guidance to family members and caregivers

OT practitioners are skilled professionals whose education includes the study of human growth and development, with special emphasis on the social, emotional, and physiologic effects of illness and injury. The aging process often leads to a variety of illnesses and injuries that can greatly affect the ability of the elderly to complete their daily living activities. OTs therefore play a vital role in the provision of skilled health care services to the geriatric population.

* Corresponding author.
E-mail address: teina.daley@bronx.va.gov (T. Daley).

0749-0690/06/$ – see front matter. Published by Elsevier Inc.
doi:10.1016/j.cger.2005.12.004

A wide variety of OT services can benefit the geriatric population, including those with the following conditions:

- Chronic back pain and repetitive stress injuries
- Limitations following a stroke or heart attack
- Arthritis, multiple sclerosis, or other serious chronic conditions
- Burns, spinal cord injuries, or amputations
- Broken bones or other injuries from falls, sports, or accidents
- Vision or cognitive problems that threaten their ability to drive and/or perform home/community mobility

The OT plays an important role as a member of an interdisciplinary team. This team typically includes a doctor, nurse, social worker, physical therapist, and speech therapist. OTs are able to provide pertinent feedback to the team on the problems and goals of the elderly from a unique perspective, one that primarily focuses on the patient's functional level for performance of activities of daily living.

History of occupational therapy

OT started in the mental health system to meet the needs of returning World War I veterans. OTs worked with American soldiers, engaging them in "purposeful occupations," which at the time involved the use of craft activities. Working toward a purposeful, tangible goal was found to stimulate and contribute to the mental and physical healing of the veterans [1].

After World War II, many OTs continued to work in the growing system of Veterans Administration hospitals. Over the years, there has been an improvement in survival rates following illnesses and trauma. This improvement is primarily due to advances in medical care and public health measures. Many of the survivors required extensive rehabilitation, which included OT, and the profession continued to grow and develop, addressing the demands of the injured [1]. Today, OTs continue to play a vital role in the care of the elderly by maintaining their function and independence. A variety of OT programs may be implemented, including cognitive training, physical rehabilitation, seating and mobility evaluations, activities of daily living (ADL) groups, and home evaluations.

Patient evaluation

To perform an effective evaluation, the therapist must be knowledgeable about the dysfunction's causes, course, and prognosis; familiar with a variety of evaluation methods, including their uses and proper administration; and able to select evaluation methods that are suitable to the patient and the dysfunction. The therapist must have good observation skills, approach the patient with openness and without preconceived ideas about his or her limitations or personality, and be able to enlist the trust of the patient in a short time [2].

Once the medical doctor's orders for OT have been received, the therapist performs a chart review to gather the patient's pertinent current medical and social information. Chart review also includes gathering information about existing precautions, such as fall risk, cardiac and pulmonary issues, visual and hearing deficits, pain, and cognitive and mental status. Knowledge of premorbid status helps to set the framework of the treatment plan and realistic goals for treatment. Information on the social history of the patient is also helpful to determine the support systems that are currently available for him or her. For instance, it is important that the therapist have knowledge of living arrangements that were in place before inpatient admission (eg, living alone versus cohabiting with family or friend; living in a private house, apartment, or skilled nursing facility), because this information is helpful when making the appropriate recommendations for discharge planning.

The OT physical assessment focuses on cognition, range of motion, pain, strength of proximal and distal upper extremity joints, including grip and pinch strength, endurance, gross and fine motor coordination, hand sensation, and sitting and standing balance. Additionally, current functional level for ADL, wheelchair mobility, bed mobility, and transfers are determined.

Cognitive assessment usually includes simple questions to test short-term and long-term memory and orientation to person, time, and place. A more detailed assessment of the patient's cognition, social interaction, problem solving, memory, communication, comprehension, and expression skills may be performed and documented using the Functional Independent Measure (FIM) instrument.

Pain is typically measured using the Visual Analog Scale, a 0 to 10 scale that quantifies the patient's pain from no pain to severe pain. For patients who are unable to quantify their level of pain, the therapist may assess pain based on the patient's willingness to move body or extremities, facial grimacing, or body gestures. Range of motion of upper extremity joints may be measured with a goniometer (a tool used to measure joint motion) or documented in terms of functional limits. Muscle strength is tested using the standard definitions of muscle grades, which range from (0)—no muscle contraction may be seen or felt—to normal (5), where the part moves through complete range of motion against gravity and full resistance [2]. Endurance is typically measured as poor, fair, or good based on the patient's ability to sustain minimal to strenuous activity before fatigue. Sitting and standing balance is also typically measured as poor, fair, or good for static and dynamic activities, based on the level of support required and how well the patient is able to maintain balance when performing an activity outside of the body's center of gravity. A detailed assessment of hand sensation may be performed for the presence of pain and temperature, vibration, moving and constant touch, touch localization, two-point discrimination, and stereognosis. The patient may also be screened quickly for intact light touch and deep pressure sensation. If numbness and tingling sensation are present, they are documented. Gross coordination is assessed with "finger-to-nose" and diadokokinesis tests. Fine motor coordination may be measured using a nine-hole peg test or by checking the patient's coordination of movement in opposing thumb to digits.

ADL, which involve components of self-care such as upper body dressing, lower body dressing, grooming, self-feeding, bathing, and toileting, are measured using the FIM instrument. Transfers to bed, chair, wheelchair, toilet, and tub may also be measured with the FIM instrument. The levels of assistance required for bed mobility tasks, such as rolling to either side of the bed and sitting-to-supine transfers, are also documented on a scale that ranges from dependent to independent.

Home evaluation

In preparation for the safe and appropriate discharge to home, an OT will occasionally perform a home evaluation. The exterior of the residence is assessed for any possible safety and accessibility barriers, such as inclined or rough terrain, steps to enter the dwelling, railings for support, and distance the car is parked from home. The inside of the home is also checked for any possible problems that may increase fall risk, such as slippery or torn rugs, furniture clutter, unstable and low chairs, wet or waxed floors, slippery bathtubs, low toilet seats, inadequate or inaccessible lighting, and inadequate support in stairways. The OT then makes the appropriate recommendations for home modification and dispenses adaptive devices, which are preferably to be issued before the patient's discharge home.

Seating and mobility assessment

OTs play a vital role in ensuring that the elderly maintain access inside the home and outside in the community. The aging process can often lead to decreased ability to negotiate around the home for self-care activities and instrumental ADL as well as decreased ability to attend medical appointments. OTs are skilled professionals who use their clinical expertise to perform an assessment of the patient's seating and mobility needs and make recommendations for an appropriate seating and mobility device. The seating and wheelchair market offers a variety of technical features that can make use of these devices more comfortable and effective for the elderly patient.

This process is generally initiated by and involves a collaboration between the therapist and the physician. The patient must be cleared for any possible contraindications to use of the recommended device, such as severe cognitive deficits, dementia, or visual and hearing deficits. The OT ensures that the patient has adequate strength, endurance, and cognitive function to operate the device safely and that use of the device will enhance the patient's overall health and not encourage functional decline.

It is important to ensure that the mobility device can be used with the patient's current means of transportation. The OT may need to make appropriate recommendations for storage of the mobility device during transit, such as ramps and trunk lifts for patients who drive a car or van.

A seating device assessment is performed to address special needs for devices such as specialty cushions, backs, and lateral and head supports, which will provide comfort, postural support and stability, spinal alignment, and midline support to patients when they are seated in the wheelchair. The seated posture of the patient in a wheelchair must be addressed to ensure that the joints of the body are resting in an anatomically correct position to prevent pressure sores, contractures, and pain in the back and extremities. This assessment is necessary to identify and reduce possible pressure points, especially in areas of bony prominences that are at a higher risk for skin breakdown.

An assessment of the need for mobility devices such as wheelchairs and scooters is made based on the patient's medical condition and disease progression, other pertinent medical history, and current level of cognition and mental status. To make the appropriate recommendations and allow the patient to use these devices within the home or community, the therapist needs to assess the patient's current level of transfers, amount of time spent sitting in the wheelchair, distance he or she is able to ambulate indoors and outdoors before fatigue, weakness or respiratory distress, risk for falls, and accessibility of his or her current place of residence.

Goal setting

OT goals are established based on the problem list and mutually agreed on by therapist and patient. Based on the medical prognosis and premorbid and comorbid status of the patient, in conjunction with the clinical expertise of the therapist, the patient is informed whether the goals are realistic for the time frame established. Typically, short-term and long-term goals are determined and then reassessed weekly and biweekly, respectively, for inpatients and biweekly and monthly for outpatients. Time frames may vary from one facility to another. Patients are continually assessed for any changes in physical and functional status, and goals are adjusted accordingly.

Treatment

OT treatments include a variety of modalities, exercises, and activities to address the patient's goals appropriately. The long-term effects of medical conditions may lead to generalized deconditioning, joint stiffness and deformity, joint and soft tissue contractures, muscle weakness and imbalance, impaired sensation, impaired range of motion, and pain. These in turn may impair the patient's ability to perform ADL and participate in social and leisure activities, leading to sedentary lifestyles and isolation.

Modalities such as superficial heat and cold may be applied to address pain, stimulate muscular relaxation, increase range of motion, increase muscle strength

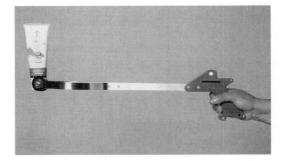

Fig. 1. Reacher.

and endurance, and decrease joint stiffness and swelling. The doctor's authorization is usually required when use of modalities is indicated; this is included as part of the prescription for therapy. Exercises for stretching and strengthening of weak and imbalanced muscles and joints are prescribed and implemented according to the patient's impairments. Modalities and exercise are applied with special attention and caution when used in elderly patients, to ensure that these media are tolerated without any adverse effects.

Therapeutic activities are often implemented as a means of stimulating interest, participation, and motivation, with the underlying benefit of achieving the desired goal of motion. A variety of activities may be used, such as sports, leisure, cooking, and table-top games, which are designed to achieve the desired goal of motion and promote healing, health, and disease prevention.

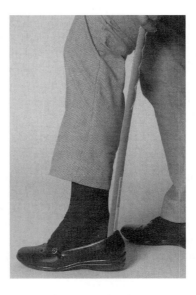

Fig. 2. Long shoe horn.

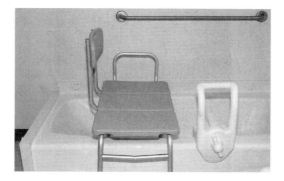

Fig. 3. Tub transfer bench and tub grab bar.

OTs also recommend alternative methods of performing daily life tasks, such as new techniques for performing ADL that promote energy conservation and protect fragile joints. OTs are instrumental in educating and prescribing adaptive devices, as appropriate, to facilitate increased independent performance of ADL tasks with reduced pain and effort. Examples of adaptive devices include (1) reacher (Fig. 1) to extend the patient's reach for objects, (2) sock aid to facilitate donning socks, (3) long shoe horn (Fig. 2) to facilitate donning and doffing shoes, (4) built-up-handled utensils to facilitate grip, (5) grab bars in the bathtub for transfer safety, (6) shower chairs for energy conservation and compensation for reduced balance, (7) raised toilet seats to facilitate sit-to-stand transfers (Fig. 3), and (8) long-handled sponges (Fig. 4).

Social support can greatly enhance one's well-being. Establishing informal or formal interactions among patients may help to effect positive functional outcomes with regard to self-care activities and to increase the individuals' self-esteem. Formal systems may include referrals to a structured stroke survivors' or amputees' group that provides continual emotional support and encouragement while expanding the patient's community resources. The therapist may also establish and promote social support by facilitating group interaction during therapy sessions among patients with shared goals. Examples may include ADL training groups or exercise groups. In conducting such programs, it is important to establish a learning objective and adapt specific aspects of the task to meet the needs of each member and further assist in guiding each individual's progress and promoting success. A group design provides a supportive atmosphere for individuals to establish leadership roles and reinforce one another with encouraging feedback.

Upper extremity splints

OTs have expertise in the assessment and fabrication of upper extremity splints. *Mosby's Medical, Nursing, and Allied Health Dictionary* defines a splint

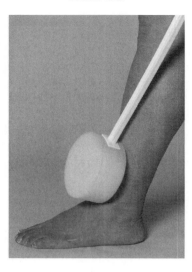

Fig. 4. Long-handled sponge.

as "an orthopedic device for immobilization, restraint, or support of any part of the body" [3]. In the health care field today, a splint refers to a temporary device that is part of a treatment program and may be used not only to immobilize but also to mobilize, position, and protect a joint or specific body part. Design and fabrication of splints ranges from simple to complex; they may be custom-made or prefabricated, depending on the needs of the particular condition. Splints can support and protect the weak, fragile, and unbalanced muscles and joints of geriatric patients who have been affected by upper extremity injuries and functional deficits. For example, a resting hand splint is a static splint that immobilizes the fingers, thumb, and wrist and may be used in inflammatory conditions to position the hand in a functional way (Fig. 5). Wrist supports are useful in conditions including but not limited to wrist sprains, cumulative trauma disorder, stable wrist fractures, and ligamentous injuries of the wrist (Fig. 6) [3].

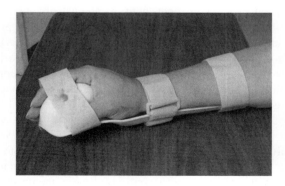

Fig. 5. Resting hand splint.

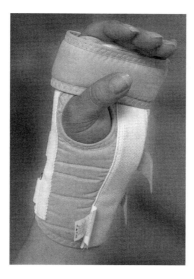

Fig. 6. Wrist brace with metacarpal support.

Finger splints may be used to correct or prevent deformities, such as the common deformities of rheumatoid arthritis, swan neck, and boutonniere deformity.

Patient and family education

Patient, family, and caregiver education is a fundamental part of an OT program. Family members and caregivers may be asked to attend therapy sessions to learn what the patient can do and may need help with. They then receive education in skills for safely instructing or assisting a patient, for example, with ADL or transfers in preparation for the return home. Educating the patient and family or caregivers on such topics as home exercise programs, energy conservation, joint protection techniques, and upper extremity exercises enables the patient to practice and reinforce skills learned in therapy sessions. Education about assistive devices and adaptive equipment increases awareness of products that may help improve independence and safety. It is important to discuss these items with the patient and make appropriate recommendations. Involving all parties in the decision-making process is vital to determining the best fit while taking into consideration factors such as the patient's skill level, the family member's or caregiver's abilities, and the space and design of the home. The therapist must assess how safely a patient can perform a task and whether the family member or caregiver may safely assist the patient or use any equipment provided. If one of these parties does not meet the requirements to complete the task safely, the therapist has the responsibility to voice such concerns to the patient and family or caregiver and to the treating team members, so that alternative means may be explored.

Summary

The OT therefore plays a vital role in the care of the geriatric population. The OT is instrumental in determining the health care needs of the older population and providing the OT services that ultimately enhance the quality of living and health of the older population as well as the functional independence for daily living activities.

References

[1] American Occupational Therapy Association. Available at: http://www.aota.org. Accessed May 6, 2005.
[2] Pedretti LW. Occupational therapy—practice skills for physical dysfunction. 4th edition. St. Louis: Mosby; 1996.
[3] Coppard BM, Lohman H. Introduction to splinting—a critical-thinking and problem-solving approach. St. Louis: Mosby; 1996.

ELSEVIER
SAUNDERS

CLINICS IN
GERIATRIC
MEDICINE

Clin Geriatr Med 22 (2006) 291–310

Speech, Language, and Swallowing Disorders in the Older Adult

Juliet Ashley, MS, CCC-SLP,
Mickey Duggan, MS, CCC-SLP,
Natalie Sutcliffe, MS, CCC-SLP*

James J. Peters Veterans Affairs Medical Center, 130 West Kingsbridge Road, Bronx, NY 10468, USA

The geriatric population has become a major component in the practice of medical speech-language pathology. According to the United States Census Bureau, as of July 1, 2003, there were 35.9 million older adults in the United States. This article discusses normal and abnormal functions of speech, voicing, language, cognition, and swallowing. Particular attention is given to disorders effecting the geriatric population. Evaluation, treatment, and ethical issues are explored, in addition to the role of the speech-language pathologist (SLP) on the interdisciplinary team.

Language and cognition

Communication is a key aspect of life whether one is using words, gestures, or signs. As Rudyard Kipling said, "Words are, of course, the most powerful drug used by mankind." Language is defined as an accepted structured symbolic system for interpersonal communication composed of sounds arranged in ordered

* Corresponding author.
  E-mail address: natalie.sutcliffe@med.va.gov (N. Sutcliffe).

0749-0690/06/$ – see front matter. Published by Elsevier Inc.
doi:10.1016/j.cger.2005.12.008

sequence to form words, with rules for combining these words into sequences or strings that expresses thoughts, intentions, experiences, and feelings [1].

Aphasia

Aphasia is a communication disorder caused by brain damage and characterized by complete or partial impairment of language comprehension, formulation, and use; excludes disorders associated with primary sensory deficits, general mental deterioration, or psychiatric disorders [1]. Aphasia is most commonly caused by a stroke. It can also be caused, however, by traumatic brain injury, brain tumors, and other sources of brain damage [2,3]. The stroke patient's ability to communicate may or may not be significantly impacted depending on the location of the lesion and the severity of the lesion or insult (injury). Recovery is also dependent on several factors including severity and size of lesion, spontaneous recovery, premorbid health status, age, prior strokes, and other social and economic factors [4].

Aphasics are generally grouped as being fluent or nonfluent (Table 1) [5]. Nonfluent aphasics exhibit impaired flow of speech, effortful speech production with usually good comprehension skills, and varying degrees of difficulty with repetition. The nonfluent aphasics tend to display agrammatical or telegraphic speech (omission of function words) and depend primarily on the use of key content words (pain... leg). Nonfluent aphasia is typically seen in Broca's, transcortical motor, and global aphasia.

Fluent aphasics exhibit a smooth flow of speech with varying degrees of deficits in comprehension and repetition. They may also exhibit circumlocution (speaking around a target word); paraphasic errors (use the word sister for mother or penkle for pencil); and neologisms (made up words [ie, gargot]). Typically Wernicke's, conduction, transcortical sensory, and anomic aphasia are grouped in the fluent category.

Table 1
Basic classification of aphasia syndromes

	Comprehension	Repetition	Fluency
Broca	+	−	−
Transcortical motor	+	+	−
Global	−	−	−
Wernicke's	−	−	+
Conduction	+	−	+
Transcortical sensory	−	+	+
Anomic	+	+	+

Each patient is individual in presentation and this table should be used as a general guideline.
+, relatively unimpaired; −, impaired.
Adapted from Kearns KP. Broca's aphasia. In: La Pointe LL, editor. Aphasia and related neurogenic language disorders. 2nd edition. New York: Thieme Medical Publishers; 1997. p. 14; with permission.

Assessment

The SLP plays a vital role on the interdisciplinary rehabilitation team. For patients who have had a stroke the SLP assesses their speech, language, and swallowing ability to identify specific deficits, their severity, and target treatment. The goal is to improve or restore functional communication and swallowing ability. Results from the evaluation and treatment goals along with the best ways to facilitate communication with the patient are conveyed to the other team members. Ways to improve communicative interaction is an important step to improve functional treatment goal outcomes for the stroke patient.

Patients may be screened initially before a complete language assessment. Choices of screening tests include the Bedside Evaluation Screening Test for Aphasia; Boston Diagnostic Aphasia Examination (short form); and shortened Porch Index of Communicative Ability. For a more detailed assessment standardized tests may include the Boston Diagnostic Aphasia Examination, the Porch Index of Communicative Ability, and The Western Aphasia Battery. For the patients who are more severely impaired the Boston Assessment of Severe Aphasia and the Communicative Activities in Daily Living maybe useful for assessment.

The SLP and other team members have to be aware of the risk for depression in the stroke patient. According to the Department of Health and Human Services an estimated 10% to 27% of first and recurrent stroke survivors experience major depression. Among the factors that affect the likelihood and severity of depression following a stroke are the location of the brain lesion, previous or family history of depression, and prestroke social functioning. Stroke survivors who are identified as being depressed, particularly those with major depressive disorder, may be less compliant with rehabilitation, more irritable, and may experience personality change [6].

Treatment

Once the areas of communication deficits have been identified treatment begins. The SLP works toward restoring and facilitating the recovery of speech-language skills. The overall goal is to improve the functional communication of the stroke patient. A spontaneous recovery period anywhere from weeks to 6 months to 1 year poststroke is documented in the literature. Bhogal and colleagues [7] analyzed clinical trials investigating the intensity and frequency of aphasia therapy in the acute-phase poststroke. They found that intense therapy for stroke patients over a short period of time can improve speech and language therapy outcomes.

Speech-language therapy can be provided in individual or group sessions. Individual treatment sessions are generally stimulus-response oriented combined with facilitative strategies. Once the patient has achieved goals or reached plateau the individual sessions are ended. The patient may then be seen in an aphasia group for therapy. Group sessions are provided to facilitate communication in a functional setting, offer support, and assist with the use and carryover of communication skills.

Augmentative-alternative communication

Depending on the severity of the language impairment, the use of an alternate or augmentative means of communication may be an option. Use of an augmentative-alternative communication system ranging from a simple picture board to a sophisticated speech-generating device and computers is available to facilitate communication if the patient is deemed able to use such a device. Factors to consider when selecting an augmentative-alternative communication device include the patient's communication skills, level of cognitive functioning, perceptual and visual skills, mobility level, and their behavioral and environmental needs.

Cognition

Assessment of the patient's ability to attend, concentrate, perform executive functions, and other higher-level cognitive skills is important to establish to what degree these skills have been impacted by the stroke. McDowd and colleagues [8] highlighted the fact that cognitive function is importantly related to successful rehabilitation. The study compared attentional functioning (divided attention and switching attention) in older adults who had a stroke versus healthy older adults. Results revealed deficits related to the stroke in both types of attention with significant associations between attentional functioning and physical and social outcome measures. Poorer attentional functioning was associated with a more negative impact of stroke on daily functioning. The Cognitive Linguistic Quick Test is one relatively quick way to assess a patient's cognitive-linguistic functioning. Another quick screen is the Mini Mental Status Examination, which assesses orientation, attention, language, concentration, word recall, calculation, and drawing.

Therapy for the cognitively impaired focuses on areas identified during the evaluation. Attention and concentration skills are needed for all aspects of the retraining and learning process during rehabilitation. Compensatory techniques, self-regulation, coping strategies, and visual, verbal, and tactile cueing may be used during the rehabilitation process.

Dementia

In the early stages of dementia the language is characterized by a decline in the use of content words (anomia); difficulty in confrontation naming; reduced fluency in speech; and use of circumlocution (speaking around an intended word). As the dementia progresses, there is a decline in ability to recall the names of family members, anomia increases, and a more dysfluent speech pattern is exhibited with increased use of circumlocution and irrelevant utterances. Psychometric screening tests, such as the Mini Mental Status Examination, are used for cognition and language. Other tests, such as the Dementia Rating Scale, and the Neurobehavioral Cognitive Status Examination, include other areas of cognitive screening, such as initiation, verbal reasoning, and memory. The Arizona Battery for Communication Disorder of Dementia assesses receptive and expressive language, orientation, and memory. In severe dementia the language resembles more that of the global aphasic. The patient has little to no language for communicative intent and requires total care.

For the dementia patient, speech-language intervention focuses on providing ways for retaining effective communication skills, providing compensatory strategies and stabilizing the patient's environment by keeping a set routine, and reducing environmental distractions. Therapy should focus on what is present in their surroundings (objects and topics); structured activities; and the use of reality orientation. Staff and caregiver training should be provided in how to increase effective communication by enhancing verbal messages with gestures, visual cues, and a reduced speech rate. As the dementia progresses modification of the aforementioned interventions is needed.

Speech and voice

Speech and voice production in the older adult can be affected by physiologic and anatomic changes that can occur with age, trauma, injury, or damage to central or peripheral nervous systems. The parameters that contribute to speech and voice production are respiration (breath support for speech); phonation (voicing produced by the larynx); resonance (quality of sound shaped by the vocal tract); prosody (intonation-stress patterns); articulation (production of speech sounds by the tongue, lips, palate); and intelligibility [9,10]. Problems or deficits in any of these areas can affect the speech and voice of an older adult.

Dysarthria

Dysarthria is a motor speech disorder caused by many different conditions that involve the nervous system. These include stroke, brain injury, Parkinson's disease, amyotrophic lateral sclerosis (ALS), multiple sclerosis, Huntington's disease, cerebral palsy, and tumors [11]. The prominent symptoms are imprecise articulation (slurred speech); abnormal rate of speech; low volume; and impaired vocal quality. The problems in oral communication are caused by paralysis, weakness, or incoordination of the speech musculature [12,13]. There are five types of dysarthria, differentiated by which area of the nervous system is affected.

Flaccid dysarthria is mainly characterized by weakness in the muscles of articulation (lips, tongue, soft palate) [14]. The resultant speech is characterized by imprecise sound production, low volume, and hypernasality. This type of dysarthria can be seen in brain stem stroke and progressive bulbar palsy [14].

Ataxic dysarthria is mainly characterized by decreased rate of speech, inappropriate stress, fluctuating volume, and poorly controlled coordination of respiration and phonation. This type of speech is commonly seen in multiple sclerosis [14].

In spastic dysarthria prominent characteristics include harsh, strained, or strangled vocal quality; imprecise articulation; and irregular prosody. The most common cause is stroke [14].

The characteristics of hyperkinetic dysarthria, common in Huntington's chorea, seem to parallel the hyperkinetic physical movements of these individuals. Speech characteristics include tremulous voice; variation in rate, pitch, and volume; and imprecise articulation [14].

Hypokinetic dysarthria, associated mainly with Parkinson's disease, is characterized by monotony of loudness and pitch; reduced stress; imprecise articulation; inappropriate silences; short spurts of speech; variable rate; and a breathy, harsh vocal quality [12,13].

Assessment

Assessment of dysarthria involves a complete oral-peripheral examination of the speech musculature at rest and during movement. The SLP assesses the facial muscles and the muscles of mastication, looking at structure, symmetry, strength, precision, and speed. The patient is asked to imitate the labial and lingual movements of the SLP in both nonspeaking and speaking tasks. For example, using diadochokinetic tasks, such as pa-pa-pa, ta-ta-ta, ka-ka-ka, and pa-ta-ka, the SLP can assess the speed, precision, and rhythm control for the respiratory, phonatory, and articulatory structures involved [15]. Respiration should be observed at rest and during phonation and speech.

In patients with ALS, measures of vital capacity can help the SLP determine severity of disease and if alternative means of communication are appropriate [15]. In Parkinson's disease, the perceptual features of dysarthria (reduced loudness, monotone, imprecise articulation, hoarse vocal quality) have been correlated with the physiologic and neuromuscular characteristics of the disease (rigidity, bradykinesia, tremor) [10,16].

Objective measurements, such as speech instrumentation, are used to evaluate dysarthria, in addition to standardized tests of intelligibility (ie, Assessment of Intelligibility of Dysarthric Speech and the Frenchay Dysarthria Assessment [10]).

Treatment

Treatment for dysarthria depends on the cause, type, severity of the symptoms, and communication needs of the patient. Interventions that modify the patient's speech or speaking environment can improve overall intelligibility [16]. Goals usually include improving articulation through increasing lip, tongue movement, and strength so speech is clearer; reducing the rate of speech [17]; and increasing breath support. Treatment strategies that increase vocal loudness through increased phonatory effort, such as the Lee Silverman Voice Treatment, have been effective in working with individuals with hypokinetic dysarthria associated with Parkinson's disease [18]. Improved intelligibility is a perceptual benefit of both rate reduction techniques and increased vocal loudness techniques [17].

Preliminary investigations into the effects of neurosurgery (ie, pallidotomy, thalamotomy, and deep brain stimulation) on the perceptual speech dimensions and oromotor functions of individuals with Parkinson's disease indicate no significant changes in these areas [10].

The SLP also works with the patient's caregiver or family so they can understand the person's communication impairment and learn compensatory techniques that facilitate improved communication, especially if the dysarthria is a result of a degenerative disease. As the disease progresses, the patient might not be able to speak at all so an augmentative-alternative communication system might be appropriate [9].

Apraxia

Apraxia is a motor speech disorder characterized by difficulty in sequencing sounds in the correct order for syllables and words. Unlike dysarthria, apraxia does not result from weakness or paralysis of the speech musculature [19]. Apraxia may result from stroke, tumor, head injury, or other disorders involving the brain [20]. One can have an oral apraxia or a verbal apraxia. Oral apraxia is a motor planning impairment that occurs when nonspeech volitional movements are attempted. For example, a patient with oral apraxia has difficulty puckering their lips or puffing out their cheeks when asked to do so [19]. With verbal apraxia, patients know what they want to say but the brain has difficulty coordinating the muscle movements necessary to say words [21]. The longer or more complex the word, the harder it is for an apraxic to say. Articulation errors usually consist of substitutions and omissions with some distortions. Initial consonants are more difficult as are clusters [19]. Mistakes are inconsistent or random. Patients with apraxia usually struggle and exhibit searching behavior (groping for the right sound or word), making several attempts to get it right [20]. The patient usually recognizes that they have made an error and try to correct it. Another characteristic of apraxia is inappropriate use of prosody. A patient with apraxia can have fairly intact "automatic speech" (ie, counting, naming the days of the week, use of social greetings). A patient can have both apraxia and dysarthria. Apraxia can also co-occur with aphasia [19].

Assessment

Assessment of apraxia is based on the observation of some or many of the previously described symptoms. A standardized test that is often used is Apraxia Battery for Adults (ABA-2) [22]. The SLP first rules out muscle weakness or language impairment. The SLP has the patient perform various speech tasks to see if any of the previously described symptoms occurred. These speech tasks might include repeating a set of words of increasing length (ie, dare, daring, daringly) or reading sentences of increasing length and complexity [20]. The patient's ability to describe a picture, write, and read a passage are also assessed. The impact of the patient's apraxia on their everyday life and interactions should be part of the assessment.

Treatment

Treatment of apraxia and dysarthria is developed specifically for the patient's needs. Such factors as the severity of the disorder, the underlying etiology, the amount of time since onset, coexisting problems, and the patient's level of motivation and own personal goals need to be taken into consideration [19]. The goal of apraxia therapy is to improve voluntary control of specific articulator movements through nonspeech exercises and speech exercises (ie, repeating sounds, sequencing sounds into words); reducing the rate of speech so the person has the time to produce all the sounds necessary to communicate their message; and reducing the groping and struggling behaviors [19,20]. In severe cases, if oral communication is not a viable goal then augmentative or alternate communication can be explored.

Voice disorders

Many older adults have voice problems [23]. Changes in the voice after age 65 occur because of physiologic changes in the body [24]. Aging itself does not necessarily result in voice problems, but those older adults who are in poor physical condition may experience more voice problems. Some common changes in the voice might be decreased loudness; a decrease or increase in vocal pitch; and changes in vocal quality, which correlate somewhat to the physiologic changes that occur in the larynx with aging. The cartilages, connective tissue, blood supply, and secretions can all be affected. Common symptoms of voice problems include hoarseness, breathiness, reduced loudness, vocal fatigue, pitch breaks or inappropriate pitch, and strain or struggle [24].

It is the SLP's role to assess the voice production, determine the cause and severity of the voice problem, and develop an appropriate treatment plan [25]. The voice evaluation should encompass a complete history, perceptual and acoustic assessment using instrumentation [25], and the impact the voice problem has on the person's quality of life and daily functions [26]. Perceptual characteristics are those characteristics that are perceived by the listener and are used to describe the vocal qualities. Some of the perceptual signs include pitch (reduced pitch variability, inappropriate pitch, pitch breaks); loudness (reduced loudness variability, reduced range and control); quality (hoarse or rough, breathy, tense, strained, tremulous); aphonia (loss of voice intermittently or consistently); and other (eg, stridor [noisy breathing] excessive throat clearing) [24]. These perceptual signs are not necessarily indicative of how an individual coordinates the respiratory, laryngeal-phonatory, or articulatory parameters of voice production. One also has to know the underlying pathophysiology [25].

Voice is produced by movements of the vocal folds, which interrupt the expiration of air [24]. The power source for voicing is respiration. Any pathology of the vocal folds or respiratory process can result in the perceptual symptoms of a voice problem. A SLP should collaborate with an otolaryngologist to assess the anatomy and physiology of the larynx, in addition to using instrumentation objectively to measure vocal function [9]. Examples of instrumentation that are used for assessing the acoustic aspects of voice disorders include Visi-Pitch (Kay Elemetrics, Lincoln Park, New Jersey); videostroboscopy; electroglottography; acoustic reflection technology [27]; and aerodynamic measures. For example, an older adult might complain of a weak voice ("no one can hear me") [24]. The perceptual signs might be breathiness, poor loudness variation, occasional loss of voice completely, or hoarseness. The acoustic signs measured by instrumentation might include reduced phonational (pitch) range; reduced dynamic range; increased perturbation (frequency-pitch variation); and increased shimmer (amplitude-loudness variation). The physiologic signs might be incomplete vocal fold adduction, which could be caused by a vocal fold paralysis as in ALS, Parkinson's, or myasthenia gravis, or bowing of the vocal folds, which could be caused by aging or reduced muscle tone [24].

It is also important to note that some medications can affect the voice mainly by drying out the protective mucosal layer that covers the vocal folds; by thinning the blood in the body, which could make bruising or hemorrhaging of the vocal folds occur if there is trauma; and by causing fluid retention, which could cause the vocal folds to swell [28]. Some common drugs that could cause vocal side effects include anticholinergics; antihistamines; antidepressants; antihypertensives (including angiotensin-converting enzyme inhibitors); diuretics; and stimulants (caffeine, amphetamines) [28,29].

Treatment

Treatment of voice disorders in an older patient is based on the medical history and results of the clinical assessment. The patient's daily activities should also be considered in developing the treatment plan. The needs might be different for those still working in the community and those living in an institutional setting [23,26]. Some general therapeutic interventions include education of how the voice works and good vocal hygiene; physiologic vocal exercises to improve the quality and strength of the voice; and compensatory techniques to optimize vocal function, all within the patient's limitations and functional potential [23]. Some therapeutic interventions include medications, surgery, or in the case of voice tremor treating it with botulinum toxin type A [30].

Dysphagia

Dysphagia is difficulty swallowing regardless of etiology and defines impairments of oral feeding and management of secretions [15,31]. Swallowing and the ability to take oral feeding have nutritional, emotional, and social impact on a patient [32,33]. At the least, changes in swallowing function can affect enjoyment and social interactions. At the worst, complications can include dehydration, malnutrition, weight loss, and aspiration pneumonia, and may significantly impact length of stay and cost of care for both acute and long-term patients [15,34,35]. Risk factors affecting the ability to swallow for the geriatric

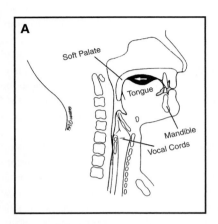

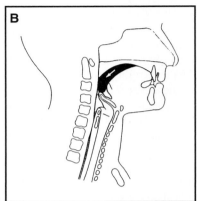

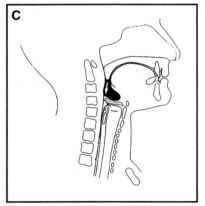

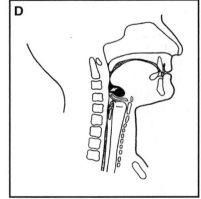

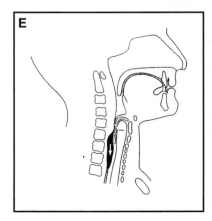

population are varied considering the mechanical, neurologic, and mental status changes common in this age group [35,36].

Normal swallow

Swallowing is a coordinated sequence of muscle movements designed to transport a bolus into the esophagus while protecting the airway. There are three stages of swallowing: (1) oral, (2) pharyngeal, and (3) esophageal. They involve parasympathetic nerves, several cranial nerves, and smooth muscle (Fig. 1) [35,36].

The oral stage begins with a preparatory phase. Labial seal allows stripping of the bolus from a utensil and contains the bolus in the oral cavity preventing leakage of intake. Food is lubricated and masticated using a rotary lateral jaw motion until a cohesive bolus is formed [35,37]. Buccal tension and grooving of the tongue contain the bolus and prevent pooling in the lateral sulcus. Posterior transport is accomplished by a rolling or sweeping movement of the tongue against the hard palate. The oral stage is terminated when the bolus passes any point between the faucial arches and the swallow reflex is triggered. The oral stage is the only voluntary phase of swallowing and transport normally takes less than 1 second for completion [36].

Triggering of the swallow reflex begins the pharyngeal stage so there is no interruption in bolus movement. Several simultaneous actions occur after the trigger. The velum elevates and retracts creating velopharyngeal closure, which prevents leakage into the nasal pathway while pharyngeal peristalsis is initiated to move the bolus. Laryngeal elevation is accomplished with contraction of three sphincters (aryepiglottic folds, false and true cords) and relaxation of the upper esophageal sphincter [36]. Sensory input is carried by cranial nerves IX, X, and XI, whereas motor control is transmitted by cranial nerves IX and X [36,37]. Duration of the pharyngeal stage is normally 1 second or less [36].

The esophageal phase begins at the cricopharyngeal juncture and ends as the bolus passes the gastroesophageal juncture [36]. Transport is accomplished by gravity and peristaltic waves [37].

Normal aging

Studies indicate minor changes in swallow function with normal aging affected by changes in dentition, salivation, loss of alveolar bone, weak oral movement, sensitivity in the trigger of the pharyngeal swallow, respiratory pattern, laryngeal, and upper esophageal sphincter tone [34,36].

Fig. 1. Lateral view of bolus propulsion during the swallow, beginning with the voluntary initiation of the swallow by the oral tongue (*A*); the triggering of the pharyngeal swallow (*B*); the arrival of the bolus in the vallecula (*C*); the tongue base retraction to the anteriorly moving pharyngeal wall (*D*); and the bolus in the cervical esophagus and cricopharyngeal region (*E*). (*From* Logemann J. Evaluation and treatment of swallowing disorders. 2nd edition. Austin: ProEd; 1998. p. 28; with permission.)

If dentition is good, masticatory function remains high but with some increased chewing necessary for bolus preparation. The oral stage is slightly extended in older adults with increased lingual gestures [35,36]. Diminished oropharyngeal sensitivity with aging has been demonstrated for both liquid and air boluses. The incidence of penetration during swallow has been noted with aging but aspiration is not shown to increase [35]. Logemann [36] documented reduced neuromuscular reserve in older men and reduced flexibility in cricopharyngeal opening as part of the normal aging of the motor system. Esophageal function shows moderate deterioration with slower transit and clearance [35].

Disorders

Several disorders with higher incidence in the geriatric population can cause dysphagia, putting the elderly patient at higher risk for aspiration [36]. Side effects of many commonly used medications can contribute to dysphagia creating dry mouth, tardive dyskinesia, drowsiness, or suppressed gag or cough reflex (Table 2) [31,34].

Cerebrovascular accident or stroke is the third leading cause of death in the United States [31]. Depending on the site of lesion, stroke patients may exhibit oral and pharyngeal stage dysphagia [31,36]. Aspiration pneumonia following a

Table 2
Common medications affecting swallowing

Product category	Examples	Common indications	Possible effects
Neuroleptics			
Antidepressants	Amitryptyle (tricyclic)	Relief of endogenous depression	Drying of mucosa, drowsiness
Antipsychotics	Haloperidol Thorazine	Management of patients with chronic psychosis	Tardive dyskinesia
Sedatives			
Barbiturates	Phenobarbital Nembutal	Treatment of insomnia	Central nervous system depressant (drowsiness causing decompensation of patients with cognitive deficits)
Antihistamines	Cold and cough preparations	Relief of nasal congestion and cough	Drying mucosa, sedative effects
Diuretics	Furosenide	Treatment of edema (eg, associated with congestive heart failure)	Signs of chronic dehydration (dryness of mouth, thirst, weakness, drowsiness)
Mucosal anesthetics	Benzocaine Cetacaine Lidocaine	Topical anesthetics used to aid passage of fiberoptic nasopharyngoscopes, control of dental pain	Suppresses gag and cough reflex
Anticholinergics	Cogentin	Adjunct in Parkinsonism therapy	Dry mouth and reduced appetite

From Murry T. Clinical manual for swallowing disorders. San Diego: Singular; 2001; with permission.

stroke results in 50,000 deaths each year [35] and risk of aspiration is highest during the first week postonset [37]. Early identification of dysphagia can reduce this risk, shorten length of stay, and improve the patient's quality of life [37,38].

Parkinson's disease is characterized by loss of striatal dopamine and can be an indirect cause of dysphagia affecting all three stages of swallowing [31]. Hand tremors can make self-feeding difficult or impossible. Repetitive or "festinating" movements typical in Parkinson's and rigidity can affect the oral stage resulting in difficulty moving the bolus posteriorly. The trigger can be delayed and strength of the pharyngeal walls decreased. This results in pooling in the valleculae and pyriform sinuses. Reduced laryngeal elevation and movement of the base of tongue can cause dysfunction at the cricopharyngeal juncture or upper esophageal sphincter. This creates risk for aspiration after the completion of the swallow [35]. With all degenerative diseases, continued monitoring of dysphagia is recommended [35].

ALS is a progressive disease involving upper and lower motor neuron degeneration. Dysphagia has been shown in 73% of ALS patients [31]. Spasticity, flaccidity, or atrophy of the face or tongue can affect lingual and labial movements resulting in impairments of bolus control especially with solids. Management of secretions may also become difficult and present risk for aspiration [31,36].

The autoimmune disorder myasthenia gravis reduces muscle activating neurotransmitters. This causes rapid muscle fatigue affecting masseter, facial, and palatal movement. One third of myasthenia gravis patients experience dysphagia [31]. Patients may fatigue before completing a meal, which negatively impacts on the adequacy of intake for nutritional support. This population may tolerate liquids more easily than solids because lower density requires less bolus preparation [36].

Dementia is a major risk factor for both feeding problems and dysphagia. Physiologic changes can cause reduced tongue movement, delayed pharyngeal trigger, or abnormalities in pharyngeal movements [36]. Diminished sensorium and changes in the cognitive control of the skeletal musculature component of swallowing are also contributing factors [35]. Even when the swallow is functional, dementia patients may be unable to sustain nutrition with oral feeding.

Diagnosis

A multidisciplinary approach is necessary for effective diagnosis and treatment of dysphagia in the elderly whether they are living in the community or an extended care facility. This holistic approach to diagnosis and management should include the physician, SLP, dietitian, nursing staff and caregivers, dentist, pharmacist, occupational therapist, and social worker [15,36,37].

While reviewing the history, physicians should note indicators of dysphagia (weight loss, aspiration pneumonia, recurrent urinary tract infection, and so forth). The examination should include testing of cranial nerves, an otolaryngology examination, blood work to detect early signs of malnutrition or dehydration, and a review of all drugs and their effect on the swallowing mechanism [31,34,35]. Assessment of mobility should consider the patient's ability to shop, prepare meals, and self-feed. If dysphagia is suspected, the SLP should be consulted.

Speech-language pathologist clinical examination

The SLP initially reviews the patient's chart and medical history for dysphagia risk factors, such as diagnosis of neurologic impairment, degenerative disease, pulmonary disease, gastrointestinal disorders, head and neck cancer, dementia, history of aspiration pneumonia, or weight loss [34,35].

A clinical examination provides evidence of dysfunction and indirect signs of aspiration and determines the need for further work-up. Initially, the patient's mental status, respiratory function, ability to manage secretions, and general physical condition are informally assessed. Careful attention is paid to the patient's description of his or her dysphagia, food consistencies that are problematic, and onset pattern [32]. Patients commonly use phrases like "It gets stuck in my throat," or "I just can't get it down." They should be asked to indicate where they feel food "sticking" and generally give an accurate indication of the site of pooling (valleculae, pyriform sinus, or upper esophagus). Patients are also asked about odynophagia (pain during swallowing) and appetite [31,34,36].

An oral peripheral examination is completed to evaluate dentition; reflexes; oral sensitivity; range of motion; strength, and precision of labial, lingual, and velar movements. Attention to vocal quality gives an indication of vocal cord function and the need for examination by an otolaryngologist [31,34,36].

If the patient is considered a candidate for trial with oral feeding, small amounts of puree, solid, thick, and thin liquid consistencies are given. The reaction to food and willingness to eat are also noted. Observation during the oral stage provides information about containment, ability to form bolus, oral transit time, struggle behavior, oral clearance, or presence of residue after completion of swallow [31,34]. The clinician positions fingers lightly at four points (behind mandible, thyroid bone, and above and below the thyroid cartilage) to assess movement during the swallow and give a rough estimate of the pharyngeal trigger [36].

Throat clearing and coughing before, during, or after completion of swallow provides indirect evidence of aspiration and pooling. For instance, "wet" vocal quality after completion of swallow is a soft sign of aspiration or pooling at level of the larynx [31,34,36]. The amount of energy expended during the feeding process and signs of fatigue are also noted because they may affect the amount of intake during a meal.

Direct examination of swallowing mechanism

If aspiration is suspected, a modified barium swallow, also known as "videofluoroscopic swallowing study," may be requested to verify and assess the

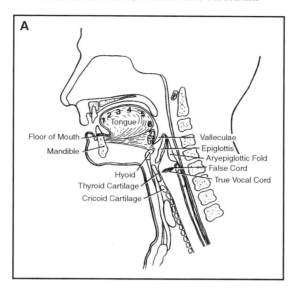

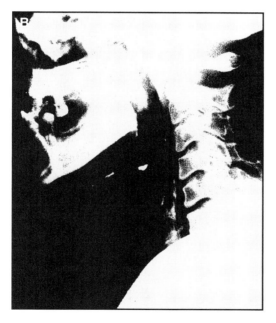

Fig. 2. (*A*) Lateral view of the oral cavity with the parts of the oral tongue labeled: tip (*1*), blade (*2*), front (*3*), center (*4*), and back (*5*). The tongue base (*6*) extends from the circumvallate papillae or approximately the tip of the uvula to the hyoid bone. (*B*) Lateral radiographic view of the oral cavity and pharynx. (*From* Logemann J. Evaluation and treatment of swallowing disorders. 2nd edition. Austin: ProEd; 1998. p. 16, 60; with permission.)

amount of aspiration or to rule out "silent" aspiration (aspiration in the absence of a cough reflex) [34,35]. Videotaping allows a frame-by-frame analysis of motility, residue, and aspiration [36].

The SLP assists the radiologist during the study. The patient is seated in an upright position. Mediums of varying viscosity are given including liquid; a puree, such as pudding mixed with powdered barium; and a cracker coated with barium. Bolus sizes are measured by syringe into a teaspoon. At least two boluses of each consistency are attempted. A lateral image is used to ensure clear detail of the dynamics of both the oral and pharyngeal stages of swallowing (Fig. 2). An anterior plane may also be taken to isolate pooling and identify unilateral paresis. Treatment techniques may be attempted for direct examination of their effect [36].

The SLP's report describes any abnormality of structures or movement, adequacy of valving, aspiration, efficacy of treatment techniques, and ultimately the patient's candidacy for oral feeding. Recommendations for diet modification, feeding procedures, positioning, and use of adaptive feeding devices are also included [31,34,36].

Videoendoscopy or fiberoptic endoscopic evaluation of swallowing is also used to evaluate structures and image the pharynx before and after a swallow. Closure of the pharyngeal walls around the lens eliminates the image during the swallow. A flexible scope is inserted through the nose after application of a light topical anesthetic. The oral stage of swallow cannot be observed. A good image of the velopharyngeal closure and the pharynx, however, can be obtained (Fig. 3). Pooling of secretion or residue can be seen and pharyngeal sensitivity can also be assessed by the flexible endoscopic evaluation of swallowing with sensory testing [31,36].

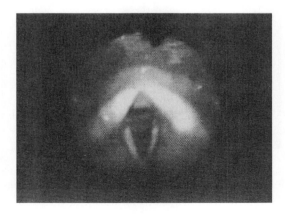

Fig. 3. The image of the larynx as viewed with the tube in the position behind the tip of the epiglottis. (*From* Logemann J. Evaluation and treatment of swallowing disorders. 2nd edition. Austin: ProEd; 1998. p. 59; with permission.)

Treatment

Based on the results or the dysphagia work-up treatment may include a variety of compensatory techniques. Positioning the patient can compensate for weak structures and increase airway protection (Table 3). Use of the supraglottic swallow increases airway protection as does a chin tuck position. Adaptive equipment (small-bowled spoon, shortened straw, cups with extended lip, and so forth) is used to control bolus size and allow midline introduction of bolus decreasing labial leakage. Modification of food consistencies and viscosity of liquids may also be recommended (eg, puree, soft mechanical, thickened liquids) [31,34,36,38].

If it is determined that a patient is not a candidate for oral feeding, alternate means of nutritional support must be considered (nasogastric tube, percutane-

Table 3
Postural techniques successful in eliminating aspiration or residue resulting from various swallowing disorders and the rationale for their effectiveness

Disorder observed on fluoroscopy	Posture applied	Rationale
Inefficient oral transit (reduced posterior propulsion of bolus by tongue)	Head back	Utilizes gravity to clear oral cavity
Delay in triggering the pharyngeal swallow (bolus past ramus of mandible, but pharyngeal swallow not triggered)	Chin down	Widens valleculae to prevent bolus entering airway; narrows airway entrance; pushes epiglottis posteriorly
Reduced posterior motion of tongue base (residue in valleculae)	Chin down	Pushes tongue base backward toward pharyngeal wall
Unilateral laryngeal dysfunction (aspiration during swallow)	Head rotated to damaged side; chin down	Places extrinsic pressure on thyroid cartilage, increasing adduction
Reduced laryngeal closure (aspiration during swallow)	Chin down; head rotated to damaged side	Puts epiglottis in more protective position; narrows laryngeal entrance; increases vocal fold closure by applying extrinsic pressure
Reduced pharyngeal contraction (residue spread throughout pharynx)	Lying down on one side	Eliminates gravitational effect on pharyngeal residue
Unilateral pharyngeal paresis (residue on one side of pharynx)	Head rotated to damaged side	Eliminates damaged side from bolus patch
Unilateral oral and pharyngeal weakness on the same side (residue in mouth and pharynx on same side)	Head tilt to stronger side	Directs bolus down stronger side
Cricopharyngeal dysfunction (residue in pyriform sinuses)	Head rotated	Pulls cricoid cartilage away from posterior pharyngeal wall, reducing resting pressure in cricopharyngeal sphincter

From Logemann J. Evaluation and treatment of swallowing disorders. 2nd edition. Astin: ProEd; 1998. p. 181; with permission.

ous endoscopic gastrostomy, or percutaneous endoscope jejunostomy) [36,39]. Enteral feeding has four commonly accepted objectives: (1) improving nutritional status, (2) decreasing risk of disease, (3) increasing length of survival, and (4) improving quality of life [40]. Based on diagnosis, prognosis, and premorbid level of functioning, however, these goals may not be attainable and tube feeding may need to be addressed as an end-of-life issue [40,41].

For the geriatric patient with advance dementia informed consent involves a proxy. Information about the anticipated results of artificial hydration and nutrition must be provided and the approach differs from the traditional rehabilitation model [40,41].

Human rights issues preclude controlled studies on the effects of enteral feeding, leaving literature review as the best means of assessment [40]. In an extensive review, Angus and Burakoff [42] showed no proved weight gain or improved nutrition in the tube-fed geriatric population with acute neurologic deficits. Ashford and coworkers [40] also failed in their literature review to substantiate attainment of the acknowledged goals of enteral feeding with severely demented patients. Nor has improvement in other outcomes, such as prevention of aspiration pneumonia or infection, been documented [40].

Ciocon and coworkers [43] studied 70 patients receiving tube feeding over an 11-month period and found that weight loss increased with the duration of tube feeding with only 6% showing consistent weight gain. Across 24 studies, Finucane and Bynum [44] found that aspiration rates ranged from 1% to a high of 54.4% and noted that tube feeding does not eliminate aspiration of secretions or gastroesophageal reflux.

Sufficient evidence to support the contention that enteral feeding affects length of survival was not found in the literature and the mortality rate for tube-fed elderly patients is high. The implication is that tube feeding does not ensure stable weight or decreased rates of aspiration of feedings or secretions [40,44].

Comfort is also questionable with enteral feeding. Thirty-three percent of dementia patients self-extubate and discomfort must be considered as a possible factor. Whatever the motivation, repeated self-extubation necessitates use of physical or chemical restraints, which are recognized as having a negative impact on the patient's quality of life [40]. The impact of tube feeding on a patient's social, religious, and personal values must also be considered, in addition to the economic and legal issues and the burden on caregivers [41].

An ethical decision-making model must balance benefit to the patient against minimizing unnecessary harm [41]. Hunger and thirst diminish in the advanced stage of dementia and suffering is not increased when tube feeding is withheld [45,46]. Caregivers may choose to focus on palliative care. The Alzheimer's Association's position states "Severely and irreversibly demented patients need only care given to make them comfortable. If such a patient is unable to receive food and water by mouth, it is ethically permissible to choose to withhold nutrition and hydration artificially administered" [47]. An ethical standard of care requires that those exercising substituted judgments for the severely demented patient must be aware of these facts to make a truly informed decision [39,46].

Acknowledgments

Special thanks to Samantha Procaccini for assistance in obtaining several reference materials for this project.

References

[1] Nicolosi L, Harryman E, Kresheck J. Terminology of communication disorders: speech-language-hearing. 3rd edition. Baltimore: Williams & Wilkins; 1989.

[2] Davis GA. A survey of adult aphasia. Englewood Cliffs (NJ): Prentice Hall; 1983.

[3] National Institute on Deafness and Other Communication Disorders updated February 23, 2005. Available at: http://www.nidcd.nih.gov/health/voice/aphasia.asp. Accessed May 26, 2005.

[4] Kramer A, Coleman E. Stroke rehabilitation in nursing homes: how do we measure quality? Clin Geriatr Med 1999;15:869–84.

[5] Kearns KP. Broca's aphasia. In: La Pointe LL, editor. Aphasia and related neurogenic language disorders. 2nd edition. New York: Thieme Medical Publishers; 1997. p. 1–34.

[6] Depression Guideline Panel. Clinical practice guideline, number 5. Depression in primary care: Volume 1. Detection and diagnosis. AHCPR Pub. No. 93–0551. Rockville (MD): US Department of Health and Human Services, Agency for Health Care Policy and Research; 1993.

[7] Bhogal SK, Teasell R, Speechley M. Intensity of aphasia therapy, impact on recovery. Stroke 2003;34:987–93.

[8] McDowd J, Filion D, Pohl P, et al. Attentional abilities and functional outcomes following stroke. J Gerontol B Psychol Sci Soc Sci 2003;58:45–53.

[9] Wheeler D, editor. Geriatric communication disorders. Prepared by the Task Force on Geriatric Communication Problems, New York State Speech-Language-Hearing Association and the Brookdale Center on Aging. New York: The Brookdale Center on Aging; 1993. p. 31–2.

[10] Farrell A, et al. Effects of neurosurgical management of Parkinson's disease on speech characteristics and oromotor function. J Speech Lang Hear Res 2005;48:5–20.

[11] American Speech-Language-Hearing Association. Dysarthia. Available at: http://www.asha.org/public/speech/disorders/dysarthria.htm. Accessed May 12, 2005.

[12] Darley F, et al. Clusters of deviant speech dimensions in the dysarthrias. J Speech Lang Hear Res 1969;12:462–9.

[13] Darley F, et al. Differential diagnostic pattern of dysarthria. J Speech Lang Hear Res 1969;12: 246–69.

[14] Heir DB. Disorders of speech. In: Stein JH, Eisenberg JM, Hutton JJ, et al, editors. Internal medicine. 5th edition. St. Louis: Mosby Year Book; 1998.

[15] Miller RM, Groher ME. Medical speech pathology. Rockville (MD): Aspen; 1990.

[16] Ramig LO. Treatment of speech and voice problems associated with Parkinson's disease. In: Cherney LR, Lewis CB, editors. Facilitating communication in the older person (topics in geriatric rehabilitation, vol. 14). Frederick: Aspen; 1998. p. 28–43.

[17] Tjaden K, Wilding G. Rate and loudness manipulations in dysarthria: acoustic and perceptual findings. J Speech Lang Hear Res 2004;47:766–83.

[18] Kleinow J, et al. Speech motor stability in IPD: effects of rate and loudness manipulation. J Speech Lang Hear Res 2001;44:1041–51.

[19] Dworkin JP. Motor speech disorders: a treatment guide. St Louis: Mosby Year Book; 1991.

[20] National Institute on Deafness and Other Communication Disorders. Apraxia of speech updated February 23, 2005. Available at: http://www.nidcd.nih.gov/health/voice/apraxia.asp. Accessed May 12, 2005.

[21] American Speech-Language-Hearing Association. Apraxia in adults. Available at: http://www.asha.org/public/speech/disorders/apraxia_adults.htm. Accessed March 25, 2005.

[22] Dabul BL. Apraxia battery for adults. 2nd edition. King of Prussia (PA): Merion Publications; 2000.

[23] Mosheim J. Voice disorders. ADVANCE for speech-language pathologists and audiologists. April 18, 2005.

[24] Colton RH, Casper JK. Understanding voice problems: a physiological perspective for diagnosis and treatment. 2nd edition. Baltimore: Williams and Wilkins; 1996.

[25] Behrman A, Orlikoff R. Instrumentation in voice assessment and treatment: what's the use? Am J Speech Lang Pathol 1997;6:9–16.

[26] Ma E, Yiu E. Voice activity and participation profile: assessing the impact of voice disorders on daily activities. J Speech Lang Hear Res 2001;44:511–24.

[27] Xue S, Hao G. Changes in the human vocal tract due to aging and the acoustic correlates of speech production: a pilot study. J Speech Lang Hear Res 2003;46:689–701.

[28] American Academy of Otolaryngology-Head and Neck Surgery. Fact sheet: Medications and voice problems–could your medications be affecting your voice? Updated 2002. Available at: http://www.entnet.org/healthinfo/throat/medications-and-voice-problems.cfm. Accessed March 25, 2005.

[29] Vogel D, Carter PB. Pharmacology and the older person: effects on communication. In: Cherney LR, Lewis CB, editors. Facilitating communication in the older person (topics in geriatric rehabilitation, vol. 14). Frederick: Aspen; 1998. p. 76–86.

[30] Adler CH, et al. Botulinum toxin type A for treating voice tremor. Arch Neurol 2004;61: 1416–20.

[31] Murry T, Carrau R. Clinical manual for swallowing disorders. San Diego: Singular; 2001.

[32] Ekberg O, Hamdy S, Woisard V, et al. Social and psychological burden of dysphagia: its impact on diagnosis and treatment. Dysphagia 2002;17:139–46.

[33] Pelletier C. What do certified nurse assistants actually know about dysphagia and feeding nursing home residents? Am J Speech Lang Pathol 2004;13:99–113.

[34] Cefalu C. Appropriate dysphagia evaluation and management of the nursing home patient with dementia. Annals of Long-Term Care 1999;7:447–51.

[35] Friedel D, Fisher R. Gastrointestinal motility in the elderly. Clinical Geriatrics 2000;8:30–42.

[36] Logemann J. Evaluation and treatment of swallowing disorders. 2nd edition. Austin: ProEd; 1998.

[37] Crary M, Groher M. Introduction to adult swallowing disorders. St. Louis: Butterworth Heinemann; 2003.

[38] Rumeau P, Vellas B. Dysphagia, a geriatric point of view. Rev Laryngol Otol Rhinol (Bord) 2003;124:331–3.

[39] Wells JL, Seabrook JA, Stolee P, et al. State of the art in geriatric rehabilitation. Part II: clinical challenges. Arch Phys Med Rehabil 2003;84:898–903.

[40] Ashford J, Janes R, McKinzie M, et al. Use of enteral feeding with patient in the advanced stages of dementia. Presented by members of an interdisciplinary ad hoc group of the VA Tennessee Valley Healthcare System; May 3, 2001.

[41] Sharp H, Genesen L. Ethical decision-making in dysphagia management. Am J Speech Lang Pathol 1996;5:15–22.

[42] Angus F, Burakoff R. The percutaneous endoscopic gastrostomy tube: medical and ethical issues in placement. Am J Gastroenterol 2003;98:272–7.

[43] Ciocon J, Silverstone M, Graver M, et al. Tube-feeding in elderly patients. Arch Intern Med 1988;148:429–33.

[44] Finucane T, Bynum J. Use of tube-feeding to prevent aspiration pneumonia. Lancet 1996; 348:1421–4.

[45] Scott L. The PEG "consult". Am J Gastroenterol 2005;100:740–3.

[46] Levy A, Dominguez-Gasson L, Brown E, et al. Technology at end of life questioned. The ASHA Leader 2004;1–14.

[47] Alzheimer's Association. Fact sheet: assisted oral feeding and tube feeding, 2000. Available at: http://www.alz.org/Resources/FactSheets/FSOralfeeding.pdf. Accessed June 29, 2005.

ELSEVIER
SAUNDERS

Clin Geriatr Med 22 (2006) 311–330

CLINICS IN
GERIATRIC
MEDICINE

Neurogenic Bowel and Bladder in the Older Adult

Michelle Stern, MD

*Department of Clinical Rehabilitation Medicine,
Columbia University College of Physician and Surgeons, 180 Fort Washington Avenue,
HP1-194, New York, NY 10032, USA*

Special skills are needed in caring for an elderly patient with a neurogenic bowel and bladder. One not only has to take into account the age-related changes that occur, but also how these changes impact on a patient already struggling with bowel and bladder issues because of various neurogenic causes. Incontinence of bowel and bladder leads to a loss of quality of life and physicians should be educated on the treatment available to provide the best care for their patients.

Neurogenic bladder in the older adult

Urinary incontinence (UI), no matter what the cause, is a major public health problem facing the aging population. A recent study revealed that over 200 million adults are incontinent. UI imposes high economic costs, with two thirds of these costs deriving from UI in the elderly. UI increases with age, but among adults over age 60 women are almost twice as likely as men to suffer from incontinence. It is not the process of aging itself that causes the incontinence, but rather the age-related changes caused by additional anatomic or physiologic insults to the lower urinary tract or by systemic disturbances, such as chronic illnesses common in the elderly. Untreated UI leads to a decreased quality of life, decreased participation in activities, increased caregiver assistance, and increased costs of care. Despite the negative impact on quality of life and the existence of effective treatments, more than half of those with problems of in-

E-mail address: ms1127@columbia.edu

0749-0690/06/$ – see front matter © 2006 Elsevier Inc. All rights reserved.
doi:10.1016/j.cger.2005.12.014   *geriatric.theclinics.com*

continence do not seek treatment mostly because of embarrassment. Older incontinent patients also may not report symptoms because they perceive it to be a normal part of the aging process. It is incumbent on the physician to inquire about the voiding habits of their elderly patient regardless of whether or not they suffer from a known neurologic disease. Risk factors for UI in women include increasing age, childbirth, the presence of lower urinary tract symptoms, obesity, and decreased mobility. Risk factor for UI in men includes increasing age; lower urinary tract symptoms, such as cystitis or bladder outlet obstruction; decreased mobility; and radical prostatectomy [1–9].

The lower urinary tract consists of the bladder and the urethra. The bladder can be divided into the bladder body or the detrusor and the bladder base (composed of the bladder neck and the trigone). The urethra contains the internal and external sphincter. The internal sphincter and the bladder are composed of smooth muscle, whereas the external sphincter is striated muscle. The internal smooth muscle sphincter is at the proximal urethra and the bladder neck, whereas the external sphincter encompasses the membranous urethra and is attached to the pelvic floor. The pelvic floor musculature, ligaments, and neural control also play an important role in micturition. In the female urethra the external sphincter is situated in the middle third of the urethra, whereas in males it is located at the most inferior aspect of the prostate around the membranous urethra [10,11].

The parasympathetic system is carried by the pelvic nerve that originates at the sacral level (S2–S4) (Fig. 1). Parasympathetic stimulation is responsible for detrusor contractions and is mediated by cholinergic (muscarinic M2) fibers. Parasympathetic stimulation leads to bladder emptying, and the receptors are primarily located in the body of the bladder than at its base. The sympathetic system is carried by the hypogastric nerve, which originates in the intermedial lateral cell column of the spinal cord at the T10 to L2 region. The sympathetic system consists of the α- and the β_2-adrenergic (norepinephrine) receptors. The α receptors are located at the base of the bladder and cause constriction of the internal sphincter, whereas the β_2 receptors are located in the body of the bladder and cause bladder relaxation. Stimulation of the sympathetic system promotes urine storage. The somatic system is carried by the pudendal nerve, which innervates the striated muscles of the external sphincter and is located in the nucleus of Onufrowicz (Onuf) at the sacral ventral horns (S2–S4). The external sphincter is closed with normal tone to prevent urine leakage, but can be opened passively by forceful urinary flow with contraction of the detrusor and of the abdominal muscle [10–12]. The many pathways of neural control are not fully understood because the bladder, the urethra, and the pelvic floor are innervated by a number of neurotransmitters and neuropathways. In addition to acetylcholine and norepinephrine, there is also a role for serotonin, glutamate, γ-aminobutyric acid, and dopamine. Sensory information is carried by afferent fibers that originate from the detrusor muscle stretch receptors, external anal and urethral sphincters, perineum, and genitalia and are carried along with pelvic, hypogastric, and pudendal nerves but the exact physiology is not yet completely understood [13].

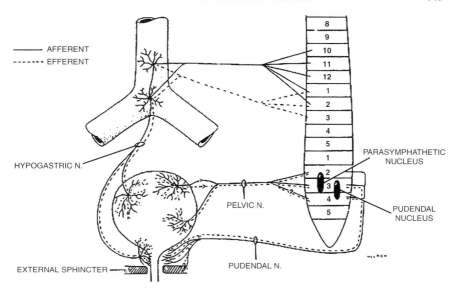

Fig. 1. Parasympathetic, sympathetic and somatic nerve supply to the bladder, urethra, and the pelvic floor. (*From* Cardenas DD, Mayo ME, King KC. Urinary tract and bowel management in the rehabilitation setting. In: Braddom RL, editor. Physical medicine and rehabilitation. Philadelphia: WB Saunders; 1996. p. 556.)

The urodynamic study is the best method to evaluate the bladder pressure-volume relationships during filling and voiding and is an important evaluation tool for patients with a neurogenic bladder. There is the gradual instillation of carbon dioxide or water into the bladder through a catheter while pressure-volume relationships and muscle activity is recorded with the intravesical pressure transducer and surface electromyograph electrodes. During this procedure, the volume at the first desire to void, the total bladder capacity, the presence of uninhibited contractions, the completeness of bladder emptying, and the ability voluntarily to interrupt voiding is examined. Usually, there is the storage of urine at low pressure (less than 10 cm H_2O) with a quiet detrusor muscle, and with voluntary bladder emptying there is low resistance urine passage with reflex detrusor contraction synchronized with voluntary sphincter relaxation. The first sensation of filling usually occurs around 100 mL with the desire to void around 250 mL. A strong urgency to void normally occurs at a urinary volume of 300 to 500 mL. Voiding pressure should be around 20 cm H_2O and the maximum flow rate is about 15 mL per second. After voiding, the amount of urine that is left in the bladder should be less than 50 mL (the older adult is normally 50–100 mL) [10–12].

Changes in the bladder with aging include the following:

Decreased bladder capacity and compliance
Impaired contractility of the bladder wall

Decreased urinary flow rates and sensation of filling

Increase in involuntary bladder contractions

Increased susceptibility to urinary tract infection (UTI)

Increase in the postvoiding residual urine volume to 50 to 100 mL

Loss of functional glomeruli, which leads to a decrease in renal function

Higher rates of urinary excretion at night because of changes in the circadian sleep-awake pattern of urine production and variation in arginine vasopressin and atrial natriuretic hormone and a decline in renal sodium-conserving mechanisms, impaired tubular sodium, and water reabsorption

Decreased ability to delay voiding

Increased prevalence in bladder outlet obstruction caused by prostatic enlargement in men

Decline in the maximal urethral closure pressure and length in women

In women, the lower urinary tract is partially supported by the vagina and the striated muscles of the pelvic floor, which can be weakened because of the effects of childbirth, age, and significant weight gain. This causes the abdominal pressure to be transmitted more to the bladder than to the urethra. In addition, a woman's urethra is only 3 to 5 cm, compared with 23 cm to a man's urethra. The decrease in estrogen levels in an aging female also diminishes the urethra's ability to compress. Detrusor overactivity from a neurologic cause is referred to as "detrusor hyperreflexia," and overactivity caused by changes in the bladder is referred to as "detrusor instability" [14–16].

The objectives of therapy for neurogenic bladder dysfunction are well defined: protecting the kidneys from progressive damage by reducing the intravesical pressure during both filling and emptying, and improving the quality of life by providing urinary continence. Individuals with neurogenic bladder are prone to bacterial colonization of the urinary tract. UTI are a common cause of morbidity in the elderly. Repeated UTI can also lead to bladder wall changes with a marked reduction in the compliance of the bladder. At this time the prophylactic use of antibiotics to prevent UTI in neurogenic bladder is not routinely recommended [11,17–19].

There are three micturition centers: (1) the sacral, (2) the pontine, and (3) the cerebral cortex. The sacral micturition center coordinates the sacral micturition reflex that is caused by the parasympathetics at S2-S4. Lesions in the sacral micturition center, such as conus and cauda equina injuries, L4-L5 or L5-S1 disk herniations, peripheral neuropathies (diabetes), and pelvic injury, lead to the loss of the sacral micturition reflex and result in urinary retention with an areflexic or atonic bladder. Urodynamics typically show diminished sensation during filling cystometry; increased capacity; detrusor underactivity; inability to initiate flow; reduced flow with increased detrusor pressure (obstruction); and increased postvoid residuals. This population most likely needs to use intermittent catheterization (IC) or an indwelling catheter. Timed voiding combined with increasing intravesical pressure either manually (Credé maneuver) or by increasing intra-abdominal pressure (Valsalva maneuver) can be tried. These maneuvers can cause exacerbation of hemorrhoids, rectal prolapse, and hernia and are contra-indicated in patients with vesicoureteral reflux. Cholinergic agents have not been shown to be effective. There are limited surgical options at this time, but the use of neurostimulation is being investigated [10–12,18,19].

Pontine micturition center (also known as the Barrington's nucleus) coor-dinates sphincter-detrusor interaction. Lesions at or below the pontine micturition center and above the sacral cord (suprasacral lesions), such as in a spinal cord injury or multiple sclerosis, have detrusor hyperreflexia and sphincter detrusor dysnergia and lead to bladder contraction with a closed sphincter. This ineffi-cient voiding pattern leads to vesicoureteral reflux or hydronephrosis. Medi-cations used include the anticholinergics to relax the bladder (see later) and the α-adrenergic blockers (antagonists) to relax the sphincter. α-Adrenergic blocking agents include terazosin, prazosin, doxazosin, and tamsulosin. These medica-tions block $\alpha_1 A$ fibers at the bladder neck and sphincter, decreasing tone and improving voiding. Side effects include postural hypotension; syncope; and faint-ing (especially with first dose). Tamsulosin has a reduced risk of hypotension and is generally better tolerated. Surgical treatment if required can include sphinc-terotomy incision, bladder neck incision, prostate resection, and stent placement. The use of botulism toxin into the urethral sphincter is also under investigation. Supportive treatment includes the use of clean IC and indwelling Foley cathe-ter. Medications to relax the striated muscles, such as baclofen, diazepam, and dantrolene, have not been proved to be clinically effective to improve voiding [10–12].

Cerebral cortex micturition center originates from the frontal lobe and exerts inhibitory influence on the sacral micturition center. Lesions above the pontine micturition center (suprapontine lesion) can lead to a hyperreflexic detrusor with a resulting small bladder capacity with urinary urgency and incontinence [10–12]. Disease states associated with detrusor hyperreflexia include strokes; masses (tumor, aneurysm, and hemorrhage); demyelinating disease (multiple sclerosis); Alzheimer's disease; and Parkinson's disease. Urodynamics show detrusor over-activity (involuntary detrusor contraction); inability to inhibit detrusor contrac-tion; and a low-capacity bladder. The postvoid residual urine volume is typically normal. Behavioral treatments include the use of bladder training, timed voiding, pelvic exercises, biofeedback, fluid restrictions, constipation management, and caffeine avoidance. Bladder training can be used with cognitively intact and cognitively impaired patients. Cognitively impaired patients can be started on a scheduled voiding regimen, every 2 to 3 hours with prompted voiding. Studies of nursing home patients placed on a toileting schedule have shown that a substantial proportion respond well to prompted voiding and a sign of those who will respond to this technique is usually seen in the first 3 days [20,21]. A recent Cochrane review looked at bladder training for UI in adults. Their conclusions regarding bladder training was that the limited evidence available suggests that bladder training may be helpful for the treatment of UI, but this conclusion can only be tentative because the trials were of variable quality and of small size with wide confidence intervals around the point estimates of effect. There was also not enough evidence to determine whether bladder training was useful as a supplement to another therapy. More research was recommended. Few of these studies looked solely at patient population over the age of 65 and most studies looked at patients with any type of incontinence, stress or urge, and not just neurogenic causes [22].

The most commonly used medication to help with bladder hyperreflexia is the anticholinergic agents. Imipramine and other tricyclics can also be used but the tricyclics are more likely to be poorly tolerated in the older population. Orthostatic blood pressure should be checked in the elderly patient on these agents. Anticholinergics are used to relax a hyperreflexic bladder by blocking acetylcholine receptors at the postganglionic cholinergic receptor sites. Oxybutynin is available in immediate release, extended release, and transdermal formulation. Side effects can include constipation; dry mucosa (mouth, vagina, eyes); confusion, impaired cognition in elderly; blurred vision; and urinary retention. The postvoid residual should be monitored in the elderly because worsening UI can result from subclinical retention that requires lower dosage of the drug. Dry mouth may be less symptomatic in the extended release and the transdermal preparation. Tolterodine is similar to oxybutynin but may be better tolerated in the elderly. Trospium is an anticholinergic agent that has a high affinity to muscarinic receptors and does not cross the blood-brain barrier in significant amounts. Studies have shown that it is at least as effective as oxybutynin and tolterodine. Solifenacin and darifenacin are recently approved anticholinergic agents with more selectivity for the receptors in the bladder. More studies are needed to determine if the newer anticholinergic agents are better tolerated in an aging population with a neurogenic bladder [23–26]. Botulinum toxin type A injection into the hyperreflexic detrusor muscle is currently under investigation. It has been used in patients with spinal cord injury with relative success. The use of botulinum toxin may be useful in the elderly to help reduce side effects that are associated with the anticholinergics but more research is needed [27,28]. Intravesical capsaicin installation has also been used for urge incontinence caused by neurologic disease. Capsaicin is thought to work by desensitizing the C fiber afferent neurons, which may be responsible for signals that trigger detrusor overactivity. Because of side effects associated with capsaicin, resiniferatoxin, which is 1000 times more potent than capsaicin but with minimal excitatory effects, has also been studied. Further studies are needed to evaluate the use of these medications [29]. Serotonin norepinephrine reuptake inhibitors, such as duloxetine, are currently under investigation to help improve symptoms of stress UI, but further research is needed [30].

Surgical options are generally thought of as a last resort if UI does not respond to behavioral methods or drugs, especially in the elderly. Procedures can include bladder augmentation; continent diversion; sacral posterior rhizotomy; denervation procedures and electrostimulation (for complete lesions); and sacral nerve neuromodulation (for incomplete lesions) [31–35]. Supportive treatment includes the use of undergarment or pads, condom catheters, Foley catheter, clean IC, bedside commode, and urinals. If the patient is voiding, postvoid residuals should be checked and ideally be less than 100 mL to confirm adequate emptying. The condom catheter is useful in men with detrusor hyperreflexia but it caries an increased risk for UTI and the potential for penile skin breakdown. To obtain continence for a patient with detrusor hyperreflexia, anticholinergics sometimes can be used to the point of urinary retention and the patient can then perform IC.

If the patient is performing clean IC target volumes should be 400 to 500 mL. If the patient is unable to perform clean IC, then the use of an indwelling catheter, such as a Foley catheter, or suprapubic tube may be required. Complications can include bladder stones, hematuria, bacteremia, prostatitis, epididymitis, meatus erosions, penile and scrotal fistulas, urethral strictures, and bladder cancer in long-term use. To help reduce the risk of complications, patients should have the catheters changed every 2 to 4 weeks, consume at least 2 L a day of fluid, detrusor hyperreflexia should be controlled with anticholinergics, and the collecting bag should remain below the level of the bladder to prevent reflux or urine in the bladder. Bacterial colonization with an indwelling catheter or suprapubic tube does not need to be treated, unless there is an associated increase in the white blood cell count in the urine or the patient is febrile [10–12].

A recent Cochrane review looked at the effects of using different types of urinary catheters and external catheters in managing the neurogenic bladder, compared with alternative management strategies or interventions. Their conclusions were that despite a comprehensive search no evidence from randomized or quasi-randomized controlled trials was found. It was not possible to draw any conclusions regarding the use of different types of catheter in management of neurogenic bladder [36]. IC in the elderly population may be a difficult option to introduce. There are limited studies, but it has been demonstrated that older adults were able to learn IC with careful education and support. Many individuals may be uncomfortable with touching the urethra, however, and older women may be less likely to understand the anatomy of the female genitalia. Sterile or clean technique can be used and most individuals reuse catheters washed with soap and water and air-dried. If urethral irritation occurs, a single-use hydrophilic catheter is available that provides an evenly lubricated mucoid surface and can be more comfortable than a standard plastic catheter inserted with a water-soluble lubricant. The aging patient with neurogenic bladder may have difficulty with their IC program because of changes that occur in mobility and vision, and other techniques need to be explored, such as chronic indwelling catheter or suprapubic tube [37–40].

Even in patients with neurologic diseases, evaluation of reversible causes of urinary dysfunction needs to be explored and treated. Reversible causes of incontinence in the elderly can be remembered by the pneumonic "diapers" listed in Box 1. Medications that reduce detrusor activity (urinary retention) include anticholinergics; antidepressants (especially tricyclics); antiparkinsons; antipsychotics; β-adrenergic agents; calcium channel blocking agents; opioid analgesics; prostaglandins inhibitors; and sedatives. Medications that increase detrusor activity (urinary frequency) are β-blockers and diuretics. Psychologic disorders

---

Box 1. Reversible causes of incontinence in the elderly

Delirium or confusional state
Infections
Atrophic vaginitis or urethritis
Pharmaceuticals (especially long-acting agents)
Psychologic disorders
Endocrine disorders
Reduced mobility
Stool impaction

---

and chronic anxiety and learned voiding dysfunction can cause symptoms of overactive bladder. Cognition in the elderly can also be impaired by the use of narcotics, sedatives, and so forth, and by polypharmacy. Poor bowel habits and constipation can cause urinary symptoms and an appropriate bowel regimen is required. Impaired mobility in the elderly can be caused by a number of conditions, such as motor weakness, sensory loss, amputation, cardiopulmonary diseases, balance impairment, rigidity, painful conditions, or orthostatic hypotension that can interfere with toileting ability and precipitate urge incontinence. This can be treated with physical therapy, bedside commodes, urinals, or bedpans. Clothing should be easy to remove. Fluid intake can also affect the bladder with excess intake of caffeine, alcohol, and polydipsia leading to polyuria and urinary frequency. Hyperglycemia and hypercalcemia can lead to increased nocturia and polyuria and should be investigated. Congestive heart failure and venous insufficiency can cause volume overload and can contribute to urinary frequency and nocturia when the patient is supine. This can be treated with leg elevation, support hose, salt restriction, and proper timing of diuretics. Desmopressin diacetate arginine vasopressin has been used for nocturia, but its benefit in the elderly patient may be outweighed by the risk of hyponatremia [17,39–44].

For an elderly patient with a neurourologic disease (without spinal cord involvement) it is usually sufficient to evaluate only the lower tracts. The first step in the work-up includes postvoid residual measurement, urinalysis and urine culture, and a frequency volume chart. If the urologic status cannot be managed by these simple tests the next step is an urodynamic study. For atypical symptoms consider the addition of ordering as the clinical picture dictates urine cytology; cystoscopy; ultrasound; intravenous pyelogram; 24-hour urine creatinine clearance; and radiograph of the kidney, ureters, and bladder. If there is spinal cord involvement, the upper tracts in addition to the lower tracts need a yearly evaluation in the first 5 to 10 years and then if stable every other year. Patients with a chronic indwelling suprapubic or Foley catheter should have yearly cystoscopy to rule out stones or bladder tumors [18,44,45]. Box 2 lists organizations clinicians can refer patients to for voiding disorders.

Box 2. Organizations for voiding disorders

National Association for Continence: 1-800-252-3337, http://www.nafc.org

Simon Foundation for Continence: 1-800-237-4666, http://www.simonfoundation.com

Let's Talk about Bladder Control for Women, from the National Institute of Diabetes and Digestive and Kidney Disease: 1-800-891-5388, http://www.niddk.nih.gov

Take Control Again, a new campaign on overactive bladder from the American Foundation for Urologic Disease: 1-877-846-3222, http://www.afud.org

---

Neurogenic bowel in the older adult

People with neurologic disease have a much higher risk of both constipation and fecal incontinence (FI) than the general population. Functional bowel complaints have been shown to diminish the quality of life and the feeling of well-being and cause social isolation. Common neurologic diseases with bowel dysfunction include dementia, stroke, multiple sclerosis, spinal cord injury, cauda equina injury, diabetes mellitus, and Parkinson's disease. There is a broad range of reported prevalence in the literature because of varying definitions used for FI and constipation and the selection of differing populations with a range of disabilities. There is often a fine line dividing constipation and incontinence; any management intended to reduce one may cause the other. Current bowel management is largely empirical with a limited research base and mostly based on clinical experience [46].

There are many age-related changes that occur in the bowel, but before one can understand the changes that occur with aging or the dysfunction that occurs with neurologic diseases, the physiology of the gastrointestinal (GI) tract should be explored (Fig. 2). Food is digested in the stomach and further processed in the small intestine, with absorption occurring in the small intestine and the proximal half of the colon. The colon is responsible for absorbing water, electrolytes, and short-chain fatty acid from the stool. Propagation through the colon takes >1 day in most individuals. The colon is essentially a closed tube that is bound proximally by the ileocecal valve and distally by the anal sphincter. Continence is maintained by the anal sphincters. The anal sphincter mechanism is composed of the internal anal sphincter, which is composed of smooth muscle arranged in an inner circular and outer longitudinal layers, and the external anal sphincter (EAS), comprised of striated, voluntary muscle. The puborectalis muscle also plays a role and the tone of the puborectalis muscle is responsible for maintaining the anorectal angle that is vital for continence. The internal anal sphincter is the major contributor of pressure in the anal canal at rest, whereas the EAS contracts

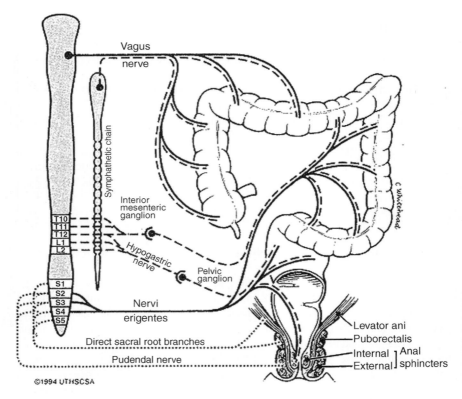

Fig. 2. Neurologic levels and pathways for the sympathetic, parasympathetic, and somatic nervous system innervation of the colon and anorectum. (*From* Cardenas DD, Mayo ME, King KC. Urinary tract and bowel management in the rehabilitation setting. In: Braddom RL, editor. Physical medicine and rehabilitation. Philadelphia: WB Saunders; 1996. p. 570.)

to retain stool if the rectum is rapidly dilated. The defecation process normally starts when stool is pushed into the rectum by peristalsis. The volume of stool stretches the puborectalis muscle and the rectal wall, stimulating the urge to defecate. Voluntary relaxation of the EAS and the puborectalis muscle straighten the anorecutm, allowing the passage of stool. Stool is pushed out with a combination of continued peristalsis and increased intra-abdominal pressure by the Valsalva maneuver. The function of the gut requires coordinated contraction between the two muscle layers with two basic types of movements: segmental contractions and high-pressure peristaltic waves. Segmental contractions impede propulsion to permit mixing and water absorption from colonic contents, whereas the high-pressure peristaltic waves produce movement toward the rectum. The peristaltic smooth muscle contractions are caused by the intrinsic innervation from the enteric nervous system [12,47].

The enteric nervous system of the GI tract is a collection of highly organized neurons in two primary layers: the myenteric or Auerbach's plexus and the submucosal or Meissner's plexus. The larger, myenteric (Auerbach's) plexus, lies between the longitudinal and circular layers of muscle and contains the neurons responsible for motility and for mediating the enzyme output of adjacent organs. The smaller, submucosal (Meissner's) plexus, is located in the submucosa between the circular muscle layer and the muscularis mucosa and contains sensory cells that communicate with the neurons of the myenteric plexus, and motor fibers that stimulate secretion from epithelial crypt cells into the gut lumen. The enteric neurons secrete a wide variety of neurotransmitters [48,49]. The colon and the pelvic floor muscles also receive input from the parasympathetic, sympathetic, and somatic nerve system. Normal colonic peristalsis and defecation occur under the combined autonomic and voluntary somatic control. The parasympathetic supply to the gut is from the vagus nerve and from the pelvic nerve (S2–S4). The vagus descends from the brainstem to innervate the distal two thirds of the esophagus and ends at the splenic flexure of the colon, whereas the lower GI tract is innervated by the pelvic nerve. The parasympathetic system inhibits the EAS and increases GI motility. Sympathetic innervation to the gut is from the mesenteric (T5–T12) and the hypogastric (T12–L3) nerves. Sympathetic stimulation relaxes the gut wall, ileocecal valve, and the internal anal sphincter. Somatic nerve supply is from the pudendal nerve (S2–S4) that supplies the EAS and the pelvic floor muscles [47]. Bowel reflexes include the holding reflex (EAS contracts to retain stool if the rectum is rapidly dilated); gastrocolic reflex (defecation after eating a meal caused by distention of the stomach stimulating evacuation of the colon); rectocolic reflex (stool can be stimulated to be released by digital stimulation either by inserting a lubricated finger in the rectum or by a suppository); and the recto-anal inhibitory reflex (stool approaching the internal sphincter causes it to relax while the EAS is voluntarily contracted to maintain continence) [11,12,47].

Constipation occurs commonly in persons 65 years and older. As a result, an estimated $400 million is spent on laxatives annually in the United States. In the elderly the transit time in the GI tract is increased. This leads to excessive water reabsorption that can lead to a dilated or enlarged colon, rectal fissures, and hemorrhoids. In addition, constipation can lead to serious complications, such as fecal impaction, FI, dilatation, and even perforation of the colon. Medication absorption is also affected with incomplete absorption of some medications and overabsorption of others. A decreased force and coordination of smooth muscle contraction in the colon is associated with aging. Other factors likely contributing to the development of constipation in elderly persons include chronic disease, medications, decreased mobility, dietary habits, and altered patterns of intake of fluids. Incontinence in the elderly can be attributed to numerous processes including local trauma (birth trauma, episiotomy, anorectal surgical procedure, or complete rectal prolapse); systemic diseases (eg, diabetes mellitus); neuronal disorders (pudendal nerve neuropathy and tumors or injury to the cauda equina); and progressive dementia, including Alzheimer's disease [50]. A bowel program for the older adult with a neurogenic bowel needs to be tailored to the patient. It is important to assess the level of disability and cognition because this might impair a bowel program. This includes the ability to learn or to direct others, sitting balance and tolerance, upper-extremity strength, fine motor skills and sensation, the degree of spasticity, transfer skills, and home accessibility and equipment needs [11,12,46,47]. Patients may need help from another person, adaptations to the home may be required to allow access to the toilet, and the use of a footstool while sitting on the toilet can facilitate evacuation by increasing the anorectal angle. Bowel programs developed for evacuation in the morning may help to prevent incontinence later in the day [46,47].

Lower motor neuron or an arelexic bowel is caused by lesions affecting the conus or cauda equina, injury to the pelvic nerves or the pudendal nerve, and so forth. This causes the descending colon wall to have a lower resting tone with no spinal cord–mediated reflex peristalsis. There is slow stool propulsion, with segmental colonic peristalsis coordinated by the myenteric plexus alone while water absorption continues. The EAS does not have reflex sphincter contraction, which increases the risk for incontinence. In addition, the pelvic floor laxity and decreased puborectalis tone contribute to a loss of the anorectal angle and the loss of the holding reflex. The EAS, which is normally puckered, becomes flattened or scalloped. Lower motor neuron impairment is manifested by reduced or absent rectal tone [46,47,51,52].

For lesions between the pons and above the conus, an upper motor neuron or a hyperreflexic bowel occurs. The EAS cannot be voluntary relaxed and the pelvic floor muscles become spastic. The nerve connections between the spinal cord and the colon and the myenteric plexus remain intact, however, and the stool can be propelled by reflex activity. Upper motor neuron lesion manifests as underactive propulsive peristalsis, overactive segmental peristalsis, or rectal distention [52–54]. Supraspinal bowel dysfunction can also occur because voluntary defecation depends on an accurate perception of the need to evacuate and the required motor function to reach the bathroom [47].

Neurogenic bowel with constipation and potential exacerbating factors

Poor dietary and behavioral habits

The elderly may especially have poor eating habits that can worsen the symptoms of a neurogenic bowel. Dietary review reveals that most of these patients do not consume adequate fiber and fluids. Ingestion of 10 to 12 g of fiber per day is useful. At least one or two glasses of fluid should be taken with meals. A diet high in fiber-containing foods, such as wheat bran, fruits, and vegetables (eg, beans, lentils, peas, and squash), retains water thereby softening the stool and fecal bulk is increased. Patients may complain of bloating, abdominal distention, and flatulence when beginning fiber supplements. These symptoms can be minimized by starting with a low dose of fiber and gradually increasing [54,55].

Structural abnormalities

Patients with a neurogenic bowel should have regular stool guaics and colonoscopy when they are past the age of 50. A sudden change in bowel habit or rectal bleeding also warrants investigations. Other causes of constipation include painful anal conditions (eg, hemorrhoids, anal fissure); rectocele; intussusception or rectal prolapse; diverticulitis; and bowel ischemia [50].

Systemic diseases

In addition to their neurologic dysfunction, the elderly are also at increased risk for endocrine and electrolyte abnormalities, such as diabetes, hypercalcemia, hypothyroidism, or hypokalemia. Hypothyroidism can cause hypomotility and slow transit in the gut. Congestive heart failure may cause bowel edema or the use of diuretics that may lead to electrolyte disorders. The autonomic or sensory neuropathies associated with diabetes can predispose to the development of constipation. Metabolic disturbances, such as hypercalcemia and hypokalemia, can affect smooth muscle function, and metabolic diseases, such as hyperparathyroidism and Addison's disease, can also affect bowel function [50,54].

Medications

Medications that can cause constipation are opioid medications, anticholinergic medications, calcium-channel blockers, iron, antidepressants, antiparkinsonian medications, aluminum antacids, and calcium products [54–57].

A recent Cochrane review concludes that it is not possible to draw any recommendation for bowel care in people with neurologic diseases from the current literature. Bowel management for these people must remain empirical until well-designed controlled trials with adequate numbers and clinically relevant outcome measures become available [46].

Medications and the bowel program

The four main categories of medications are stool softeners, colonic stimulants, contact irritants, and bulk formers (Table 1). An example of a stool softener is docusate sodium, which emulsifies fat in the GI tract and leads to stool softening. Senna tablets are colonic stimulants that stimulate Auerbach's plexus to induce peristalsis. Bisacodyl tablets and suppositories act as contact irritants in the mucosa of the colon and produce peristalsis. Psyllium is a type of bulk former. A bowel care regimen should be maintained for at least 3 to 5 days before considering possible modifications. A typical bowel program for a neurogenic bowel with constipation may consist of the daily use of a stool softener three times per day with two senna tablets and a bisacodyl enema daily or every other day (usually required only for patients with spinal cord involvement). The times that the senna and enema should be given depends on the time of day the bowel movement is desired. If a morning bowel program is desired, the senna tablets should be given at night and the enema in the morning; if a nighttime regimen is desired, then the senna tablets should be taken in the morning and the enema at night. It should be noted that for an areflexic bowel a chemical stimulant is needed to produce a bowel movement. Medication and diet are needed to produce a soft, formed stool that can be evacuated with rectal stimulation. Firm,

Table 1
Types of medication used in bowel care

Medication	Dosages
Stool softeners	
Docusate sodium	100 mg one–three times a day
Mineral oil	15–45 mL once or twice daily
Fiber laxatives	
Psyllium	1 tsp once or twice daily
Methylcellulose	1 tsp once or twice daily
Calcium polycarbophil	1 or 2 tablets once or twice daily
Osmotic laxatives	
Magnesium salts	15–30 mL once or twice a day
Lactulose or 70% sorbitol	15–60 mL one to three times a day
Polyethylene glycol	17 g in 8 oz of water once or twice a day
Stimulant laxative	
Bisacodyl	5–15 mg orally or 10 mg per rectum
Cascara	4–8 mL or 2 tablets as needed
Senna	1–2 tablets orally
Glycerin suppositories	
Enemas	
Tap water	
Phosphate enema	
Soapsuds enema	
Mineral oil enema	
Enemeez	

formed stool allows the stool to be retained between bowel regimens and to be manually evacuated easily. The stimulant (eg, a glycerin suppository or a mini enema) is placed into the rectum with the patient in the upright or left lateral decubitus position, and digital stimulation is performed until evacuation. Digital stimulation increases peristalsis and relaxes the EAS. It is performed by inserting a gloved, lubricated finger into the rectum and slowly rotating the finger in a circular movement. Other assistive techniques, such as the Valsalva maneuver, push-ups, abdominal massage, or leaning forward, may also be used. The Valsalva maneuver should not be used in patients with a cardiac condition [11,12,47,53].

Even in a neurogenic bowel, changes in fecal continence or diarrheal-like stool should be explored for other causes. A total of 90% of the deaths from acute diarrheal diseases occur in the elderly. Infectious diarrheas, especially *Clostridium difficile* infection, may cause symptoms from the chronic use of antibiotics used to treat multiple UTI in this population and from the relatively reduced cell-mediated immunity in old age. Diarrhea in older patients is also commonly caused by medications, such as antimicrobials, magnesium-containing antacids, digitalis, quinidine, hydralazine, methyldopa, propranolol, guanethidine, indomethacin, cholinergic agents, colchicine, theophylline, and cholestyramine. Diarrhea can also be caused by diabetes, disaccharidase deficiencies, caffeine, artificial sweeteners, spicy foods, fruit juices, fatty food, or enteral feedings. An underlying malnutrition may also be contributing to diarrhea because of gut wall edema and malabsorption. To avoid bowel incontinence, the bowel needs to be cleared of stool regularly, patients should avoid increased abdominal pressure, and wearing tight undergarments may help retain stool by supporting the pelvic floor [58–60].

There is little known about which outcomes of bowel controls are important goals for the aging adult with FI or their caregivers. A bowel symptom questionnaire has been developed for older people, but its use as an outcome measure for research and practice has not been reported. A start has been made in defining symptoms and quality of life issues of adults with FI, but an examination of their relevance to an older or frail population is needed [61–63].

Fecal impaction is the presence of hard stools in the rectum, oozing of liquid stools without the passing of fecal mass, and the absence of a bowel movement for over 3 days. Clinical presentation includes decreased appetite, nausea and vomiting, and abdominal pain and distention. There may be paradoxical "diarrhea" as liquid stool leaks around the impacted feces. Firm feces are palpable on digital examination of the rectal vault. Initial treatment is directed at relieving the impaction with enemas (saline or mineral oil) or digital disruption of the impacted fecal material. Fecal impaction is much more common in the elderly and in the patient with a neurogenic bowel, so a high index of suspicion is needed to avoid complications [47].

Biofeedback has been used to treat FI in people with some rectal sensation and voluntary anal sphincter contraction [64]. When no satisfactory answers to leakage are found, pads or anal plugs might be necessary.

Bowel habit training and toileting programs

Unlike the literature on UI, there have been virtually no reports of bowel retraining or toileting programs for FI. There is no report of urge resistance training or deferment of defecation for people with urgency, the most common precursor to episodes of FI. Investigators of one study designed to address UI using a prompted voiding program made an incidental finding that, although actual episodes of FI were not reduced, bowel frequency increased and so did the proportion of stools passed continently in the toilet. They concluded, unsurprisingly, that increasing opportunities to use the toilet increases bowel frequency and continence. Only one study has ever addressed the role of muscle exercises and biofeedback in an older population. Seventy-seven percent of elders who failed to show an improvement in FI frequency using sphincter exercises alone had a 75% decrease after biofeedback training. There is good evidence from clinical series that biofeedback and exercises may be effective in the general adult population, but evidence from randomized controlled studies is scarce for all age groups. Recent studies revealed there was no adjunctive benefit of using biofeedback over digital guidance for pelvic floor retraining and similar bowel continence outcomes were achieved with or without pelvic floor muscle exercises. The role of electrical stimulation of the external sphincter muscle on continence enhancement is unanswered in all age groups [65].

Box 3. For further support for patients the clinician can refer their patients to the following sites

1. American Gastroenterological Association
   National Office
   4930 Del Ray Avenue
   Bethesda, MD 20814
   Phone: 301–654–2055
   Fax: 301–652–3890
   E-mail address: webinfo@gastro.org
   Internet: www.gastro.org
2. International Foundation for Functional Gastrointestinal Disorders
   PO Box 170864
   Milwaukee, WI 53217
   Phone: 1–888–964–2001 or 414–964–1799
   Fax: 414–964–7176
   E-mail address: iffgd@iffgd.org
   Internet: www.iffgd.org
3. National Digestive Diseases Information Clearinghouse
   2 Information Way
   Bethesda, MD 20892–3570
   Phone: 1–800–891–5389
   Fax: 703–738–4929
   E-mail address: nddic@info.niddk.nih.gov
4. Digestive Disease National Coalition
   507 Capitol Court NE, Suite 200
   Washington, DC 20002
   Phone: 202–544–7497
   Fax: 202–546–7105
5. The Simon Foundation for Continence
   PO Box 815
   Wilmette, IL 60091
   Phone: 1–800–23–SIMON or 847–864–3913
   Fax: 847–864–9758
   Internet: www.simonfoundation.org
6. National Association for Continence (NAFC)
   (formerly Help for Incontinent People [HIP])
   PO Box 1019
   Charleston, SC 29402–1019
   Phone: 1–800–BLADDER or 843–377–0900
   Fax: 843–377–0905
   E-mail address: memberservices@nafc.org
   Internet: www.nafc.org

Surgical options for neurogenic bowel

Surgery is rarely required in the elderly neurogenic bowel but is an option if there is a lack of response to conservative treatments or for severely disabled patients, in whom surgical options can markedly improve quality of life. In patients in whom the delay in transit can be demonstrated to be in the distal large bowel a colostomy can be performed. If transit is slow throughout the whole colon, then an ileostomy may be preferable. The time spent in bowel care has been reported to decrease from 11 hours to 4 hours per week with ostomies, and FI is prevented. Other surgical options include the placement of a stoma; anal sphincter repair; post anal repair (puborectalis muscle is sutured to decrease the anorectal angle and the length of the anal canal is increased); dynamic graciloplasty; sacral nerve stimulation; and artificial bowel sphincter. Another surgical option mostly used in children with spina bifida is the Malone procedure. This involves bringing out the appendix or a neoappendix created from the cecum to the abdominal wall creating a stoma to use as a channel for antegrade colonic irrigation. Few studies have evaluated adults with neurogenic bowel and those adults who were studied were not in the geriatric population [47,66,67].

There is still much more to learn about the neurogenic bowel at any age. A recent Cochrane review concluded that there is not enough evidence on which to judge the benefits and disadvantages of any bowel program in people with neurologic diseases. Although there is considerable literature on the causes of bowel dysfunction in people with neurologic diseases, there are few studies that focus on the practical management. Recommendations for a bowel program are based on the personal experience of professionals rather than on findings from well-designed studies There is a need for well-designed randomized controlled trials to assess the effects of fiber intake, use of laxatives, rectal stimulants (suppository), and facilitative techniques (abdominal massage, Valsalva) for neurologic diseases and evaluating the quality of life, cost analysis, the methods for teaching bowel management, and the effects of aging with a neurogenic bowel.

Box 3 lists organizations to which clinicians can refer patients with bowel disorders.

References

[1] Abrams P, Kelleher CJ, Kerr LA, et al. Overactive bladder significantly affects quality of life. Am J Manag Care 2000;6:S580–90.
[2] Wilson L, Brown JS, Shin GP, et al. Annual direct cost of urinary incontinence. Obstet Gynecol 2001;98:398–406.
[3] Roe B, Doll H, Wilson K. Help seeking behaviour and health and social services utilisation by people suffering from urinary incontinence. Int J Nurs Stud 1999;36:245–53.
[4] Wagner TH, Hu T-W. Economic costs of urinary incontinence in 1995. Urology 1998;51:355–61.
[5] Burgio KL, Ives DG, Locher JL, et al. Treatment seeking for urinary incontinence in older adults. J Am Geriatr Soc 1994;42:208–12.

[6] Thom D. Variation in estimates of urinary incontinence prevalence in the community: effects of differences in definition, population characteristics, and study type. J Am Geriatr Soc 1998;46: 473–80.

[7] Goldstein M, Hawthorne ME, Engeberg S, et al. Urinary incontinence: why people do not seek help. J Geron Nurs 1992;18:15–20.

[8] Cassells C, Watt E. The impact of incontinence on older spousal caregivers. J Adv Nurs 2003; 42:607–16.

[9] Hunskaar S, Burgio K, Diokno A, et al. Epidemiology and natural history of urinary incontinence in women. Urology 2003;62(Suppl. 1):16–23.

[10] Tan J. Voiding dysfunctions. In: Tan J, editor. Practical manual of physical medicine and rehabilitation. St Louis: Mosby; 1998. p. 538–52.

[11] Linsenmeyer TA, Stone JM. Neurogenic bladder and bowel. In: Delisa JA, Gans BM, editors. Rehabilitation medicine: principle and practice. 3rd edition. Philadelphia: JB Lippincott; 1998. p. 1073–93.

[12] Cardenas DD, Mayo ME, King KC. Urinary tract and bowel management in the rehabilitation setting. In: Braddom RL, editor. Physical medicine and rehabilitation. Philadelphia: WB Saunders; 1996. p. 555–79.

[13] Thor KB. Targeting serotonin and norepinephrine receptors in stress urinary incontinence. Int J Gynaecol Obstet 2004;86(Suppl 1):S38–52.

[14] Wagg A, Malone-Lee J. The management of urinary incontinence in the elderly. Br J Urol 1998; 82:11–7.

[15] Miller M. Nocturnal polyuria in older people. J Am Geriatr Soc 2000;48:1321–9.

[16] Elbadawi A, Diokno A, Millard R. The aging bladder: morphology and urodynamics. World J Urol 1998;16:S10–34.

[17] Fantl JA, Newman DK, Colling J, et al. Urinary incontinence in adults: acute and chronic management. Clinical practice guideline No. 2, 1996 update. Rockville: Agency for Health Care Policy and Research; 1996.

[18] Rivas DA, Ditunno JF. The management of neurogenic bladder and sexual dysfunction after spinal cord injury. Spine 2001;26:S129–36.

[19] Aslan AR, Kogan BA. Conservative management in neurogenic bladder dysfunction. Curr Opin Urol 2002;12:473–7.

[20] Resnick M, Yalla SV. Management of urinary incontinence in the elderly. N Engl J Med 1985; 313:800–5.

[21] Ouslander JG, Schnelle JF, Uman G, et al. Predictors of successful prompted voiding among incontinent nursing home residents. JAMA 1995;273:1366–70.

[22] Wallace SA, Roe B, Williams K, et al. Bladder training for urinary incontinence in adults. Cochrane Database Syst Rev 2004;1:CD001138.

[23] Weiss BD. Selecting medications for the treatment of urinary incontinence. Am Fam Physician 2005;71:315–22.

[24] Giannitsas K, Perimenis P, Athanasopoulos A, et al. Comparison of the efficacy of tolterodine and oxybutynin in different urodynamic severity grades of idiopathic detrusor overactivity. Eur Urol 2004;46:776–82 [discussion: 782–3].

[25] Rovner ES. Trospium chloride in the management of overactive bladder. Drugs 2004;64:2433–46.

[26] Kershen RT, Hsieh M. Preview of new drugs for overactive bladder and incontinence: darifenacin, solifenacin, trospium, and duloxetine. Curr Urol Rep 2004;5:359–67.

[27] Schurch B, Stohrer M, Kramer G. Botulinum A toxin for treating detrusor hyperreflexia in spinal cord injured patients: a new alternative to anticholinergic drugs? J Urol 2000;164:692–7.

[28] Flynn MK, Webster GD, Amundsen CL. The effect of botulinum-A toxin on patients with severe urge urinary incontinence. J Urol 2004;172:2316–20.

[29] Chancellor M, deGroat W. Intravesical capsaicin and resiniferatoxin therapy: spicing up the ways to treat overactive bladder. J Urol 1999;162:3–11.

[30] Norton PA, Zinner NR, Yalcin I, et al. Duloxetine versus placebo in the treatment of stress urinary incontinence. Am J Obstet Gynecol 2002;187:40–8.

[31] Madersbacher H. Neurogenic bladder dysfunction. Curr Opin Urol 1999;9:303–7.

[32] DeLancey JOL. The pathophysiology of stress urinary incontinence in women and its implications for surgical treatment. World J Urol 1997;15:268–74.

[33] The American Urological Association Female Stress Urinary Incontinence Clinical Guidelines Panel. The surgical management of female stress urinary incontinence. Clinical Practice Guidelines. Baltimore: American Urological Association; 1997.

[34] Ruud Bosch J, Groen J. Sacral nerve neuromodulation in the treatment of refractory motor urge incontinence. Curr Opin Urol 2001;11:399–403.

[35] Chartier-Kastler EJ, Bosch JLHR, Perrigot M. Long term results of sacral nerve stimulation for the treatment of neurogenic refractory urge incontinence related to detrusor hyperreflexia. J Urol 2000;164:1476–80.

[36] Jamison J, Maguire S, McCann J. Catheter policies for management of long term voiding problems in adults with neurogenic bladder disorders. Cochrane Database Syst Rev 2004; 2:CD004375.

[37] Bennett CJ, Diokno AC. Clean intermittent self-catheterization in the elderly. Urology 1984; 24:43–5.

[38] Prashar S, Simons A, Bryant C, et al. Attitudes to vaginal/urethral touching and device placement in women with urinary incontinence. Int Urogynecol J Pelvic Floor Dysfunct 2000; 11:4–8.

[39] Goode PS, Burgio KL. Pharmacological treatment of lower urinary tract dysfunction in geriatric patients. Am J Med Sci 1997;314:262–7.

[40] Jamison J, Maguire S, McCann J. Catheter policies for management of long term voiding problems in adults with neurogenic bladder disorders. Cochrane Database Syst Rev 2004; 2:CD004375.

[41] Ouslander JG, Johnson II TM. Continence care for frail older adults: it is time to go beyond assessing quality. J Am Med Dir Assoc 2004;5:213–6.

[42] Ouslander JG. Management of overactive bladder. N Engl J Med 2004;350:786–99.

[43] Wagg A, Cohen M. Medical therapy for the overactive bladder in the elderly. Age Ageing 2002;31:241–6.

[44] Tannenbaum C, Perrin L, DuBeau C, et al. Diagnosis and management of urinary incontinence in the older patient. Arch Phys Med Rehabil 2001;82:134–8.

[45] Scientific Committee of the First International Consultation on Incontinence. Assessment and treatment of urinary incontinence. Lancet 2000;355:2153–8.

[46] Coggrave M, Wiesel PH, Norton C, et al. Management of faecal incontinence and constipation in adults with central neurological diseases. Cochrane Database Syst Rev 2005;1:CD002115.

[47] Tan J. Bowel dysfunction. In: Tan J, editor. Practical manual of physical medicine and rehabilitation. St Louis: Mosby; 1998. p. 553–79.

[48] Gershon MD. The enteric nervous system: a second brain. Hosp Pract (Off Ed) 1999;34:31–2, 35–8, 41–2.

[49] Goyal RK, Hirano I. The enteric nervous system. N Engl J Med 1996;334:1106–15.

[50] Romero Y, Evans J, Fleming K, et al. Constipation and fecal incontinence in the elderly population. Mayo Clin Proc 1996;71:81–92.

[51] Stiens SA, Bergman SB, Goetz LL. Neurogenic bowel dysfunction after spinal cord injury: clinical evaluation and rehabilitative management. Arch Phys Med Rehabil 1997;78:S86–102.

[52] Benevento BT, Sipski ML. Neurogenic bladder, neurogenic bowel, and sexual dysfunction in people with spinal cord injury. Phys Ther 2002;82(6):601–12.

[53] Consortium for Spinal Cord Medicine. Neurogenic bowel: what you should know. Washington: Paralyzed Veterans of America; 1999.

[54] Camilleri M, Bharucha AE. Gastrointestinal dysfunction in neurologic disease. Semin Neurol 1996;16:203–16.

[55] Lembo A, Camilleri M, et al. Chronic constipation. N Engl J Med 2003;349:1360–8.

[56] Odegard PS, Burke C. Management of opioid-induced constipation in the elderly patient. Consult Pharm 1996;11(Suppl C):17–22.

[57] Schiller LR. Constipation and fecal incontinence in the elderly. Gastroenterol Clin North Am 2001;30:497–515.

[58] Schiller LR. Fecal incontinence. Clin Gastroenterol 1986;15:687–704.

[59] Bliss DZ, Fischer LR, Savik K. Self-care practices for managing fecal incontinence by elders at managed care clinics. Gerontologist 2001;41:188.

[60] Bliss DZ, McLaughlin J, Jung HJ, et al. Comparison of the nutritional composition of diets of persons with fecal incontinence and that of age- and gender-matched controls. J Wound Ostomy Continence Nurs 2000;27:90–7.

[61] O'Keefe EA, Talley NJ, Tangalos EG, et al. A bowel symptom questionnaire for the elderly. J Gerontol 1992;47:M116–21.

[62] Bugg GJ, Kiff ES, Hosker G. A new condition-specific health-related quality of life questionnaire for the assessment of women with anal incontinence. Br J Obstet Gynaecol 2001;108:1057–67.

[63] Rockwood TH, Church JM, Fleshman JW, et al. Fecal Incontinence Quality of Life Scale: quality of life instrument for patients with fecal incontinence. Dis Colon Rectum 2000;43:9–17.

[64] Norton C, Chelvanayagam S, Wilson-Barnett J, et al. Randomized controlled trial of biofeedback for fecal incontinence. Gastroenterology 2003;125:1320–9.

[65] Hosker G, Norton C, Brazzelli M. Electrical stimulation for faecal incontinence in adults (Cochrane Review). The Cochrane Library, Issue 3. Chichester, UK: John Wiley & Sons; 2004.

[66] Wiesel PH, Norton C, Glickman S, et al. Pathophysiology and management of bowel dysfunction in multiple sclerosis. Eur J Gastroenterol Hepatol 2001;13:441–8.

[67] Teichman JM, Harris JM, Currie DM, et al. Malone antegrade continence enema for adults with neurogenic bowel disease. J Urol 1998;160:1278–81.

ELSEVIER
SAUNDERS

Clin Geriatr Med 22 (2006) 331–354

CLINICS IN
GERIATRIC
MEDICINE

A Geriatrician's Guide to the Use of the Physical Modalities in the Treatment of Pain and Dysfunction

Danielle Marie Perret, MD[a], Josephine Rim, MD[b],
Adrian Cristian, MD[c],*

[a]*Department of Rehabilitation Medicine, The Mount Sinai Medical Center, 1425 Madison Avenue,
Box 1240, New York, NY 10029-6574, USA*
[b]*Department of Anesthesiology, The State University of New York Health Sciences Center at Brooklyn,
450 Clarkson Avenue, Box 6, Brooklyn, NY 11203-2098, USA*
[c]*Department of Rehabilitation Medicine, James J. Peters Veterans Affairs Medical Center,
Room 3D-16, Route #526-117, 130 West Kingsbridge Road, Bronx, NY 10468, USA*

Modalities are physical agents that are used to produce a therapeutic response in tissues. The major modalities used in common practice are heat, cryotherapy, and electrotherapy. The use of these physical forces to lessen pain and to speed healing is a centuries-old practice that is still appropriate today. Particularly in the spectrum of pain management, multimodal forms of therapy—including patient education, exercise, physical, occupational, and kinesiotherapy, the use of the physical modalities, and psychosocial, medical, pharmacologic, and surgical interventions—must supplement one another for maximum benefit to the patient [1]. In fact, the 1992 Agency for Health Care Policy and Research clinical practice guideline on pain management recommends both cognitive-behavioral approaches (patient education, simple relaxation, imagery, hypnosis, and biofeedback) and physical therapeutic agents and modalities (superficial heat, cold, massage, exercise, immobility, electro-analgesia) as essential in the management of acute pain [2]. Furthermore, various guidelines for the management of osteoarthritis, including those of the American College of Rheumatology [3], the European League Against Rheumatism [4], Algorithms for the Diagnosis and

* Corresponding author.
E-mail address: acristianmd@msn.com (A. Cristian).

0749-0690/06/$ – see front matter. Published by Elsevier Inc.
doi:10.1016/j.cger.2005.12.005

geriatric.theclinics.com

Management of Musculoskeletal Complaints [5], and the Institute for Clinical Systems Improvement [6], feature recommendations for the use of heat, ice, and electrical stimulation.

In the elderly, the sole reliance on pharmacotherapy to manage pain and dysfunction has many disadvantages. With analgesic use, there is an increased incidence of anticholinergic side effects in the elderly, including glaucoma and urinary retention; dysrhythmias are also more common [7,8]. The elderly also have an increased sensitivity to the neurologic side effects of antiepileptics and benzodiazepines [7]. Commonly prescribed in the elderly for pain, nonsteroidal anti-inflammatory medications (NSAIDs) have gastrointestinal side effects, including dyspepsia, ulcers, perforation, bleeding, and liver dysfunction; bleeding especially may occur when the NSAID is coupled with daily aspirin or another anticoagulation that is commonly prescribed in the elderly [1]. Hypersensitivity reactions and central nervous system effects are also common [1]. Opiate derivatives, such as acetaminophen with codeine and oxycodone, cause side effects that are often prominent in the elderly. These include sedation, mental clouding, confusion, respiratory depression, nausea, vomiting, constipation, pruritus, and urinary retention [1]. The use of nonpharmacologic approaches to pain management, including the physical modalities, offers many advantages, especially in the geriatric patient. This approach can improve mood, reduce anxiety, increase a patient's sense of control, strengthen coping abilities, relax muscles, and improve attention to ergonomics, body mechanics, sleep, limb or joint function, and performance of activities of daily living, thus enhancing overall quality of life [1].

In the geriatric population, physical modalities, when prescribed with a therapy program, should be the cornerstone of treatment of pain and dysfunction, especially when the cause is a musculoskeletal condition. Because the elderly typically have multiple medical comorbidities and multiple foci of pain, conditions that would ordinarily not be a cause of dysfunction may have a cumulative effect and cause a patient to become severely disabled. In the context of spinal stenosis and osteoarthritis, an added insult such as a carpal tunnel syndrome may severely limit a patient. It might even precipitate a major functional breakdown [7].

This article introduces the reader to the major physical modalities, when they should be considered for use, and the contraindications or precautions for each. In the appendix, three clinical vignettes illustrate the use of the physical modalities in caring for a geriatric patient with shoulder, knee, and hand disabilities.

Prescription for a modality

The elements in the prescription for a modality should include indication or diagnosis, choice of modality, location, intensity, and duration and frequency specifications. Before selecting a modality, one must understand the physiologic effects each exerts on tissues. The target tissue, the depth and intensity of heat or cooling desired, and patient characteristics are all factors to consider when writing the prescription. The patient's body habitus (amount of adipose tissue), comorbid conditions (eg, cancer, neuropathy, peripheral vascular disease), implants (eg, pacemaker, metallic implants), age, and sex (during pregnancy) should all be considered in the equation. Sample modality prescriptions are included in the Appendix.

Especially in the elderly, the use of modalities is not without limitations. Careful attention must be paid to reduced mental status, circulatory impairment, local malignancy, or sensory impairment. Temperature sensation in the elderly has been shown to be reduced [9], so the elderly may be particularly susceptible to burns. Coronary artery disease or congestive heart failure may be aggravated by the increases in cardiovascular demand and cardiac output that heating modalities may cause. In a patient who has vascular compromise, heat may precipitate gangrene and subsequent limb loss. Even body temperature may be dangerous enough to cause a burn, especially in the patient with peripheral vascular disease. Deep-heat diathermy modalities may cause increased heating of metal sutures, clips, pacemakers, and artificial joints, resulting in local tissue damage that may be catastrophic. Necrosis and gangrene may result from cold modality treatments in patients with dysproteinemia. Cold therapy should be avoided with cold intolerance or hypersensitivity, arterial insufficiency, impaired sensation or cognition, and cryopathies such as Raynaud's disease—all of which are commonplace in the geriatric patient [10]. Electrotherapy should be avoided near cardiac pacemakers or defibrillators, over the carotid sinuses, and when patients cannot report the effects. For a summary of the indications, precautions, and contraindications to the major physical modalities, please refer to Tables 1, 2, and 3.

The physician should remember that patient education is always paramount to success when using the physical modalities. The patient should be taught that heat alone will most likely not provide long-term or long-lasting relief of pain. Greater and longer-lasting relief of pain and stiffness and overall im-

Table 1
Uses of, precautions for, and contraindications to thermal therapy

Uses	Precautions and contraindications
General: musculoskeletal conditions (tendonitis, tenosynovitis, bursitis, capsulitis), pain (neck, low back, myofascial, postherpetic neuralgia), arthritis, contractures, muscle relaxation, chronic inflammation	General: acute trauma, inflammation, impaired circulation, bleeding diatheses, edema, large scars, impaired sensation, malignancy, cognitive or communication deficits that preclude reporting of pain
Superficial heat to heat joints	The thermal pain threshold is 45°C.
Deep heat to large joints, tissue contractures, chronic phase of injury, or disease states	Superficial heat: circulatory impairment, poor sensation, obtundment, sedation
Hydrotherapy for joint contractures, stiffness, systemic or local arthritis, soft tissue lesions, large areas of limbs, trunks (ie, sprains, strains, burns, postoperative pain, stiffness, chronic ulcers)	Deep heat: local malignancy, bleeding diathesis, metal implants, postlaminectomy, obtundment, sedation, poor sensation
	Hydrotherapy: poor cardiac function, adrenal insufficiency, poor sensation, obtundment, sedation

Table 2
Uses of, precautions for, and contraindications to cryotherapy

Uses	Precautions and contraindications
Initial management of acute musculoskeletal and soft tissue injuries, including strains and sprains	Cold intolerance
Spasticity management	Cryotherapy-induced neuropraxia/axonotmesis
Myofascial pain syndrome	Arterial insufficiency
Postoperative pain	Impaired sensation
Tendonitis, bursitis, trigger points, tenosynovitis, capsulitis	Cognitive or communication deficits that preclude reporting of pain
Emergent treatment of minor burns	Cryopathies
	Cryoglobulinemia
	Paroxysmal cold hemoglobinuria
	Cold hypersensitivity
	Raynaud's disease/phenomenon

provement in function will occur when, for example, heat is used in conjunction with an exercise program.

Superficial heating modalities

Heat has been used for centuries to provide relief of pain, to reduce muscle spasticity, and to promote the feeling of tranquility. Heat is known to have several physiologic effects on tissue, including hemodynamic, neuromuscular, and joint and connective tissue effects. It also decreases pain and provides a sense of general relaxation. The physiologic effects of heat are summarized in Table 4. Heat can increase acute inflammation and edema but decreases chronic inflammation [11,12]. It decreases joint stiffness and provides analgesia [13,14]. The analgesic effect of heat may be explained by a cutaneous counterirritant effect, by vasodilation wash-out of pain mediators, by the release of endogenous endorphins, and by the "gate theory" of pain modulation. In the gate theory, the transmission of pain via small unmyelinated nerve fibers is blocked at the level of the spinal cord by the stimulation of large myelinated afferent fibers whose impulses arrive at the "gate" more quickly and block out the unmyelinated fiber impulses. An afferent thermal signal inhibits the transmission of nociceptive

Table 3
Uses of, precautions for, and contraindications to electrotherapy

Uses	Precautions and contraindictions
Musculoskeletal pain	Avoid stimulation over the carotid sinuses.
Posttraumatic pain	Cardiac pacemakers or implanted cardiac defibrillators
Postsurgical pain	Pregnancy
Peripheral nerve injury	Inability to report effects or discomfort
Peripheral neuropathy	Atrophic skin
Phantom limb pain	Allergy to electrodes or gels
Sympathetically mediated pain	Avoid extremities with an intravenous Line.
Total joint arthroplasty	

Table 4
Physiologic effects of heat

Hemodynamic effects of heat	Increased blood flow
	Decreased chronic inflammation
	Increased acute inflammation
	Increased edema
	Increased bleeding
Neuromuscular effects of heat	Increased group Ia fiber firing rates (muscle spindle)
	Decreased group II fiber firing rates (muscle spindle)
	Increased group Ib fiber firing rates (Golgi tendon organ)
	Increased nerve conduction velocity
Joint and connective tissue effects of heat	Increased tendon extensibility
	Increased collagenase activity
	Decreased joint stiffness
Other physiologic effects of heat	Decreased pain
	Cutaneous counterirritant effect
	Endorphin-mediated response
	Vasodilation washing out pain mediators
	Alteration of nerve conduction
	Alteration of cell permeability
	General relaxation

signals through the spinal cord to higher centers and the consequent recognition of pain [15,16]. Heat also alters nerve conduction and cell permeability. Secondary effects on the Golgi tendon apparatus and local muscle spindles translate into muscular relaxation [17], greater tendon extensibility [18], and increased collagenase activity [19]. These features make the thermal modalities useful in the treatment of contractures and the arthritides. Heat should generally be avoided in the treatment of acute conditions, because it can exacerbate edema [12].

Heating modalities may be classified as superficial or deep heat. Table 5 summarizes the heating modalities in these classifications. In general, moist heat penetrates more deeply into the underlying tissue [20]. Dry heat is known to cause a greater elevation in surface temperature [20]. Superficial heating agents (eg, heat lamps, hot packs, paraffin, fluidotherapy, hydrotherapy) heat the skin and subcutaneous fat (perhaps therapeutically cooling deeper tissues) and are applied for 15 to 20 minutes at temperatures of 40°C to 45.5°C (104°F to 113.9°F). Superficial heat may also affect underlying tissues via reflex pathways.

Table 5
Types of thermal therapy

Modality	Depth
Hot packs and heating pads	Superficial
Paraffin baths	Superficial
Fluidotherapy	Superficial
Whirlpool baths	Superficial
Radiant heat	Superficial
Ultrasound	Deep
Shortwave diathermy	Deep
Microwave	Deep

Some evidence suggests that optimal biophysical effects (eg, muscle length-ening) may require intramuscular temperatures of at least 40°C, which necessitate at least a 3°C to 4°C increase in surface temperature [21]. This process may require continuous topical heat application at low levels for 8 hours or more [15], comparable to continuous transcutaneous electrical nerve stimulation application. In one study, low-level heat worn directly on the skin for 8 hours per day in ambulatory patients was randomized against ibuprofen and acetaminophen in the treatment of acute, nonspecific low back pain [22]. Heat wrap was shown to provide significantly better pain relief on Day 1 and extended pain relief on Days 3 and 4 [22]. Another study compared overnight heat use with ibuprofen and placebo and proved statistical significance over placebo for morning pain relief (Days 2 to 4), daytime pain relief (Days 2 to 4), and extended pain relief (Days 4 to 5) [23]. Furthermore, heat-wrap therapy considerably reduced morning muscle stiffness (Day 4), increased lateral trunk flexibility (Day 4), and decreased low back disability (Day 4) [23]. The positive effect of heat therapy persisted for more than 48 hours after treatment was discontinued [23]; this may be a unique feature of continuous heat application.

Other clinical trials have generally shown that superficial heat provides pain relief. In patients who have myofascial pain with at least one trigger point, su-perficial heat increased the pressure pain threshold over approximately 50% of trigger points immediately after treatment [24]. An increase in the pressure pain threshold has also been noted in patients who have temporomandibular joint dysfunction [25]. When whirlpool or paraffin baths were applied, alone or with exercise, all study groups showed significant pain relief [26]. In a study involving patients who had Colles' fractures and comparing warm whirlpool baths with exercise versus exercise alone, however, both groups had significantly increased range of motion and decreased pain [27]. When superficial heat is compared with cryotherapy, no difference between groups is observed [28,29], indicating that both modalities may be good adjunctive treatments.

Superficial heat is useful for osteoarthritis, rheumatoid arthritis, neck pain, low back pain, and other muscular syndromes. No particular superficial heating agent is considered more beneficial than others.

Hot packs

Hot packs, such as the commercially available Hydrocollator packs (Chatta-nooga Group, Hixson, Tennessee), are a commonly prescribed superficial heating modality. The packs are bags filled with silicon dioxide sand that can absorb many times its weight in water. Their temperature is maintained in water baths between 70°C and 80°C (168°C to 175°F). When used, the packs are drained of excess water, wrapped in several layers of insulating towels, and laid on—never under—the body (compression under the body greatly increases the risk of burn). The application time is 15 to 20 minutes, and the therapeutic temperature is maintained for 20 to 30 minutes. Studies document a 3.3°C temperature rise at 1 cm depth and a 1.3°C temperature rise at 3 cm depth in the posterior thigh after a 30-minute application of a Hydrocollator pack [30].

Heating pads

Heating pads are also commonly prescribed. These may be electric or composed of a circulating fluid. Both reach peak temperatures of 52°C (125°F) but may have wide (5°C) temperature fluctuations [31]. As in application of hot packs, because of the potential for burn, the patient should not lie on the pad. Heating pads may present a greater risk for electric shock, especially when moist toweling is used [32].

Heating lamps

Heating lamps are less commonly used superficial heating modalities. Some use special infrared heat sources, whereas others use standard incandescent light as a source of heat, which is produced by molecular vibration [33]. The heating effectiveness decreases with the square of the distance between the lamp and the patient. Most clinic lamps use 100- to 150-W incandescent lights placed 50 to 75 cm away from the patient. The patient should be warned that the heat could produce a reddish or brownish skin mottling. A 1.3°C temperature rise has been documented at depths of 2 cm [30]. Radiant heat is often preferred in patients who cannot tolerate the weight of the hot packs. Skin drying and dermal photo-aging are significant disadvantages [13,33]. One of the great benefits of radiant heat is that it permits direct observation of the area being treated.

Fluidotherapy

Fluidotherapy (Fig. 1) is a popular dry-heat superficial heating modality that employs forced hot air to circulate a bed of finely divided solid particles

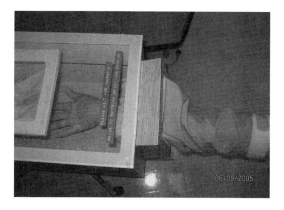

Fig. 1. Fluidotherapy.

(generally composed of corn husk) [34]. Both the temperature and agitation level may be controlled. The temperature used ranges from 46.1°C to 48.9°C (115°F to 120°F) with application for 15 to 20 minutes. Hand muscle and joint capsule may be heated to 42°C (107.6°F); foot muscle and joint capsule may be heated to 39.5°C (103.1°F) after a 20-minute application at 47.8°C (118°F) [34]. Some physicians even consider superficial heating modality treatments to the hands and feet effectively to be deep heating modalities, because of the paucity of subcutaneous tissues. A great benefit of fluidotherapy is the patient's freedom to perform range-of-motion exercises during the heat application [35]. General heat precautions should be followed; infected wounds can cause cross-contamination in such a setting, and use in their presence should be avoided [32].

Paraffin

Paraffin (Fig. 2) is a mixture of paraffin wax and mineral oil in a 6:1 ratio, which is kept at a temperature of approximately 52.2°C to 54.4°C (126°F to 129.9°F) and applied for 15 to 20 minutes [13]. The paraffin application temperature is able safely to exceed the thermal pain threshold of 45°C because of the low heat conductivity of the paraffin mixture. Treatments consist of repeatedly dipping the part to be treated, usually the hand, in the paraffin bath, then letting the wax harden briefly while removed from the bath. This cycle is repeated 10 times; an insulating mitt is then placed on the hand for an additional 20 minutes [36]. Immersion dipping in the paraffin for 20 minutes is a more vigorous route of application; a brush may also be used to paint portions of the body that cannot be dipped. Paraffin baths are highly effective for rheumatoid arthritis and treatment of contractures, especially those involving the hands, such as in scleroderma. Open wounds and infected areas should be avoided. In a study

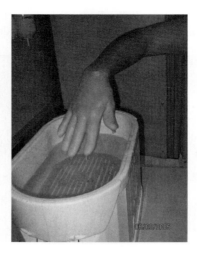

Fig. 2. Paraffin.

of scleroderma patients, paraffin bath applications in conjunction with friction massage and active range-of-motion exercises resulted in an improvement in skin compliance and overall hand function [37]. In studies done on patients with rheumatoid arthritis, improvements in range of motion and grip function were found following treatment with paraffin and active range-of-motion exercises. Notably, paraffin baths alone had no statistically significant effect on these outcomes [38]. This point should emphasize once again that modalities are supplemental treatments in a multimodal management program that should always include exercise or physical, occupational, or kinesiotherapy regimens.

Hydrotherapy

Hydrotherapy is a superficial heating modality wherein whirlpools are used to provide heat, massage, and gentle debridement over a larger body surface. Overall water temperature should not exceed 38°C to 39°C when most of the body is submerged. When only a local area is submerged, such as a hand or foot with intact temperature sensation, a temperature as high as 45°C may be tolerated. Elderly patients should be treated cautiously, especially those with congestive heart failure, poor cardiac function, adrenal insufficiency, obesity, or respiratory difficulties. Although it is mainly used for wound care, hydrotherapy may be employed for contractures and treatment of muscle spasms [39]. In the use for debridement, special solutions may be added to the hydrotherapy tub.

Ultrasound: a deep heating modality

The deep heating modalities or diathermies can heat the skin and underlying tissue to as deep as 8 cm [40]. Deep heat maximizes heating to the muscles, tendons, ligaments, and bones. Ultrasound (Fig. 3) is commonly used for application to deep joints, tendon sheaths, fibrous scars, and myofascial interfaces

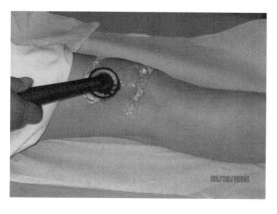

Fig. 3. Ultrasound.

[41]. Deep heat such as ultrasound is especially useful when there is an underlying tissue contracture, such as in chronic disease or injury states. When deep heating is done by ultrasound waves, pain is used to measure deep tissue temperature elevation; nerve endings around the bone are sensitive to the ultrasonic waves. Microwave and short-wave diathermy are also deep heating modalities, but these are less commonly used. Short-wave diathermy can heat a larger area and volume of tissue than ultrasound in the same period [42]; it has been shown in a double-blinded repeated-measures study to increase tissue extensibility more than did superficial heating or no heating [42]. Common indications for the deep heating modalities include contractures, tendonitis, myofascial and musculoskeletal pain, arthritis, and carpal tunnel syndrome.

Ultrasound is energy in the form of acoustic vibration above audible range (>20,000 Hz). It is generated when an electric current is passed around certain quartz crystals, causing them to vibrate and produce energy in the form of ultrasonic waves. Ultrasound energy is absorbed by the tissue and then converted into heat. The tissue medium, frequency of the ultrasound waves, and direction of application are all important in determining the tissue penetrance of ultrasound. Adipose tissue, for example, is penetrated more easily than bone; a beam applied parallel to the muscle fibers will penetrate that tissue much more than would a beam applied perpendicularly. Frequencies used in common practice are generally 0.8 to 3 MHz, with intensities of 0.5 to 2.0 W/cm^2. The most common frequency used is 1 MHz. The bone–soft tissue interface develops the highest temperatures, so ultrasound should be avoided at laminectomy sites to avoid direct heating of the spinal cord. Besides heat, ultrasound has some nonthermal effects. These may be disruptive to the tissue and may be used in scar or fibrous tissue breakdown or minimized by different application techniques. Ultrasound is applied by moving the applicator in a 25-cm^2 area in a circular or longitudinal manner [43], as in stroking. Treatments usually last for 8 to 10 minutes and may cause 4°C to 5°C temperature elevations at depths as great as 8 cm [40].

More than 35 clinical trials have tested the efficacy of ultrasound [44]. A literature review reveals both support and lack of support for ultrasound use. One literature summary demonstrates that pain and range of motion improve in both osteoarthritis and acute periarticular inflammatory conditions, but not in chronic periarticular inflammatory conditions [45]. Two meta-analyses conclude that there is not enough evidence to support either the use or the avoidance of ultrasound for pain control in a variety of musculoskeletal conditions [46,47]. In a double-blind randomized controlled trial in patients with shoulder pain, no difference was observed in pain relief, range of motion, or functional activities between patients treated with ultrasound and sham ultrasound [48]. Nonrandomized trials with blind evaluators exist, however, that show differences between ultrasound and no ultrasound [49,50] or sham ultrasound [50] for patients with shoulder pain [49] and low back pain [50]. Significant pain relief also occurs with ice [51], transcutaneous electrical nerve stimulation [52,53], superficial heat [53], and massage [54], however, and there was no difference between groups. Ultrasound has been shown to make a significant improvement, when combined with exercise and massage, in treating trigger points, providing pain relief, and reducing analgesic intake, although even a sham ultrasound group demonstrates a significant improvement over the control group that does not receive treatment [55]. Large trials are necessary for a more definitive answer about the benefit of ultrasound. Overall, evidence exists to support its use for pain relief, even if its benefit is similar to those of other heating modalities.

In a review of 23 randomized controlled trials, ultrasound was found to have statistically significant treatment effects as an intervention for lateral epicondylitis [56]. In 2003, the Australian Cochrane Centre conducted a review of trials using physiotherapy techniques for shoulder disorders, which are common in the geriatric population. Patients who had trauma and systemic inflammatory disorders, such as rheumatoid arthritis, were excluded from the analysis. Laser therapy was found to be more effective than placebo for adhesive capsulitis; both ultrasound and pulsed electromagnetic field therapy showed improvement compared with placebo in calcific tendonitis shoulder pain (mixed diagnosis), adhesive capsulitis, and rotator cuff tendonitis [57]. Ultrasound, however, resulted in no additional improvement over exercise alone [58]. The Philadelphia Panel guidelines [59], formulated in 2002 as evidence-based guidelines for the management of low back, knee, neck, and shoulder pain, recommend the use of therapeutic ultrasound in the treatment of calcific tendonitis of the shoulder [59]. Overall, despite the recommendations, there is still a lack of evidence regarding the beneficial effects of ultrasound intervention in the management of soft tissue problems and the arthritides. Further randomized controlled trials, perhaps conducted in the geriatric population, are warranted even today. Ultrasound, despite the lack of definitive evidence, continues to be a favorite modality among physicians, therapists, and patients alike.

Ultrasound should not be used near the brain, eyes, or reproductive organs, near a pacemaker, near the spine or a laminectomy site, or in the case of a malignancy or arthroplasty (any cement present will be dislodged or destroyed). There have been reports of increased radicular pain with the use of ultrasound [60,61]. The uses of, precautions for, and contraindications to both the superficial and deep heating modalities are summarized for review in Table 1.

Cryotherapy

Traditionally, heat has been used as a physical modality to treat stiffness, and cold therapy has been used as a treatment for pain. Great debate exists over these two modalities. Cold is more commonly used for acute conditions and for analgesia. Cryotherapy has long been a method of effecting fever reduction, control of bleeding, and control of pain, owing to both its analgesic properties and its capacity to reduce or moderate inflammation [12,41]. The analgesic properties result from the release of endogenous endorphins, altered local blood flow, and subsequent alteration of neural transmission [1,41,62]. Spasticity is reduced by means of prolonged cooling to the level of the muscle spindles. The physio-

Table 6
Physiologic effects of cold

Hemodynamic effects of cold	Immediate cutaneous vasoconstriction
	Delayed reactive vasodilation
	Decreased acute inflammation
Neuromuscular effects of cold	Slowing of conduction velocity
	Conduction block and axonal degeneration with prolonged exposure
	Decreased group Ia fiber firing rates (muscle spindle)
	Decreased group II fiber firing rates (muscle spindle)
	Decreased muscle stretch reflex amplitudes
	Increased maximal isometric strength
	Decreased muscle fatigue
	Temporarily reduced spasticity
Joint and connective tissue effects of cold	Increased joint stiffness
	Decreased tendon extensibility
	Decreased collagenase activity

logic effects of cold are summarized in Table 6. Cryotherapy is used mostly to treat acute conditions, such as in the initial management of postoperative pain or in the management of acute soft tissue strains and sprains. Cryotherapy may also be used to treat spasticity [63,64], myofascial pain syndrome, and other chronic conditions, including bursitis and tendonitis, and for desensitization of persistent trigger points [62,65–68]. The physician must be cognizant of the many contraindications to the use of cryotherapy, namely cold intolerance, cryotherapy-induced neuropraxia, arterial insufficiency, impaired sensation, cognitive or communication deficits that preclude the reporting of pain, cryopathies, cryoglobulinemias, paroxysmal cold hemoglobinuria, cold hypersensitivity, and Raynaud's disease or phenomenon [40,69].

The cold modalities are all superficial modalities and are summarized in Table 7. Cold packs, available as Hydrocollator packs, endothermic chemical gel packs, and ice packs, are applied for 15 to 20 minutes (but not longer) and can cool tissue approximately 5°C to a depth of 2 cm [70]. The use of ice packs is the most common form of cryotherapy, framed in the acronym RICE for "rest, ice, compression, and elevation." Hydrocollator packs are commercially available ice packs that are cooled in a freezer to −12°C and then applied over a moist towel. External compression can increase their effectiveness. In the elderly, ice massage, as with ice frozen in a cup, may be used for localized areas, such as

Table 7
Types of cryotherapy

Modality	Depth
Cold packs	Superficial
Ice massage	Superficial
Cold water immersion	Superficial
Cryotherapy compression units	Superficial
Vapocoolant spray	Superficial
Whirlpool baths	Superficial

in epicondylitis [32]. Ice massage is applied with gentle stroking motions at 5 to 10 minutes per site and has satisfaction ratings as great as 80% when combined with active range-of-motion exercises [65,71]. Vapocoolant sprays may be used in the treatment of trigger points. Fluorimethane spray or ethyl chloride may be applied in a unidirectional manner parallel to the muscle fibers while passively stretching the muscle [68]. Cutaneous freezing should be avoided. Hydrotherapy may also be used as a form of cryotherapy, although this is not recommended in the care of the geriatric patient.

The analgesia that cryotherapy provides has its greatest accomplishment in permitting movement which would otherwise be too painful for the patient. This virtue is enshrined in a more contemporary acronym for the management of acute pain: MICE, for "movement, ice, compression, and elevation." It is the emphasis on movement that cryotherapy's analgesia can provide. The uses, precautions, and contraindications to the use of cryotherapy are summarized in Table 2.

In clinical studies, ice has provided immediate and short-term reduction in pain in patients with rheumatoid arthritis [28,72] and low back pain [52]. In a study comparing ice with exercise versus heat packs with exercise for patients who had rheumatoid arthritis of the shoulder, significant reductions in pain occurred in both groups, with no difference between the groups [29]. In another study involving patients who had rheumatoid arthritis, no difference was noted between the analgesic effects of heat and ice [73]. Ice has also been compared with transcutaneous electrical nerve stimulation (TENS). In a study of patients who had low back pain, a significant reduction in pain was found with ice and TENS, but TENS showed longer-lasting relief (23 hours) than ice (12 hours) [52]. Cold clearly provides short-term analgesia; there may be some longer benefits as well. If the analgesia provided allows the patient to exercise with reduced pain, then cold is a useful adjunct therapy in the pain management program.

Electrotherapy: transcutaneous electrical nerve stimulation

Electrical stimulation has many uses in humans. It has been used in prevention of cardiovascular deconditioning, osteoporosis, deep venous thrombosis, and neuromuscular complications associated with spinal cord injury. It can aid in the conservative treatment of urinary incontinence, help manage spasticity, improve hemiplegic gait, and promote wound and bone healing [32].

TENS (Fig. 4) is a physical modality in which electrical signals are transmitted to the body by electrodes placed on the skin. These may be placed on peripheral nerves or nerve roots proximal, distal, or contralateral to or over painful areas. The production of analgesia has various success rates, ranging from placebo to 95%, depending on the study [32]. The analgesia may result from different mechanisms. One explanation involves changes in neuronal activity and the gate theory of pain modulation. This explanation may not account for the prolonged pain relief produced, however. Alteration of endogenous cerebrospinal fluid endorphins most likely plays a role: it has been shown that endorphins can

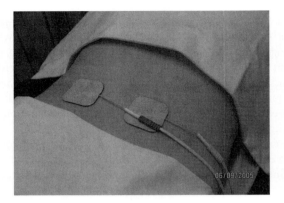

Fig. 4. Transcutaneous electrical nerve stimulation.

be released by electrical stimulation of supraspinal brainstem sites [10]. These endorphins block transmission of pain centrally by binding to opiate sites. Naloxone has been shown to inhibit TENS analgesia [74]. Also of note, the primary precursor of endogenous endorphins is adrenocorticotropic hormone; electroacupuncture has been shown to increase blood plasma corticosteroid levels by as much as 50% [75].

TENS is commonly used for musculoskeletal pain, posttraumatic and postsurgical pains, peripheral nerve injury, peripheral neuropathy, phantom limb pain, and sympathetically mediated pain, as in complex regional pain syndrome. However, several contraindications to its use should be reviewed. TENS should not be used when the patient is unable to report the effects or unable to report any discomfort, when the skin is atrophic, or when there is an allergy to the electrodes or gel. TENS should not be used when a pacemaker or implanted cardiac defibrillator is present. In the elderly, one must pay careful attention to neck stimulation, because the risk for vagal effects is high. Despite these cautions, TENS is highly acceptable and useful in the geriatric population for both acute and chronic conditions.

In a study involving chronic pain patients, a patient survey of pain relief was used to extrapolate treatment outcomes [76]. TENS was prescribed for an average of 40 months, and the patients reported a statistically significant reduction in their use of opiate analgesics, tranquilizers, muscle relaxants, NSAIDs, and steroids. Physical and occupational therapy use were also significantly reduced [76]. The cost stimulations indicate that long-term TENS use is associated with a cost reduction of as much as 55% for medications and as much as 69% for physical or occupational therapy [76]. With regard to most clinical studies, however, TENS stimulus parameters are not standardized, and interpretation of studies may be difficult across groups. In a study involving patients with chronic low back pain, TENS effects were the same as those of placebo TENS [77]. However, other modalities such as hot packs were allowed during the study, again making interpretation difficult. By contrast, high-frequency TENS has been shown significantly to reduce the affective component of pain; this TENS effect was also cumulative across treatments [78]. No long-term effects after discontinuation of therapy were observed, however [78]. Long- and short-term effects pertaining to relief of pain were demonstrated using TENS compared with placebo TENS for patients who had chronic low back pain [79]. Several other studies failed to show a difference between TENS and placebo TENS for pain relief in patients who had acute low back pain [80], chronic low back pain [81], temporomandibular joint disorders [82], or osteoarthritis [83]. Thus, the current clinical data are in conflict. In animal studies, TENS has been shown partially to reduce hyperalgesia at the site of injury [58] and completely to reduce the hyperalgesia surrounding the site [56,84,85]. TENS has been recommended in the 2002 Philadelphia Panel evidence-based guidelines for management of knee osteoarthritis [59].

Several studies using TENS have been done in the geriatric population, particularly studying alleviation of pain in osteoarthritis of the knees. In a study involving elderly subjects (mean age 85) who were randomly assigned to electro-acupuncture, TENS, or a control group for the treatment of osteoarthritis-induced knee pain, both electro-acupuncture and TENS treatments were found to be effective in reducing the knee pain [86]. Patients in the TENS group received low-frequency TENS (2 Hz) with a pulse width of 200 micros on acupuncture points for 20 minutes per session; treatment was continued for a total of eight sessions in 2 weeks [86]. Another study evaluated the cumulative effect of 4 weeks of TENS treatments on chronic osteoarthritic knee pain compared with placebo stimulation. The patients were aged 50 to 75. Visual Analog Score (VAS) was used to measure pain before and after each treatment session. A significant cumulative reduction in the VAS scores was observed across the four treatment sessions in the TENS group and in the placebo group [87]. Linear regression of the daily recordings of the VAS indicated that the slope in the TENS group was similar to that in the exercise group; these slopes were steeper than those of the other groups [87]. The reduction in osteoarthritic knee pain was maintained at the 4-week follow-up session in the TENS group and in the TENS-plus-exercise group, but not in the other two groups [87]. In a randomized controlled trial involving some patients older than 65, one-time TENS treatment provided immediate pain relief for low-back pain patients [88]. Finally, in the setting of carpal tunnel syndrome, a randomized double-blind placebo-controlled cross-over trial was conducted among United States veterans, all of whom had mild to moderate carpal tunnel syndrome. Significant decreases in the McGill Pain Questionnaire score, median nerve sensory latency, and Phalen and Tinel signs resulted after the real but not after the sham treatment series [89]. Patients were able to perform their previous work, and their carpal tunnel syndrome remained stable for 1 to 3 years [89]. These studies indicate that, within the geriatric population, TENS can be effective for carpal tunnel syndrome, low back pain, and osteoarthritis-induced pain. Because of the convenience of application and the low frequency of side effects, TENS is often a recommended physical modality intervention.

A TENS unit consists of a battery, electrodes, and one or more generators that produce the electrical signal. Signals may be pulsed, burst, or ramped, and the amplitudes, rates, and widths of the pulses may vary. In common practice, asymmetric and biphasic waveforms are used. These limit the electrolysis and skin irritation that may result when a single polarity is used. Frequencies are commonly high, from 60 to 80 Hz, because lower frequencies (<8 Hz) are generally more uncomfortable. The units are convenient, small, and programmable and may fit in one's pocket. Generally, they can be purchased for less than $100 and are covered by insurance companies. Several manufacturers lend TENS machines to patients for a trial. Before purchase, patients should have had several therapy sessions with the TENS unit to establish the electrode placement, stimulator settings, and benefits. After several months of consistent stable use with benefits, purchase may be recommended. The uses of, precautions for, and contraindications to the use of TENS are summarized in Table 3.

Electrotherapy: percutaneous electrical nerve stimulation

Percutaneous electrical nerve stimulation (PENS) uses electrical stimulation in conjunction with acupuncture. When low-frequency electrical stimulation is used (2 to 4 Hz), an endorphin-dependent analgesia has been identified. This response is characterized by a slow onset with a peak at about 30 minutes and a long duration with effects usually lasting many hours. This analgesia also exhibits potentiation, with a second treatment having a greater effect than the first and cumulative effects seen after several treatments [40]. Other frequencies, including intermediate (10 to 30 Hz) and high (75 to 200 Hz) may also produce this effect. Treatments generally last 30 minutes each, one to three times per week.

PENS has some good clinical trials to support its use. In a randomized controlled trial involving adults who had type II diabetes mellitus and complained of lower extremity neuropathic pain for at least 6 months, PENS treatment done at alternating 15-Hz and 30-Hz frequencies for a total of 3 weeks was compared with sham PENS treatment [90]. VAS for pain measurement was impressively reduced following the PENS treatment but not the sham treatment (6.2 ± 1.0 to 2.5 ± 0.8 and 6.4 ± 0.9 to 6.3 ± 1.1, respectively). VAS Activity and Sleep scores also improved in the PENS treatment group (5.2 ± 1.0 to 7.9 ± 1.0 and 5.8 ± 1.3 to 8.3 ± 0.7, respectively), whereas the sham PENS group did not show any changes from baseline. Daily nonopioid analgesia requirements decreased by 49% in the PENS group but only decreased by 14% in the sham treatment group. Furthermore, significant improvement was demonstrated in other outcome measurements, including the medical outcomes study 36-Item Short-Form Health Survey, the Beck Depression Inventory, and the Profile of Mood States.

In a randomized cross-over study involving patients with low back pain secondary to degenerative disc disease, PENS treatment was compared with sham PENS, TENS, and exercise therapy [91]. The PENS group showed a decrease in VAS pain scores and a decrease in the average daily intake of nonopioid analgesics. Compared with the other three modalities, 91% of patients reported that PENS was the most effective treatment for reducing their low back pain. The

PENS treatment group also showed a statistically significant increase in physical activity, quality of sleep, and sense of well-being.

In a randomized, controlled, sham-controlled study involving patients who had sciatica, PENS was shown to be more effective than TENS at a stimulation frequency of 4 Hz for the short-term relief of pain and improvement in function [92].

Contraindications to PENS are the same as those for electrical stimulation in general: avoid pregnant patients, patients who have carcinoma, and stimulation over the thorax in patients with pacemakers [40].

Summary

The treatment of pain and dysfunction in the geriatric population is a challenge. As Gerald Felsenthal [7] eloquently concludes in his 1994 textbook *Rehabilitation of the Aging and Elderly Patient*: "To simply ascribe pain in the elderly to arthritis and to merely prescribe medication without giving thought to the full impact that the pain may have on the patient's function is a disservice. An aggressive multidisciplinary approach may ultimately help the patient to continue or resume a productive and functional existence." A conclusion written today, more than a decade since the book's publication, is an echo of his wisdom. This multimodal approach to the management of pain and dysfunction has since been broadcast by the American Pain Society and the Agency for Health Care Policy and Research. Its message is perhaps most applicable to the geriatrician. In this unique population, the physician has the opportunity to restore function and thus independence and sanctity. By learning and employing a multimodal approach to the management of pain and dysfunction with a concentration on the use of the physical modalities, the physician may restore, preserve, and perhaps even enhance functionality.

Appendix: clinical vignettes

The following clinical vignettes are designed to show how modalities may be used. The modalities chosen are not necessarily required, nor should they be the sole treatment for the named conditions. They should be used together with other therapies, including medical treatments.

To communicate formally with rehabilitation personnel, the authors recommend using the following prescription as a guideline. Formal consultation or referral to a physiatrist, if available, might be warranted if further expertise is needed.

- Diagnosis: This should include the diagnosis for which the modality (or physical, occupational, or other therapy) is prescribed, as well as other relevant medical, surgical, and psychiatric diagnoses.
- Impairment: loss of range of motion, strength, endurance, or balance

- Disability: loss of activities of daily living (ADL) or ambulation
- Precautions: sensory or cognitive deficits, minimum and maximum cardiac and respiratory parameters, hypoglycemic precautions (if applicable), fall precautions (if applicable), and specific weight-bearing status of each limb. Open wounds, metal, pacemakers, cardiac defibrillators, joint precautions (eg, hip precautions after total joint arthroplasty), and cancer diagnoses should be incorporated as well.
- Goals: These may be short-term, usually about 4-week goals, long-term, usually about 6-month goals, or both and may include ADL and ambulation goals.
- Treatment: should specify physical therapy, occupational therapy, and modalities chosen. Ideally, a stretching and strengthening program should be included with the modality prescription as part of a multimodal therapy approach. The sample prescriptions focus only on the modality chosen, because prescription writing for the entire stretching and strengthening program is beyond the scope of this article.

1. Adhesive capsulitis

An 81-year-old woman reports an 8-month history of decreased ability to abduct the right shoulder. She is right-hand dominant and complains of difficulty with washing and combing her hair and reaching into cabinets. Her past medical and surgical history is significant for atrial fibrillation and episodic congestive heart failure. She is not on any anticoagulation. She denies peripheral vascular disease, malignancy, and open wounds and has intact cognition and sensation. Sedimentation rate is within normal limits. Physical examination reveals limited passive and active shoulder abduction to 100°. MRI shows a chronic partial rotator cuff tear.

- Diagnosis: right shoulder adhesive capsulitis; right rotator cuff tear; history of atrial fibrillation, congestive heart failure
- Impairment: decreased range of motion (ROM)
- Disability: decreased ADL
- Precautions: cardiac
- Goals: increase shoulder abduction to 120° short-term, 150° long-term

Occupational therapy:

Hydrocollator pack to right shoulder ×15 minutes (followed by active ROM)
Ultrasound at 1.5 W/s × 6 minutes (followed by active ROM)
Ice pack after ROM × 15 minutes
ADL evaluation for reacher device and other devices for the home
Home exercise program: prescribe pulley for home use

Note: Deep heat would be contraindicated in a patient receiving anticoagulation therapy.

2. Knee osteoarthritis

A 65-year-old man reports difficulty in walking secondary to bilateral knee pain. His knee pain has worsened in the past 1 month. He has a past medical and surgical history of emphysema, obesity, sleep apnea, and decreased left ventricular function on echocardiogram. He does not have a pacemaker or cardiac defibrillator. He can only ambulate for two blocks secondary to pain. Physical examination reveals enlarged arthritic knees with valgus deformities and joint line tenderness bilaterally. Knee radiographs reveal severe arthritic changes with loss of joint space. He is not an operative candidate. He has previously received cortisone intra-articular injections with some improvement in pain.

- Diagnosis: bilateral knee osteoarthritis, obesity, chronic obstructive pulmonary disease, sleep apnea, diminished cardiac function
- Impairment: decreased ROM, pain, decreased endurance
- Disability: decreased ambulation
- Precautions: cardiac precautions
- Goals: decrease knee pain by 50%

Physical therapy:

Traditional TENS to bilateral knees for pain control (80 Hz, shortest duration, with increased frequency for effect, to a minimally perceptible sense of electricity) × 20–30 minutes to cover the duration of the therapy session
Cold pack × 15 minutes to bilateral knees for analgesia
Quadriceps and hamstring strengthening
Evaluation for offloading knee braces and possible shoe wedges to offload valgus deformity
Gait training with appropriate assistive device for antalgic gait

3. Hand rheumatoid arthritis

A 74-year-old woman reports decreasing strength, increasing pain, and increasing stiffness in her hands that has worsened in the past 3 months. She has difficulty buttoning clothes, opening jars, and turning doorknobs. She has a past medical and surgical history of recently diagnosed lung cancer, myocardial infarction, and depression. Physical examination reveals deformed hands with flexion contractures and ulnar deviated fingers and poor hand grip and pinch strengths. There is no sensory loss. Her cognition is intact.

- Diagnosis: rheumatoid arthritis affecting both hands, depression, lung cancer (no known metastases)
- Impairment: decreased ROM, decreased strength
- Disability: decreased ADL
- Precautions: cardiac

- Goals: increased strength by one grade for hand grip and pinch, independence in ADL by means of increasing ROM and stretching shortened muscles

Occupational therapy:

Fluidotherapy at 104°F × 15 minutes with simultaneous active assisted ROM

or

Paraffin dipping × 10, then insulation glove × 15 minutes

or

Whirlpool hydrotherapy at 102°F × 10 minutes
ROM and strengthening exercises to the bilateral hands
ADL and adaptive equipment evaluation and training for larger-handled utensils, tools to assist with buttons and zippers, pens with larger grip, and so on

References

[1] Berry P, Chapman R, Covington E. Pain: current understanding of assessment, management and treatments. American Pain Society. July 2004. Available at: http://www.ampainsoc.org/ce/npc. Accessed March 2005.
[2] Jacox AK, Carr DB, Chapman CR, et al. Acute pain management: operative or medical procedures and trauma clinical practice guideline no. 1. Rockville (MD): US Department of Health and Human Services, Agency for Health Care Policy and Research; 1992. AHCPR publication #92-0032.
[3] Anonymous. Recommendations for the medical management of osteoarthritis of the hip and knee: 2000 update. Arthritis Rheum 2000;43:1905–15.
[4] Pendleton A, Arden N, Dougados M, et al. EULAR recommendations for the management of knee osteoarthritis: report of a task force of the Standing Committee for International Clinical Studies Including Therapeutic Trials (ESCISIT). Ann Rheum Dis 2000;59:936–44.
[5] Lipsky PE, Alarcon GS, Bombardier C, et al. Algorithms for the diagnosis and management of musculoskeletal complaints. Am J Med 1997;103(6A):49S–85S.
[6] Lee JA. Adult degenerative joint disease of the knee: maximizing function and promoting joint health: Institute for Clinical System Integration. Postgrad Med 1999;105:183–97.
[7] Felsenthal G, Garrison S, Steinberg F. Rehabilitation management of pain in the elderly—rehabilitation of the aging and elderly patient. Williams & Wilkins; 1994. p. 311–8.
[8] Felsenthal G, Cohen BS, Hilton EB, et al. The physiatrist as primary physician for patients on an inpatient rehabilitation unit. Arch Phys Med Rehabil 1984;65:375–8.
[9] Sherman ED, Robillard E. Sensitivity to pain and relationship to aging. J Am Geriatr Soc 1964; 12:1037–44.
[10] Gloth MJ, Matesi AM. Physical therapy and exercise in pain management. Clin Geriatr Med 2001;17(3):525–35 [vii].
[11] Guy AW, Lehmann JF, Stonebridge JB. Therapeutic applications of electromagnetic power. Proc IEEE 1974;62:55–75.

[12] Schmidt KL, Ott VR, Rocher G, et al. Heat, cold and inflammation (a review). Z Rheumatol 1979;38:391–404.

[13] Lehmann JF. Therapeutic heat and cold. 4th edition. Baltimore (MD): Williams & Wilkins; 1990.

[14] Stelian J, Gili Habot B. Improvement of pain and disability in elderly patients with degenerative osteoarthritis of the knee treated with narrow band light therapy. J Am Geriatr Soc 1992;40: 23–6.

[15] Harden N, McCarberg B, O'Connor A. A new look at heat treatment for pain disorders, part I. American Pain Society. November/December 2004. Available at: http://www.ampainsoc.org/ pub/bulletin/nov04/inno1.htm. Accessed March 2005.

[16] Harden N, O'Connor A, McCarberg B. A new look at heat treatment for pain disorders, part II. American Pain Society. Winter 2005. Available at: http://www.ampainsoc.org/pub/bulletin/ win05/inno1.htm. Accessed March 2005.

[17] Mense S. Effects of temperature on the discharge of muscle spindles and tendon organs. Pflugers Arch 1978;374:159–66.

[18] Lehmann JF, Masock AJ, Warren CG, et al. Effect of therapeutic temperatures on tendon extensibility. Arch Phys Med Rehabil 1970;51:481–7.

[19] Harris ED, McCroskery PA. The influence of temperature and fibril stability on degradation of cartilage collagen by rheumatoid synovial collagenase. N Engl J Med 1974;290:1–6.

[20] Michlovitz SL. Biophysical principles of heating and superficial heat agents. In: Michlovitz SL, editor. Thermal agents in rehabilitation. Philadelphia: F.A. Davis Co.; 1986. p. 99–118.

[21] Kankaanpaa M, Taimela S, Airaksinen O, et al. The efficacy of active rehabilitation in chronic low back pain. Effect on pain intensity, self-experienced disability, and lumbar fatigability. Spine 1999;249(10):1034–42.

[22] Nadler SF, Steiner DJ, Petty SR, et al. Continuous low-level heat wrap therapy provides more efficacy than ibuprofen and acetaminophen for low back pain. Spine 2002;27(10):1012–7.

[23] Nadler SF, Steiner DJ, Petty SR, et al. Overnight use of continuous low-level heatwrap therapy for relief of low back pain. Arch Phys Med Rehabil 2003;84:335–42.

[24] McCray RE, Patton NJ. Pain relief at trigger points: a comparison of moist heat and short wave diathermy. J Orthop Sports Phys Ther 1984;5:175–8.

[25] Nelson SJ, Ash Jr MM. An evaluation of a moist heating pad for the treatment of TMJ/muscle pain dysfunction. Cranio 1988;6:355–9.

[26] Hoyrup G, Kjorvel L. Comparison of whirlpool and wax treatments for hand therapy. Physiother Can 1986;38:79–82.

[27] Toomey R, Grief-Schwartz R, Piper MC. Clinical evaluation of the effects of whirlpool on patients with Colles' fractures. Physiother Can 1986;38:280–4.

[28] Kirk JA, Kersley GD. Heat and cold in the physical treatment of rheumatoid arthritis of the knee. A controlled clinical trial. Ann Phys Med 1968;9:270–4.

[29] Williams J, Harvey J, Tannenbaum H. Use of superficial heat versus ice for the rheumatoid arthritic shoulder: a pilot study. Physiotherapy 1986;38:8–13.

[30] Lehmann JF, Silverman DR, Baum BA, et al. Temperature distributions in the human thigh, produced by infrared, hot pack and microwave applications. Arch Phys Med Rehabil 1966;47:291–9.

[31] Diller KR. Analysis of burns caused by long-term exposure to a heating pad. J Burn Care Rehabil 1991;12:214–7.

[32] Braddom RL. Physical agent modalities. Electrical stimulation. In: Buschbacher RM, Dumitru D, Johnson EW, et al, editors. Physical medicine and rehabilitation. 2nd edition. Philadelphia: WB Saunders; 2000. p. 440–87.

[33] Dover JS, Phillips TJ, Arndt KA. Cutaneous effects and therapeutic uses of heat with emphasis on infrared radiation. J Am Acad Dermatol 1989;20:278–86.

[34] Borrell RM, Parker R, Henley EJ, et al. Comparison of in vivo temperatures produced by hydrotherapy, paraffin wax treatment, and fluidotherapy. Phys Ther 1980;60:1273–6.

[35] Borrell RM, Henley EJ, Ho P, et al. Fluidotherapy: evaluation of a new heat modality. Arch Phys Med Rehabil 1977;58:69–71.

[36] Abramson DI, Tuck S, Chu SW, et al. Effect of paraffin bath and hot fomentations on local tissue temperatures. Arch Phys Med Rehabil 1964;45:87–94.

[37] Askew LJ, Beckett VL, An K, et al. Objective evaluation of hand function in scleroderma patients to assess effectiveness of physical therapy. Br J Rheumatol 1983;22:224–32.

[38] Dellhag B, Wollersjo I, Bjelle A. Effect of active hand exercise and wax bath treatments in rheumatoid arthritis patients. Arthritis Care Res 1992;5:87–92.

[39] Hong C, Tobis J. Physiatrist rehabilitation and maintenance of the geriatric patient. In: Kottke FJ, Lehman JF, editors. Krusen's handbook of physical medicine and rehabilitation. 4th edition. Philadelphia: WB Saunders; 1990. p. 1209–16.

[40] O'Young BJ, Young MA, Stiens SA. Physical medicine and rehabilitation secrets. 2nd edition. Philadelphia: Hanley & Belfus; 2002.

[41] Schwab CD. Musculoskeletal pain. Phys Med Rehabil 1991;5(3):1.

[42] Robertson VJ, Ward AR, Jung P. The effect of heat on tissue extensibility: a comparison of deep and superficial heating. Arch Phys Med Rehabil 2005;86:819–25.

[43] Barber FA, McGuire DA, Click S. Continuous-flow cold therapy for outpatient anterior cruciate ligament reconstruction. Arthroscopy 1998;14(2):130–5.

[44] Ter Haar G, Dyson M, Oakley EM. The use of ultrasound by physiotherapists in Britain, 1985. Ultrasound Med Biol 1987;13:659–63.

[45] Falconer J, Hayes KW, Chang RW. Therapeutic ultrasound in the treatment of musculoskeletal conditions. Arthritis Care Res 1990;3:85–91.

[46] Gam AN, Johannsen F. Ultrasound therapy in musculoskeletal disorders: a meta-analysis. Pain 1995;63:85–91.

[47] van der Windt DAWM, van der Hejiden GJ, van der Berg SGM, et al. Ultrasound for musculoskeletal disorders: a systemic review. Pain 1999;81:257–71.

[48] Downing DS, Weinstein A. Ultrasound therapy of subacromial bursitis. A double blind trial. Phys Ther 1986;66:194–9.

[49] Munting E. Ultrasonic therapy for painful shoulders. Physiotherapy 1978;64:180–1.

[50] Nwuga VC. Ultrasound treatment of back pain resulting from prolapsed intervertebral disc. Arch Phys Med Rehabil 1983;64:88–9.

[51] Hammer J, Kirk JA. Physiotherapy and the frozen shoulder: a comparative trial of ice and ultrasonic therapy. N Z Med J 1976;83(560):191–2.

[52] Halle JS, Franklin RJ, Karalfa BL. Comparison of four treatment approaches for lateral epicondylitis of the elbow. J Orthop Sports Phys Ther 1986;8:62–9.

[53] Svarcova J, Trnavsky K, Zvarova J. The influence of ultrasound, galvanic currents and short-wave diathermy on pain intensity in patients with osteoarthritis. Scand J Rheumatol 1987; 67(Suppl):83–5.

[54] Stratford PW, Levy DR, Gauldie S, et al. The evaluation of phonophoresis and friction massage as treatments for extensor carpi radialis tendonitis: a randomized controlled trial. Physiother Can 1989;41:93–9.

[55] Gam AN, Warming S, Larsen LH, et al. Treatment of myofascial trigger-points with ultrasound combined with massage and exercise—a randomized controlled trial. Pain 1998;77:73–9.

[56] Smidt N, Assendelft WJ, Arola H, et al. Effectiveness of physiotherapy for lateral epicondylitis: a systematic review. Ann Med 2003;35(1):51–62.

[57] Green S, Buchbinder R, Hetrick S. Physiotherapy interventions for shoulder pain. Cochrane Database Syst Rev 2003;2:CD004258.

[58] Gopalkrishnan P, Sluka KA. Effect of varying frequency, intensity, and pulse duration of transcutaneous electrical nerve stimulation on primary hyperalgesia in inflamed rats. Arch Phys Med Rehabil 2000;81:984–90.

[59] Harris GR, Susman JL. Managing musculoskeletal complaints with rehabilitation therapy: summary of the Philadelphia Panel evidence-based clinical practice guidelines on musculoskeletal rehabilitation interventions. J Fam Pract 2002;51(12):1042–6.

[60] Gnatz SM. Increased radicular pain due to therapeutic ultrasound applied to the back. Arch Phys Med Rehabil 1989;70:493–4.

[61] Batavia M. Contraindications for superficial heat and therapeutic ultrasound: do sources agree? Arch Phys Med Rehabil 2004;85:1006–12.

[62] Meeusen R, Lievens P. The use of cryotherapy in sports injuries. Sports Med 1986;3:398–414.

[63] Hedenberg L. Functional improvement of the spastic hemiplegic arm after cooling. Scand J Rehabil Med 1970;2:154–8.

[64] Miglietta O. Action of cold on spasticity. Am J Phys Med 1973;52:198–205.

[65] Grant AE. Massage with ice (cryokinetics) in the treatment of painful conditions of the musculoskeletal system. Arch Phys Med Rehabil 1964;45:233–8.

[66] Hocutt JE, Jaffe R, Rylander CR, et al. Cryotherapy in ankle sprains. Am J Sports Med 1982;10:316–9.

[67] Melzack R, Jeans ME, Stratford JG, et al. Ice massage and transcutaneous electrical stimulation: comparison of treatment for low-back pain. Pain 1980;9:209–17.

[68] Travell J. Ethyl chloride spray for painful muscle spasm. Arch Phys Med Rehabil 1952;33:291–8.

[69] Ritzmann SE, Levin WC. Cryopathies: a review. Arch Intern Med 1961;107:186–204.

[70] Knutsson E, Mattsson E. Effects of local cooling on monosynaptic reflexes in man. Scand J Rehabil Med 1969;1:126–32.

[71] Lowdon BJ, Moore RJ. Determinants and nature of intramuscular temperature changes during cold therapy. Am J Phys Med 1975;54:223–33.

[72] Halliday SM, Littler TR, Littler EN. A trial of ice therapy and exercise in chronic arthritis. Physiotherapy 1969;55:51–6.

[73] Curkovic B, Vitulic V, Babic-Naglic D, et al. The influence of heat and cold on the pain threshold in rheumatoid arthritis. Z Rheumatol 1997;52:289–91.

[74] Cheng RSF, Pomerantz B. Electroacupuncture analgesia could be mediated by at least two pain relieving mechanisms: endorphin and non-endorphin systems. Life Sci 1979;25:1957–62.

[75] Bengston R. Physical measure useful in pain management. Int Anesthesiol Clin 1983;21:4165.

[76] Chabal C, Fishbain DA, Weaver M, et al. Long term transcutaneous electrical nerve stimulation (TENS) use: impact of medication utilization and physical therapy costs. Clin J Pain 1998; 14(1):66–73.

[77] Deyo RA, Walsh NE, Martin DC, et al. A controlled trial of transcutaneous electrical nerve stimulation (TENS) and exercise for chronic low back pain. N Engl J Med 1990;322:1627–34.

[78] Marchand S, Charest J, Li J, et al. Is TENS purely a placebo effect? A controlled study on chronic low back pain. Pain 1993;54:99–106.

[79] Thorsteinsson G, Stonnington HH, Stilwell GK, et al. Transcutaneous electrical stimulation: a double-blind trial of its efficacy for pain. Arch Phys Med Rehabil 1977;58:8–13.

[80] Herman E, Williams R, Stratford P, et al. A randomized controlled trial of transcutaneous electrical nerve stimulation (CO-DETRON) to determine its benefits in a rehabilitation program for acute occupational low back pain. Spine 1994;19:561–8.

[81] Lehmann TR, Russell DW, Spratt KF, et al. Efficacy of electroacupuncture and TENS in the rehabilitation of chronic low back pain patients. Pain 1986;26:277–90.

[82] Taylor K, Newton RA, Personius WJ, et al. Effects of interferential current stimulation for treatment of subjects with recurrent jaw pain. Phys Ther 1987;67:346–50.

[83] Lewis B, Lewis D, Cumming G. The comparative analgesic efficacy of transcutaneous electrical nerve stimulation and a non-steroidal anti-inflammatory drug for painful osteoarthritis. Br J Rheumatol 1994;33:455–60.

[84] King EW, Sluka KA. The effect of varying frequency and intensity of transcutaneous electrical nerve stimulation on the treatment of secondary mechanical hyperalgesia in an animal model of inflammation. J Pain 2001;17(3):278.

[85] Sluka KA, Bailey K, Bogush J, et al. Treatment with either high or low frequency TENS reduces the secondary hyperalgesia observed after injection of kaolin and carrageenan into the knee joint. Pain 1998;77:97–102.

[86] Ng NM, Leung MC, Poon DM. The effects of electro-acupuncture and transcutaneous electrical nerve stimulation on patients with painful osteoarthritic knees: a randomized controlled trial with follow-up evaluation. J Altern Complement Med 2003;9(5):641–9.

[87] Cheng GL, Hui-Chan CW, Chan KM. Does four weeks of TENS and/or isometric exercise produce a cumulative reduction of osteoarthritic knee pain? Clin Rehabil 2002;16(7):749–60.

[88] Hsieh RL, Lee WC. One-shot percutaneous electrical nerve stimulation vs. transcutaneous electrical nerve stimulation for low back pain: comparison of therapeutic effects. Am J Phys Med Rehabil 2002;81(11):838–43.

[89] Naeser MA, Hahn KA, Lieberman BE, et al. Carpal tunnel syndrome pain treated with low-level laser and microamperes transcutaneous electric nerve stimulation: a controlled study. Arch Phys Med Rehabil 2002;83(7):978–88.

[90] Hamza MA, White PF, Craig WF, et al. Percutaneous Electrical Nerve Stimulation: a novel analgesic therapy for diabetic neuropathic pain. Diabetes Care 2000;23(3):365–70.

[91] Ghoname EA, Craig WF, White PF, et al. Percutaneous electrical nerve stimulation for low back pain: a randomized crossover study. JAMA 1999;281(9):818–23.

[92] Ghoname EA, White PF, Ahmed HE, et al. Percutaneous electrical nerve stimulation: an alternative to TENS in the management of siatica. Pain 1999;83(2):193–9.

ELSEVIER
SAUNDERS

Clin Geriatr Med 22 (2006) 355–375

CLINICS IN
GERIATRIC
MEDICINE

Wheelchair Evaluation for the Older Adult

Timothy P. Sabol, PT, DPT, CSCS*, Evelyn S. Haley, PT

*Spinal Cord Injury Unit, James J. Peters Veterans Affairs Medical Center,
130 West Kingsbridge Road, Bronx, NY 10468, USA*

An estimated 1.6 million Americans residing outside of institutions use wheelchairs, according to the National Health Interview Survey on Disability. Most wheelchairs are manual, with only 155,000 using power wheelchairs. Wheelchair use increases sharply with age. The highest rates are found in the elderly population: 2.9% of people older than 65 years use wheelchairs, which is approximately 900,000 people. Interestingly, although most manual wheelchair users are elderly (57.5%), more than two thirds of power chair users are not elderly [1].

Given the gradual increase in life expectancy, more and more individuals need devices to facilitate improved living conditions. To ensure proper seating and mobility, clinicians performing wheelchair evaluations must consider the patient's susceptibility to skin breakdown, ability to complete activities of daily living (ADLs), endurance capacity, environmental constraints, safety, impairments, functional limitations, and disabilities. Seating and mobility can have an impact on a patient's posture, level of pain, participation, and quality of life [2–4]. Various individuals in the adult population are candidates for assisted seating and mobility. In the aging population, the various comorbidities that may exist affect the type of wheelchair selected for the patient. Some of these diagnoses include spinal cord injuries (SCI), multiple sclerosis, Parkinson's disease, cerebrovascular accidents, amputations, diabetes mellitus, orthopedic issues, cardiac conditions, and respiratory diseases. One must understand the ramifications of poorly positioning a patient in a wheelchair, especially if the wheelchair will be used for an extended period. A patient with an ill-fitting wheelchair runs the risk of shoulder injuries from repetitive stress and sacral or ischial breakdown. However, a prop-

---

* Corresponding author.
E-mail address: timothy.sabol@med.va.gov (T.P. Sabol).

0749-0690/06/$ – see front matter © 2006 Elsevier Inc. All rights reserved.
doi:10.1016/j.cger.2005.12.013   *geriatric.theclinics.com*

erly fitted wheelchair can help patients maximize their potential for a greater level of function and higher quality of life.

Evaluation

As with any patient being seen for an evaluation, it is important to gather all the background information to have a complete picture of the clinical situation. The patient is usually referred from a physician for a wheelchair and seating evaluation in an appropriate clinic. The clinic is usually composed of a physical or occupational therapist, and perhaps a physician if time permits.

For the evaluation process to be successful, the practitioner needs to address all the components of the disablement model, pathologic conditions, impairments, functional limitations, and disabilities or handicaps, keeping in mind the prognosis of the patient [5].

The first element to establish is what brought the patient to the clinic. Some helpful questions include

How is your current chair working or not working for you?
Which aspects of your current chair are you happy or unhappy with?
What would you like to do differently or keep the same?
What is the wheelchair used for primarily?

A thorough history, chart, and systems review is essential during the examination. Gathering notes from the patient, family, and caregivers may garner more information than was initially established by the other health care professionals involved in the process. Items such as the patient's living situation and home environment are important to know beforehand (Box 1).

One key step is performing a thorough mat evaluation of the patient. Information gathered from the mat evaluation is crucial to discovering any range of motion or functional mobility deficits [4,6,7].

Box 1. Sample questions regarding patient's home environment

In what type of building do you live (eg, house, apartment, nursing home)?
Are there stairs to the entrance?
Is there a ramp to enter the building?
Is there an elevator?
Do you have narrow doorways?
Are there "tight" spaces in the building?
How many levels are there?

The mat evaluation consists of taking the patient out of the wheelchair and placing him or her supine on a mat to assess for joint mobility and positioning issues. A mat evaluation is an essential component of the decision-making process for wheelchairs and cushions. A thorough mat evaluation can be used to ascertain information about flexible versus fixed pelvic obliquities and spinal asymmetries. These dysfunctions may contribute to the development of pressure sores on the seating surface and along the thorax with increased areas of pressure. This information may be used to determine the best possible intervention to address these deformities. Flexible obliquities are correctable deformities, generally addressed by building up the lower side until the pelvis is leveled. Fixed obliquities are addressed by accommodating the problem, namely by building up the higher side to provide increased contact and hence better pressure distribution across the entire seating surface. The mat evaluation typically covers pelvic and thoracic mobility, postural stability, and key measurements such as hamstring length [7,8].

The seated evaluation is another integral component of the decision-making process. Once the impairments and functional limitations have been taken into consideration, actual anatomic measurements of the patient may be obtained. Primary considerations should include seat width, seat depth, and back height. To obtain seat width, the practitioner should measure the patient's actual width by measuring the distance between the greater trochanters in the seated position. Then add a total of 1 in to that measurement. Some space is necessary for clothing and pressure reduction on the greater trochanters. In general, wheelchair users prefer a tighter-fitting seat, which will reduce the overall width of a manual wheelchair. This arrangement improves propulsion and increases overall accessibility [9]. To measure a patient's seat depth accurately, one measures the distance from the popliteal fossa to the posterior aspect of the pelvis (which includes redundant tissue). The general rule of thumb for the seat depth of the chair is to subtract 2 to 3 in from the patient's seat depth to ensure clearance between the edge of the seat and the back of the knee [10]. Finally, to obtain the seat height, one measures from the seat base to a point 1 in below the inferior angle of the scapula. If a patient prefers or requires more posterior trunk support (ie, tilt-in-space chair), then the clinician should measure 1 in or more above the inferior angle of the scapula. Other components of the wheelchair may be based on patient preference. Additional measurements may need to be taken for more complex patients, such as arm height, lateral height, and leg-rest length [11]. Contacting individual companies may provide the necessary information about additional specific measurements. Patients coming into the clinic may have existing wheelchairs that currently fit them appropriately. In this case, measurements may be taken from the existing wheelchair, eliminating the potential for measurement error.

It is important during the actual seating evaluation to attempt to correct postural problems with temporary build-ups. This process gives the patient a simulation of how the new positioning might feel. Patients may then provide the therapist with feedback as to whether they can function in this position. This measure also allows the clinician to address postural concerns, such as decreased lumbar lordosis, and determine whether the patient can tolerate the interventions. Although patients may look posturally correct to the clinician's standards, if they cannot perform daily functions, the wheelchair will not work. Probably the most difficult decision for the clinician is the determination of which components are sufficient to address the postural needs of the patient while maximizing the patient's functional independence [11]. Additionally, contacting local wheelchair representatives for trial wheelchairs may be helpful in the decision-making process. Patients can thus get a feel for their individual preferences [4].

Pressure sores are a major health care problem for patients who have decreased mobility [12]. The primary cause of wound development is the high level of contact forces [12–14]. Prevention is crucial in decreasing the incidence and recurrence of pressure sores [15]. Pressure mapping systems offer a means of measuring direct pressure (perpendicular force) of the skin against a seating surface [12,13,16]. Tools that are available to the provider will further assist in the evaluation process. Although there is no means of directly measuring skin ischemia, pressure mapping correlates potential problem areas that are likely to develop pressure sores. Pressure sore management works on the theory that if tissue compression exceeds the capillary pressure within the tissue, an ischemic response will occur in the adjacent tissue, leading to skin breakdown [13].

This tool does not address concerns related to shearing forces, moist or macerated tissue, skin breakdown due to infection (such as osteomyelitis) or poor nutrition (low albumin levels), or inadequate hydration. Other factors to consider are the patient's metabolism, the location of the wound, the chronicity of the wound, and the patient's age [17]. Studies indicate that direct pressure greater than 32 mm Hg, upward of 40 to 60 mm Hg, is indicative of a increased risk for skin breakdown [13,18]. It is important to keep in mind that pressure mapping is only a tool. In the opinion of the authors, when a patient does not map particularly well on his or her existing cushion, this does not necessarily mean that drastic changes need to be made to the seating system. If a patient does not have skin redness and has been on a particular type of cushion for some time, a change in the seating system is not always required. Identifying the cause of breakdown, which may be difficult to ascertain from the patient, is crucial in determining the best type of intervention to address the problem. Failure to investigate and identify the cause of skin breakdown may lead to chronic wounds.

Box 2. Some questions to ask patients who have skin breakdown

Has there been any recent change in your daily routine?
How often do you perform pressure relief?
Have you had a change in medical status?
Are you having difficulty with transfers?
When is the last time your cushion was replaced?

Table 1
Common areas of skin breakdown

Areas of breakdown	Possible cause	Possible corrections
Ischial tuberosities	Direct pressure	Assess cushion status; use pressure mapping as guide. Check wound status and appearance of wound. Monitor out of bed time. Increase frequency and duration of pressure reliefs.
Greater trochanters	Wheelchair too small	Reassess width of wheelchair.
Fibular head	Pressing against leg-rest	Minimal correction—placement of gel or foam padding Moderate correction—hip guides to realign femur into more adducted position off leg-rest
Sacrum	Sacral sitter	Assess pelvic positioning and correct or accommodate pelvic obliquity. Assess cushion status.

Box 2 lists some questions to assist in finding the cause of breakdown. When pressure is suspected as the culprit in the development of skin breakdown, pressure mapping is a useful tool to determine a more appropriate cushion [17]. Some common areas of skin breakdown are listed in Table 1.

Given that measurement of capillary pressure requires invasive procedures, contact pressures are the most suitable noninvasive method [13]. Information is gathered from a pressure sensing mat that is analyzed by a connected computer and may display the pressure readings with color-coded visual and numeric data (Fig. 1). This information may be used during an assessment to make an objective decision about acceptable levels of pressure for patients. Clinicians may make appropriate decisions based on the readings given by different seating surfaces [12].

Consideration of the patient's cognitive status in light of the aforementioned factors is important. A patient who is not cognizant of the environment and is unable to recognize safety problems may contribute to decreased safety in the wheelchair. Wheelchair-related falls may occur as a result of tipping and falling, propulsion over uneven terrain, poor transfer ability, reaching for objects, and poor management of curbs [19]. Careful consideration before ordering may prevent inappropriate wheelchair selection [8,19].

Once the evaluation is complete and the patient's needs and desires have been determined, the next step is to consider the product options.

Product options

Wheelchairs

Determining whether the patient needs a power chair or a manual chair is not as obvious as looking at the diagnosis. In SCI, it is common to say that a paraplegic will need a manual chair and a quadriplegic a power chair. However, the total picture of how the patient presents is important. Any condition that may preclude use of a manual wheelchair, such as paraplegia with respiratory or cardiac issues, needs to be acknowledged. Although one may think that "pushing is beneficial," the reality is that people who have such conditions will be prevented from going long distances with a manual chair, a situation that will detract from their independence [3,8]. This factor is important to consider with any

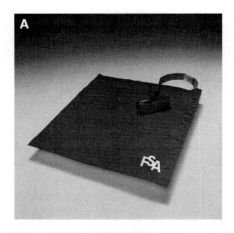

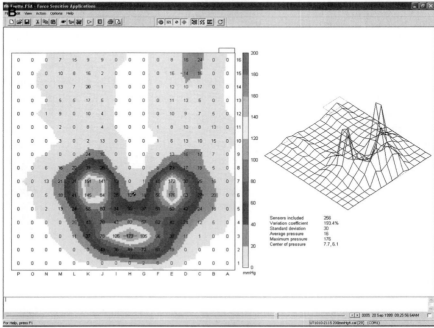

Fig. 1. (*A*) Pressure sensing mat data. (*B,C*) Pressure mat data. (*Courtesy of* Vista Medical Ltd., Winnipeg, Manitoba, Canada; with permission.)

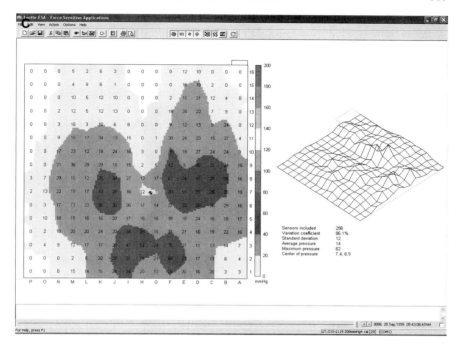

Fig. 1 (*continued*).

diagnosis in the geriatric population. The more complicated the medical picture (eg, arthritis and a cardiac condition), the more likely the patient will be to need powered mobility, depending on the severity of the condition [8].

The types of power wheelchair are front-wheel drive (Fig. 2), midwheel drive (Fig. 3), and rear-wheel drive (Fig. 4). As the name implies, front-wheel drive wheelchairs have the larger wheel in the front, midwheel drive chairs have the larger wheel in the middle, and rear-wheel drive chairs have the larger wheel posterior. In the past, rear-wheel drive wheelchairs were more frequently pre-scribed, because of the problems that resulted from midwheel drive casters' being off the ground. This arrangement often led to a rocking effect in the wheelchair, and the front casters tended to dig into the ground on softer surfaces. Recent adjustments made by manufacturers place the front and rear casters of the mid-wheel drive wheelchair onto the ground, decreasing the "see-saw effect" pre-viously encountered. This development has led to more frequent midwheel drive wheelchair orders. Midwheel drive wheelchairs offer a decrease in front turning radius, which can make this type of wheelchair more maneuverable in tight spaces (eg, apartment buildings) than its rear-wheel drive counterpart. Front-wheel drive wheelchairs offer decreased front turning radius, although this appearance may be misleading, given the increased rearward turning radius (tractor-trailer effect). A tendency can exist for rear-wheel slippage or "fish-tailing" at higher speeds in a front-wheel drive wheelchair. Rear-wheel drive

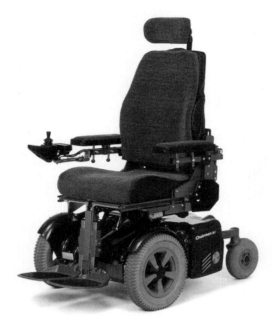

Fig. 2. Front-wheel drive power wheelchair. (*Courtesy of* Permobil, Inc., Lebanon, TN; with permission.)

wheelchairs place the rear wheel behind the center of gravity of the user, making the chair slightly longer. For people without space limitations, this is another option.

Scooters continue to be popular choices for the geriatric population because they grant impaired patients greater mobility (Fig. 5). Scooters offer trans-

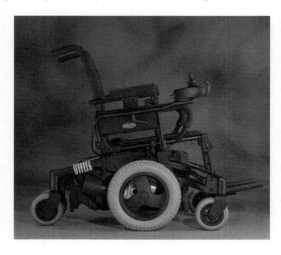

Fig. 3. Midwheel drive power wheelchair. (*Courtesy of* Invacare Corp., Elyria, OH; with permission.)

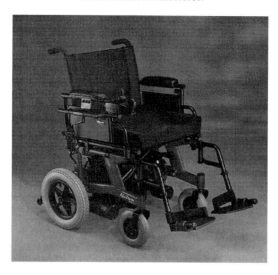

Fig. 4. Rear-wheel drive power wheelchair. (*Courtesy of* Invacare Corp., Elyria, OH; with permission.)

portability, ease of use, and often lower cost. Good candidates should be able to stand and transfer. Scooters can be tipsy (eg, unstable while turning on inclines) and difficult to maneuver indoors (eg, up to tables and desks). Scooters are not necessarily good choices for patients with postural stability needs.

Pressure relief may be provided to patients in various forms. In terms of mechanical options, the choices are tilt and recline. *Tilt* refers to an arrangement

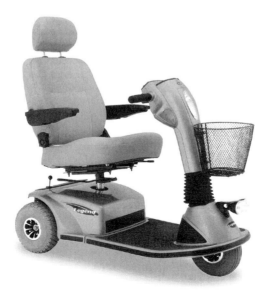

Fig. 5. Scooter. (*Courtesy of* Pride Mobility Corp., Exeter, PA; with permission.)

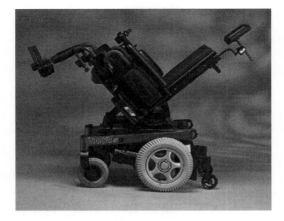

Fig. 6. Tilt. (*Courtesy of* Invacare Corp., Elyria, OH; with permission.)

where the relationship between the hips and torso remains the same and the patient's weight is transferred from the lower extremities to the torso (Fig. 6). *Recline* refers to an arrangement where the hip angle changes and the patient is moved into a supine position. Recline offers a greater amount of pressure relief because the forces are distributed across the entire portion of the body (Fig. 7). The concern that arises from the use of recline is that the patient may slide forward in the wheelchair when returning to a seated position and end up in a more sacral sitting posture. This will require frequent repositioning. Some research indicates that tilting backward to 65° is adequate in pressure reducing capacity [20] and does not require the frequent repositioning that is associated with recline. Generally speaking, tilt is more frequently ordered for patients.

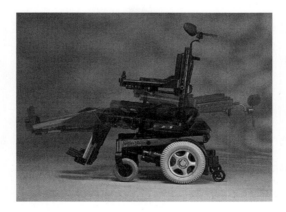

Fig. 7. Recline. (*Courtesy of* Invacare Corp., Elyria, OH; with permission.)

Frame

A folding frame wheelchair may be disassembled and folded to fit into a car, usually the trunk (Fig. 8). It can be considered heavy, however, weighing approximately 27 to 40 lbs with no accessories or wheels. The long-term wheelchair user has often become accustomed to this type of chair. Manufacturers have improved the weight of the folder by using lighter metals, but, because of the necessary cross bracing and additional hardware, these chairs are still rather heavy.

A rigid frame wheelchair includes no mechanical mechanism for horizontal folding of the chair. Rigid wheelchairs are easier to propel and lighter and offer more maneuverability than a folding frame wheelchair. In either case, given the individual's physical ability, they may require assistance for stowage in the trunk or backseat of a car. It is possible, however, to have the wheels of a rigid frame wheelchair removed and the back folded for placement in the trunk or backseat. In addition, the less energy is absorbed by the joints of the wheelchair, the more efficient propulsion is for the user. Rigid chairs can be as light as 15 lbs with no accessories. The reduced weight can make a significant difference for the elderly, especially for the wife or husband taking care of the patient. The industry is continually refining rigid chairs and removing more and more hardware, making them lighter. This lightness is advantageous to the user in that there is less stress on the shoulder and increased distance with each rotation [21].

Power-assist wheelchairs offer an alternative means of using a powered chair to patients who have limited endurance or orthopedic limitations of the upper extremity or who require wheelchair transportability. Some research indicates that power-assist wheelchairs reduce electromyographic activity in certain muscle groups, decrease stroke frequency, reduce perceived exertion, and decrease heart

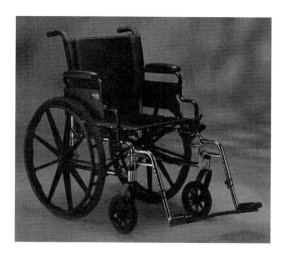

Fig. 8. Manual folding frame wheelchair. (*Courtesy of* Invacare Corp., Elyria, OH; with permission.)

rate [22,23]. The disadvantage of this type of wheelchair is the increased weight of the chair, which creates difficulty when attempting to stow it in a car. The other disadvantage is that, if the battery is not charged or the patient uses the chair over a long period, the patient may end up pushing as much as an extra 50 lbs of wheelchair when the battery has drained completely. Factors to consider before choosing this option are the weight of the patient and the type of terrain (eg, hills or rough terrain), both of which reduce battery life. The limited range capability presents problems for the active user.

Casters

Casters are the smaller wheels in the front of a wheelchair. Smaller casters offer more maneuverability but a harder ride. Larger casters offer a better ride over rougher terrain but tend to be less maneuverable. Casters come in a variety of sizes for manual wheelchairs, generally ranging from 3 to 8 in.

Tires

The tires on a chair can be crucial to maneuverability. Some tires are pneumatic (air filled), and others are solid and require no filling or maintenance. The pneumatic tire will give a smoother ride but may go flat, depending on the terrain. Pneumatic tires are lighter but require occasional maintenance (ie, filling with air). The flat free inserts give a harder ride, but this is a better option for the active user who does not want to get a flat in the middle of the street. Polyurethane and flat free tires offer durability but are also heavy. Cosmetically, this tire is less appealing for most patients. One should be sure to educate the patient and caregiver about all areas of wheelchair use, such as disassembly of the wheelchair and propulsion technique. Spokes are another option in the selection process. Spokes are lighter than mag (also known as composite or plastic) wheels.

Wheel locks

Several different wheel lock options are available for manual wheelchairs, including push-to-lock, pull-to-lock, extension handles, scissor locks, and hub locks. Push-to-lock and pull-to-lock are engaged as the name implies. Extension handles offer an easier securing of the locks for those patients who have shoulder, elbow, or wrist problems. Scissor locks are hidden beneath the seat and pose less of a concern for catching clothing when performing a transfer. Scissor locks can be problematic in that they may not secure against the tire when it has deflated. Hub locks offer a pin-style locking system attached to the hub: a secure locking system with minimal sway.

Hand-rims

Hand-rim options include aluminum or titanium, plastic coating, ergonomic grip or "foam grip," and projections. The plastic and foam grips allow for more traction to promote ease of pushing. However, when the chair is going downhill, there could be rubbing that causes a good deal of friction, potentially causing skin trauma. This may happen even when the patient is wearing wheelchair push gloves. Aluminum and titanium can be slippery to push but do not have the problems with friction associated with plastic-coated or foam rims. The ergonomic grip allows the thumb to rest comfortably while pushing.

Arm-rests

Arm-rests may be full length, for full support, or desk length, which enables the patient to access tables and desks. They may be fixed or height adjustable; may flip back or be removable. Arm-rests can provide balance for safe sitting postures. They are also important for repositioning and transferring out of the chair and in functional terms. For instance, many users require the arm-rest for pressure relief in a push-up or for use during a transfer. Additionally, arm-rests have hand-rests that act as splints for the hands in positioning and prevent contractures.

Leg-rests

A decision on the style of leg-rest is actually a decision about how the patient functions. Does he or she need to swing away so he or she can transfer and get closer to things or need rigidity for less hardware and overall lightness? Are the patient's legs rest abducted, so that getting two leg-rests might place pressure on the outer calf, causing breakdown? If so, one might consider a pedestal single flip-up plate to rest on, so there is nothing on the side of the lower leg. If the patient needs the swing away for transfer but his or her legs do lean on the leg-rests, many companies offer padding to alleviate the pressure.

The angle of the leg-rest or hanger is dependent on how the patient wants to be positioned in the chair. If patients want a tighter fit or a look of "less chair," they will go with the higher degree of foot-rest, because the angle is measured from a line coming horizontally from the seat of the chair. Therefore, a 60° leg-rest would be angled out the farthest, with an 85° leg-rest sitting almost perpendicular to the seat of the chair. Some patients have hamstring limitations in which a higher angle of hanger would help better maintain their feet on the foot-rest at a higher angle. If patients are placed in 60° leg-rests without sufficient hamstring length, they will most likely end up in a sacral sitting posture to reach the foot-rest. The foot-rest, which is at the end of the leg-rest to position the foot, can be a lightweight composite for ease of moving or a heavier, extra-large footplate for durability. Flip-up footplates may make transfers easier; if safety is a concern, swing-away leg-rests are an option. Also, one may order heel loops to prevent slipping or toe loops to prevent the foot from sliding forward in the chair.

Elevating leg-rests, like 60° leg-rests, can pull patients into sacral sitting position. Moreover, they require an increased turning space, because the chair is longer. This may be an option for patients with rigid contractures who cannot flex into traditional position or for those with comfort issues. Postorthopedic conditions are another reason patients may need an elevating leg-rest. This leg-rest makes the chair more susceptible to breakdown, because there are more moving parts. One consideration is whether the patient can independently operate, maneuver, and raise the leg-rests without falling out of the wheelchair.

Elevating leg-rests are often misconstrued as being useful for reducing edema. However, the leg is not above the level of the heart, which is necessary for venous return [7].

Wheelchair backs

The types of wheelchair backs vary. Some chairs are fitted with backs made from vinyl/material. Material backs offer low cost and, in some cases, a means of adjusting tension. The tension adjustment may be useful when one is trying to accommodate or correct kyphotic curves and other spinal malalignments. It allows one to provide a tighter fit in the lumbar region, with a looser thoracic level support, so the patient may sit in the chair with the curvature of the spine intact. Backs made from nonrigid materials may suffer from sagging, and the user may ultimately be placed in a posturally compromised position. For the patient who has advanced postural decay, an aftermarket add-on back may be beneficial. These backs are added to an existing wheelchair and offer a more aggressive approach, by way of contouring, to repositioning and stabilizing the trunk and upper body. They also offer the clinician the opportunity to make coarse and fine adjustments to the seat-to-back angle and back height and offer greater control through the addition of supplemental positioning components.

The height of a back-rest is dependent on many factors. If the patient is in a power chair with tilt, it will require a higher back for trunk support. Many elderly people feel safer with a high back, whereas some feel it pushes them forward. There are custom backs with molded supports on the side for a patient who has decreased trunk stability. This effect may also be achieved with lateral supports connected to the back canes. Backs with more padding are available for a patient who has trouble with breakdown or seeks greater comfort.

Accessories

Some accessories to the wheelchair include backpacks, seat pouches, cargo nets, luggage carriers, extension handles for the brakes, cup-holders, lap-desks, seatbelts, chest straps, and crutch holders. Wheelchairs are generally sold with the most common options in place. Patients may require additional options for purposes of improved safety or enhanced function. These additional items should not be viewed as frivolous accessories. Rather, they should be considered important components that help to define the technical configuration of the chair and the usability of the device.

Wheelchair safety

Of great concern when considering a wheelchair for a geriatric user is safety. Options such as wheel-lock extensions that extend the length of the locking handle can make it easier for the user to reach and use the locks. Safety belts come in many models with different types of buckles. Seatbelts can be a critical prevention tool for avoiding falls [19]. Depending on the user's hand and arm function, some will be easier to operate than others.

Optional upgraded electronics for a powered wheelchair can enhance use by allowing adjustments that control speed, braking distance, and turning speed and may be dampened to minimize the effects of tremors and spasms when the patient is controlling the wheelchair.

Scooter options such as full swiveling seats help a user access the device safely. Elevating seats can assist users in safely reaching for items and enable them to set the seat at safe heights for transferring to and from the device. Bags and totes play an important role in organizing the user's traveling items and keeping important items, such as medications, medical supplies, and ADL devices, from getting lost—or, worse, winding up under the user, where they may cause skin breakdown.

Any of the aforementioned options should be tailored to the patient's needs. The variables in terms of the patient's terrain, primary use, and so forth will help guide the decision-making process to suit the patient's needs. Wheelchair components and some common problems are listed in Table 2.

Cushions

Three primary types of cushions exist (Table 3): air filled, fluid filled or gel, and foam. Custom cushions and dynamic cushions may be used in specialized situations. The advantages and disadvantages of each type are discussed here.

Table 2
Wheelchair components and common problems

Wheelchair component	Intended function	Common problem	Correction
Casters	Maneuvers/pushes wheelchair.	Caster flutter	Tighten caster. Align caster angle (squaring caster).
Rear tires (manual, air-filled)	Maneuvers/pushes wheelchair.	Patient has multiple flat tires.	Consider alternative tire (eg, flat-free insert, Kik tire).
Wheel lock	Secures rear wheel during transfers.	Tire is moving with brake application. Lock is difficult to engage.	Inflate rear tire. Adjust the locks. Rear wheel may be overinflated; consider using brake extensions.
Hand-rim	Patient grasps during pushing of manual wheelchair.	Plastic-coated hand-rim causes excessive friction on patient's hands during hill descent.	Consider using wheelchair gloves or aluminum hand-rims.
Arm-rest	Provides upper extremity support surface.	Patient is unable to approach a table or desk.	Consider changing from full-length arm-rest to desk length or adjusting seat-to-floor height.

Table 3
Cushions

Cushions	General advantages	General disadvantages
Air	Good pressure relief ability	Greater instability with transfers
Fluid/Gel	Moderate pressure relief	Temperature changes can affect consistency of fluid.
Foam	More stable cushion Minimal to moderate pressure relief ability	Not good for patients at high risk for skin breakdown.

Air cushions

Air cushions are generally rubber designed cushions with multiple air bladders. These types of cushions offer good pressure relief capabilities [24]. The disadvantage is the inherent instability of the air-filled bladders. Patients who have difficulty with transfers but do not necessarily require high pressure relief characteristics may be candidates for more stable cushions. Maintenance is also required with these cushions. The user must be cognizant of when to refill and needs to be trained properly to inflate the cushion [17]. Overinflation or under-inflation could have deleterious effects [25,26]. The bladders can be punctured or burned with cigarettes, rendering the cushion unusable.

Fluid cushions

Fluid cushions offer foam in areas that are not prone to skin breakdown (mid- to distal femur) and have a fluid material in the posterior segment encompassing the sacrum and ischial tuberosities. This style offers improved stability over the air cushions but generally with fewer pressure-relief characteristics. A disadvantage of this type of cushion is that it may become too hard or soft at extremes of temperature. Another disadvantage is the increased weight.

Foam cushions

A number of variants of foam-type cushions exist, ranging from poorly pressure-reducing styles to memory-type foams that offer good pressure-reducing qualities. Generally speaking, foam cushions last 1 to 2 years before needing replacement.

Custom design cushions

Custom design cushions offer an option for patients who have chronic skin breakdown as a result of pressure. These cushions are designed to redistribute pressure away from more problematic areas, such as the ischial tuberosities, and redistribute pressure to the femurs, greater trochanters, and the sacrum. This effect is achieved with a cut-out area where the patient sits. This cushion allows for postural corrections or accommodations because it is made from an impression of the patient's seating area. The patient needs to be able to sit in the cut-out area for this type of cushion to be effective. Patients who have skin breakdown in the redistribution areas are not good candidates for this type of cushion.

Some companies offer a cushion design that allows water and moisture to pass through, which may be of benefit to patients who are incontinent. It also may help avert maceration of the skin.

Dynamic cushions

The dynamic cushion is made up of air bladders that inflate and deflate through a battery-operated pump. The air bladders are divided into sections for different problem seating areas, for example, the ischial tuberosities and the sacrum. The idea is to alternate pressure under the seating area by alternately filling and deflating the air tubes in sections. The cushion creates a circulation by acting like a muscle pump. This effect may be beneficial for wound healing, although not enough research substantiates this claim [25]. For patients who are static, cannot move, and have frequent skin breakdown, this cushion may offer the possibility of healing without staying in bed.

Even with a good cushion, patients need to be able to perform frequent pressure reliefs to prevent skin breakdown, especially those who have decreased or absent sensation.

Other considerations

More considerations warrant mention. For instance, there are wheelchair travel considerations. For the patient who travels a great deal, an important feature is how well the manual chair will disassemble. In terms of power wheelchairs, the patient will require lockdowns (to secure the chair) to be installed on the chair for riding in vehicles.

Cognitive issues play a role in determining how well the patient can control the chair. Sometimes a power chair is not a viable option for a patient who would not remember how to drive the chair or would be unsafe in the handling of power.

Common in the geriatric population is the fear of technology. A power chair and its intricacies can be overwhelming and at times intimidating. Although some individuals may easily adjust, others may remain fearful and reluctant to use the device. At these times, provider and family member support becomes important. Having access to people who understand the technology and who can work with the user in a supportive manner helps to dispel fears. An extended initial trial of the chair, before prescription and purchase, may help to acclimate the user. Geriatric users should always be given the benefit of extensive training with a clinician or caregiver who is familiar with the wheelchair. Training in the proper management of the device should also be extended to caregivers and family members who are part of the user's support system [8].

The patients living longer with complex medical issues, such as respiratory dysfunctions (eg, chronic obstructive pulmonary disease), diabetes, and cardiac issues, are in need of assistive technology that will provide greater energy conservation and thus greater ability to complete ADLs. Educating the patient on propulsion technique can lead to a more efficient stroke pattern [27,28].

Energy conservation is an important factor for this population. Often geriatric persons with limited ambulation expend a great deal of energy in getting to a destination, as do many manual wheelchair users—so much so that, when they arrive at their destinations, they are too tired to benefit from the event. Arriving in a fatigued state for a therapy session, a social event, or a recreational activity defeats the purpose. One should not confuse mobility with therapy. Struggling to ambulate is not therapy. One should afford one's patients the appropriate wheeled mobility device so that they may benefit from the activities and treatments at the end of the trek. Some research indicates that the tilt angle of the wheelchair, but not the amount of recline, can affect the amount of effort required to push a manual wheelchair [29,30].

Being comfortable in a wheelchair is a primary concern for most geriatric users. Other clinical and technical realities may be just as important but will be less upsetting to the user. Discomfort when using the wheelchair can result in the patient's rejection of the device, emotional agitation, and injury from attempts to stand up and leave the wheelchair environment. Many individuals will opt to spend extended periods of time in bed rather than suffer discomfort in a wheelchair. Poor seated and functional posture may develop from willful repositioning away from the discomfort stimuli. Repositioning in a poor position may add pressure to tissue covering an ischial tuberosity or a trochanter. The unbalanced pressure situation may then result in tissue trauma to the area.

It is always important to monitor for skin changes, although especially so in a new chair or new cushion. Areas of redness mean an increase in pressure that could lead to breakdown. When this is seen, the caregiver or patient should tell his or her physician or therapist so the problem may be corrected, if indeed it is being caused by an aspect of the wheelchair or seating surface.

When available, trialing wheelchairs may help the patient get a feel for the chair before it is ordered. A trial can also help the treating clinicians, caregivers, and family members understand the workings of the chair [11].

The patient who spends most of his or her time in a wheelchair will develop postural conditions in relation to the chair. When one is fitting the patient, starting out with good posture (so long as it renders the patient functional) will help allay these conditions. Delaying the development of orthopedic conditions will avert or reduce long-term complications.

To avoid deformities and contractures, the wheelchair should fit the user properly, and the trunk, pelvis, and extremities should be aligned as best as possible. For orthopedic purposes, a wheelchair should be viewed as an orthotic device [11]. The skeletal system should be maintained in the best seated alignment possible. Joints should not be overly extended, flexed, rotated, depressed, protracted, or retracted. The trunk, pelvis, and extremities should maintain an acceptable alignment similar to that which is demonstrated in any good seated posture, in or out of a wheelchair.

In the event that there is poor postural alignment, it should be dealt with immediately. Positioning devices, adjustment of the wheelchair components and angles, and switching to a more supportive cushion should all be considered.

Joints and extremities that are left in poor alignment or unsupported are much more likely to develop problems. Evidence suggests that, with proper positioning, mechanical strain on musculoskeletal tissue and joints may be reduced [31]. Despite corrections, long-term orthopedic problems may develop as a result of wheelchair propulsion [8].

Geri-chairs are particularly problematic in this population. Often geri-chairs are used for patients because of weakness, behavioral problems, or contractures or for lack of a wheelchair. They are frequently misused; proper positioning is difficult to maintain and may lead to detrimental effects in the long term. To compound the problem, patients in such chairs are less likely to be involved in social activities secondary to the inherent difficulty of maneuvering. This type of chair should not be for long-term use [6,7].

Future directions

No significant body of formal research covers the geriatric population and its seating and mobility needs. Much of the authors' experience and knowledge comes from seating patients who have lost significant muscular function,

---

Box 3. List of resources

www.invacare.com
www.sunrisemedical.com
www.permobil.com
www.tilite.com
www.kuschallna.com
www.falconrehab.com
www.motionconcepts.com
www.pridemobility.com
www.ridedesigns.com
www.stealthproducts.com
www.aelseating.com
www.ottobockus.com
www.rohogroup.com
www.starcushion.com
www.pressuremapping.com
www.resna.org

For the patient and clinician

www.usatechguide.org

regardless of age. Some of the research used in this article is based in the SCI population and has been extrapolated to the general geriatric population. The geriatric patient with aging components demonstrates a higher level of need for proper positioning. Research that examined wheelchair use over the long term and how being confined to a wheelchair after a life of ambulation creates special needs would be beneficial.

Summary

In a properly seated patient, mobility and function are maximized. When patients can maintain the lifestyle to which they are accustomed, overall compliance and independence are enhanced. When patients cannot do what is important to them, the wheelchair will most likely not be used. One should also keep in mind that what worked in the past for a patient may not work any longer. (See list of online resources in Box 3. The following list should not be construed as an endorsement of the following products.) Finally, one should always check areas of skin breakdown and attempt to find the cause and reduce pressure.

Acknowledgments

The authors would like to thank Ziggi Landsman, Director of Assistive Technology, United Spinal Association, for all his help and feedback on this article.

References

[1] Kaye HS, Kang T, LaPlante M. University of California, San Francisco. Disability Statistics Center. Publication abstract #23. Wheelchair use in the United States. Available at: http://dsc.ucsf.edu/publication.php?pub_id=1. Accessed July 11, 2005.

[2] Bourret E, Bernick L, Cott C, et al. The meaning of mobility for residents and staff in long-term care facilities. J Adv Nurs 2002;37(4):338–45.

[3] Brandt A, Iwarsson S, Stahle A. Older people's use of powered wheelchairs for activity and participation. J Rehabil Med 2004;36(2):70–7.

[4] Rader J, Jones D, Miller L. The importance of individualized wheelchair seating for frail older adults. J Gerontol Nurs 2000;26(11):24–32.

[5] Guide to Physical Therapy Practice. 2nd edition. Phys Ther 2001;81.

[6] Rader J, Jones D, Miller L. Individualized wheelchair seating: reducing restraints and improving comfort and function. Topics in Geriatric Rehabilitation 1999;15(2):34–47.

[7] Rappl L, Jones D. Seating evaluations: special problems and interventions for older adults. Topics in Geriatric Rehabilitation 2000;16(2):63–72.

[8] Minkel JL. Seating and mobility considerations for people with spinal cord injury. Phys Ther 2000;80:701–9.

[9] Cooper RA. Wheelchair selection and configuration. New York: Demos Medical Publishing; 1998.

[10] Batavia M. The wheelchair evaluation: a practical guide. Boston: Butterworth-Heinemann; 1998.

[11] Ham R, Aldersea P, Porter D. Wheelchair users and postural seating: a clinical approach. New York: Churchill Livingstone; 1998.

[12] Stinson MD, Porter-Armstrong AP, Eakin PA. Pressure mapping systems: reliability of pressure map interpretation. Clin Rehabil 2003;17:504–11.

[13] Sugama J, Sanada H, Takahashi M. Reliability and validity of a multi-pad pressure evaluator for pressure ulcer management. J Tissue Viability 2002;12(4):148–53.

[14] Brienza D, Karg P, Geyer M, et al. The relationship between pressure ulcer incidence and buttock-seat cushion interface pressure in at-risk elderly wheelchair users. Arch Phys Med Rehabil 2001;82:529–33.

[15] Gusenoff J, Redett R, Nahabedian M. Outcomes for surgical coverage of pressure sores in non-ambulatory, nonparaplegic, elderly patients. Ann Plast Surg 2002;48(6):633–40.

[16] van Dijk D, Aufdemkampe G, van Langeveld S. The QA pressure measurement system: an accuracy and reliability study. Spinal Cord 1999;37:123–8.

[17] Sprigle S. Effects of forces and the selection of support surfaces. Topics in Geriatric Rehabilitation 2000;16(2):47–62.

[18] Conine T, Hershler C, Daeschsel D, et al. Pressure sore prophylaxis in elderly patients using polyurethane foam or Jay wheelchair cushions. Int J Rehabil Res 1994;17:123–37.

[19] Gavin-Dreschnack D, Nelson A, Fitzgerald S, et al. Wheelchair-related falls: current evidence and directions for improved quality care. J Nurs Care Qual 2005;20(2):119–27.

[20] Henderson JL, Price SH, Brandstater ME, et al. Efficacy of three measures to relieve pressure in seated persons with spinal cord injury. Arch Phys Med Rehabil 1994;75(5):535–9.

[21] Beekman C, Miller-Porter L, Schoneberger M. Energy cost of propulsion in standard and ultralight wheelchairs in people with spinal cord injuries. Phys Ther 1999;79(2):146–58.

[22] Levy L, Chow J, Tillman M, et al. Variable-ratio pushrim-activated power-assist wheelchair eases wheeling over a variety of terrains for elders. Arch Phys Med Rehabil 2004;85:104–12.

[23] Algood S, Cooper R, Fitzgerald S, et al. Impact of a pushrim-activated power-assisted wheelchair on the metabolic demands, stroke frequency, and range of motion among subjects with tetraplegia. Arch Phys Med Rehabil 2004;85:1865–71.

[24] Yuen H, Garrett D. Comparison of three wheelchair cushions for effectiveness of pressure relief. Am J Occup Ther 2001;55(4):470–5.

[25] Hamanami K, Tokuhiro A, Inoue H. Finding the optimal setting of inflated air pressure for a multi-cell air cushion for wheelchair patients with spinal cord injury. Acta Med Okayama 2004; 58(1):37–44.

[26] Brienza D, Geyer M. Using support surfaces to manage tissue integrity. Adv Skin Wound Care 2005;18(3):151–7.

[27] de Groot S, Veeger H, Hollander A, et al. Adaptations in physiology and propulsion techniques during the initial phase of learning manual wheelchair propulsion. Am J Phys Med Rehabil 2003;82(7):504–10.

[28] de Groot S, Veeger H, Hollander A, et al. Effect of wheelchair stroke pattern on mechanical efficiency. Am J Phys Med Rehabil 2004;83(8):640–9.

[29] Aissaoui R, Arabi H, Lacoste M, et al. Biomechanics of manual wheelchair propulsion in elderly: system tilt and back recline angles. Am J Phys Med Rehabil 2002;81(2):94–100.

[30] Samuelsson K, Tropp H, Nylander E, et al. The effect of rear-wheel position on seated ergonomics and mobility efficiency in wheelchair users with spinal cord injuries: a pilot study. J Rehabil Res Dev 2004;41(1):65–74.

[31] Makhsous M, Lin F, Hendrix R, et al. Sitting with adjustable ischial and back supports: biomechanical changes. Spine 2003;28(11):1113–21.

ELSEVIER
SAUNDERS

CLINICS IN
GERIATRIC
MEDICINE

Clin Geriatr Med 22 (2006) 377–394

Prosthetics and Orthotics for the Older Adult with a Physical Disability

Bruce Pomeranz, MD[a,b,*], Uri Adler, MD[a,b],
Nigel Shenoy, MD[a], Cynthia Macaluso, PT[a],
Shailesh Parikh, MD[a]

[a]*Kessler Institute for Rehabilitation, 300 Market Street, Saddle Brook, NJ 07663, USA*
[b]*Department of Physical Medicine and Rehabilitation, University of Medicine and
Dentistry of New Jersey, New Jersey Medical School, 30 Bergen Street, Newark, NJ 07663, USA*

Prosthetics and orthotics serve many functions for the elderly and disabled. Assessment of patients in need of such devices is discussed. Prosthetic and orthotic devices are described with attention to their components, biomechanical effects, and potential value to patients. Strategies for selecting the proper device are presented. Structured rehabilitation is vital to ensure that patients maximally benefit from these devices; strategies for optimizing a rehabilitation program are discussed.

Lower-extremity amputations and prosthetic devices

Epidemiology

Most lower-extremity amputations experienced by a geriatric population are associated with vascular disease [1]. Trauma and tumor are less common reasons for amputation. Diabetics in particular are at significant risk for lower-extremity amputation. Upper-extremity amputations are significantly less common and are not discussed here in detail.

* Corresponding author. Kessler Institute for Rehabilitation, 300 Market Street, Saddle Brook, NY.
  E-mail address: bpomeranz@kessler-rehab.com (B. Pomeranz).

0749-0690/06/$ – see front matter © 2006 Elsevier Inc. All rights reserved.
doi:10.1016/j.cger.2005.12.006

The impact of lower-extremity vascular disease may lead to skin breakdown and nonhealing skin ulcers, or osteomyelitis. Gangrene may develop gradually in the foot (dry gangrene); a purple toe is a common manifestation of dry gangrene. Wet gangrene may occur rapidly followed by an urgent lower-extremity amputation to prevent life-threatening sepsis.

Surgical treatments, such as peripheral bypass surgery, offer the potential to improve circulation to the lower extremity and prevent the need for an amputation. Prognosis for lower-extremity bypass surgery is best when the bypass is proximal (iliac-femoral arteries compared with tibial arteries) and the success rate is better when grafting with an individual's own vasculature (eg, saphenous vein graft) as opposed to a synthetic vein graft [2].

The geriatric upper-extremity amputee population is different than the lower-extremity population. As a group, the amputation happens earlier in life and the patient is familiar with their prosthesis by the time they reach this stage of life. Trauma is the leading cause of acquired upper-extremity amputation. It accounts for close to 80% of all amputations. Most of these are amputations of the digits and occur in men in the 20- to 40-year-old age group. The rest of the amputations occur as a result of disease (tumors, vascular, infectious) [3]. The ratio of upper-extremity to lower-extremity amputation is approximately 1:5. As such, upper-extremity prostheses are not further discussed here.

Terminology and determination of amputation level

Amputations are typically classified based on the anatomic location of the amputation. Transtibial is an amputation below the knee, commonly referred to as a "below-knee amputation." Transfemoral is an amputation above the knee, commonly referred to as an "above-knee amputation." Foot amputations consist of (1) ray amputations, a single toe; (2) transmetatarsal, transection of the metatarsal bones (at times, some of the tarsal bones are amputated [transtarsal]); and (3) Syme's amputation, the entire foot at the ankle.

The determination of level of amputation incorporates the principle of retaining as much as possible of the limb while preserving a high likelihood of successful healing; this sets the stage for maximized independent function in the future. For example, a transtibial amputation is obviously preferable and significantly more functional than a transfemoral amputation. A toe amputation, however, followed by a transmetatarsal amputation, with subsequent revision to a transtibial and finally a transfemoral amputation is a physically and emotionally disheartening sequence of events [4].

Preprosthetic period

The period immediately following an amputation is the preprosthetic period. Typically, prosthesis is not fabricated until good healing has occurred (weeks to months later). This initiates the prosthetic period of the rehabilitation process. Issues during the preprosthetic period include edema control, skin and wound management, pain control, maintenance of range of motion and strength, and functional training.

Edema of the residual limb is expected after surgery. Reducing edema facilitates healing and helps to control pain. Edema may be controlled with elastic wrap using a figure-of-eight technique or an elastic shrinker sock. At times, a rigid, immediate postoperative or rigid removable dressing is used [5].

Pain naturally results from the surgical procedure itself. In addition, amputees often experience phantom limb sensation, and the more disturbing phantom pain. Phantom limb sensation may be described as a perception that all or part of the amputated limb is still present. This common phenomenon is generally not painful, usually improves with time, and may respond to desensitization techniques [6].

Phantom pain may be described as a perception that all or part of the amputated limb is still there and it hurts. The pain is frequently described as neuropathic in quality. Phantom pain is more likely to be a problem when chronic preoperative pain existed. Treatments include pain medications; desensitization techniques; prosthetic revisions; and pain management procedures (eg, nerve blocks).

During the preprosthetic period, individuals are vulnerable to loss in strength and range of motion (contractures). This usually does not impact significantly on an individual's daily life during the preprosthetic period. This complication may prevent optimal comfort and prosthesis use, however, during the prosthetic period.

In this period, especially for the unilateral amputee, it is also important to instruct the patient to become functionally independent with the intact limb. In upper-extremity amputees, this is especially important when the amputated side is the dominant side (as often is the case in traumatic amputees), because the patient's nondominant side will more than likely be responsible for most of the patient's activities of daily living. When the patient has a bilateral upper-extremity amputation, the side with the longer residual limb usually becomes the dominant side (even if before the injury it was the nondominant side) because of the biomechanical advantage offered by a longer residual limb.

Early acceptance and fitting of the prosthesis is essential. To ensure functional use and return to preamputation levels of function and return to occupation, Malone and coworkers [7] speaks of a 30-day "golden period" from time of amputation. After this time, the rate of successful prosthetic rehabilitation drops considerably.

Prosthetic period

Prosthetic components include the following [8]:

1. Socket: the interface between the residual limb and the prosthesis
2. Suspension: what secures the prosthesis to the body
3. Joints: depending on the level of amputation, these may include in the lower extremity the knee and ankle, and in the upper extremity the wrist, elbow, or shoulder

4. Terminal devices: in the lower extremity, the foot; in the upper extremity, the hand or the hook; unique to the lower extremity is a shank or pylon used to interface between the knee and foot

Socket

The sockets are generally total contact. This is to say that the entire surface area of the residual limb within the socket maintains contact with the internal socket wall. The lower-extremity prosthesis has to be able to bear the body weight safely and comfortably. Areas of the residual limb vary, however, with regard to pressure tolerance. Hard, bony areas, such as the anterior shaft of the residual tibia, are relatively pressure intolerant and vulnerable to skin breakdown. Soft tissue areas (eg, gastrocnemius muscle) are pressure tolerant; the socket may be designed to fit tighter in these areas. The standard transtibial socket is "patella tendon bearing." This describes the invagination in the socket at the area of the patella tendon. The fact that the patella tendon is relatively soft compared with some of the surrounding bony areas makes this a strategic design for holding the socket in place.

Suspension

The prosthetic socket may be suspended in a number of ways. These include various cuffs and sleeves, which hold the socket onto the residual limb. Suction, alone or in combination, is often a feature, which contributes to reliable suspension of the socket. Another type of popular suspension involves a pin on the bottom of a liner, which inserts and locks into a pinhole in the bottom of the socket.

Joints

The ankle joint is usually included in the foot (see terminal devices next). Depending on the level of the amputation a prosthetic knee or hip may be required. There are many different types of these joints. Discussion between the patient, therapist, prosthetist, and prescribing doctor is necessary to ensure the proper components are selected.

Terminal devices

The foot or terminal device serves as a shock absorber and provides a stable weight-bearing surface. Selection of a prosthetic foot often involves consideration of the balance between issues of mobility and stability. Dynamic feet are available, which facilitate running, jumping, and optimized activity. Although this is ideal for some amputees, a geriatric amputee or one with neurologic impairments is likely best off with a more stable, less dynamic foot.

The shank or pylon serves as a tube, which connects the socket to the prosthetic foot. Usually, these are endoskeletal in design. Endoskeletal refers to an internal, adjustable metal rod, which is typically covered with a cosmetic covering once the prosthesis is completed. An exoskeletal shank is a hard outer shell, which provides increased durability. The endoskeletal design is generally favored because they are lighter in weight, easier to adjust, and more cosmetically appealing. The exoskeletal design is used when durability is the major issue.

Rehabilitation and prosthetic training

In a rehabilitation center, a physiatrist works closely together with a physical therapist and prosthetist to optimize the outcome for an amputee. Shared information and diverse expertise frequently leads to interventions, prosthetic modifications, or training strategies that maximize an individual's comfort, endurance, and overall function with prosthesis.

Many factors impact on the capacity of an amputee to ambulate and function with prosthesis. Cardiac, neurologic, cognitive, visual, and overall medical status all impact on functional potential. Ambulation with prosthesis requires increased energy expenditure compared with that required for ambulation without a lower-extremity amputation. Oxygen consumption increases approximately 33% for a transtibial amputee and nearly doubles for a transfemoral amputee. A transfemoral amputee with severe cardiac or respiratory disease may have limited potential for functional independent ambulation with prosthesis [9].

The experience of an amputation and the associated rehabilitation process creates psychologic and emotional issues and challenges. Inclusion of a psychologist with the treatment team is an asset. The Amputee Coalition of America is a valuable resource to amputees. The Amputee Coalition of America sponsors support groups; serves as an educational resource; and provides a diversity of services to amputees, their families, and caregivers.

Spinal orthotic devices

This is a complex topic that requires a larger forum for full coverage. The following is a short synopses and coverage of a few common orthoses.

Spinal orthoses are used for many different reasons, such as pain control, protection, stabilization, immobilization, and enhancing function. Unfortunately, if complete immobilization of a segment is required, it is often very uncomfortable to the recipient. Also, these devices are often difficult to don and doff and can lead to skin breakdown, weakening of axial musculature, osteoporosis, nerve compression, and restriction in movement of the abdominal or thoracic cavities.

Nomenclature has been haphazard in the past. To standardize the nomenclature and to be more exact with the type of brace required, these braces are named by the segments they encompass and often with the description of the motion to be restricted. For example, a device that encompasses the neck only is called a cervical orthosis. If it also includes the head it is called a head-cervical orthosis. Another example is the thoracolumbosacral orthosis [10].

One can also specify in what plane to restrict the motion. A thoracic orthosis can be made only to restrict flexion. Often to immobilize a segment fully, the segment above and below also needs to be immobilized. It is for this reason that the head and sacral spine are the hardest segments to immobilize.

Some common orthoses

Cervical collars

These are either rigid or the more recognizable, soft, variety. These are poor at fully restricting motion but do provide feedback to limit motion. They also add warmth and comfort and are very well tolerated. They do not immobilize an unstable neck; however, they can be used over the short-term to relieve pain and provide partial support to soft muscle injury of the cervical spine.

Halo devices

These provide the most restriction of cervical motion. They do this by using pins to fix a metal ring to the upper portion of the head. This ring is connected to a body vest by way of metal rods. With a proper fitting vest and a tightened ring, except for a phenomenon known as "snaking," cervical spine movement is virtually eliminated.

Thoracolumbosacral orthoses flexion control

These are especially useful in the elderly population in the primary or secondary prevention, and for pain relief, of osteoporotic fractures. These devices prevent flexion, which is the spinal motion that leads to these fractures. It does allow extension of the thoracolumbar spine, which provides comfort and allows for proper strengthening to prevent further fractures. These devices can be tailored to fit many different needs. The degree of mobilization and location of the mobilization dictate which of these orthoses are needed. There are many other spinal orthoses beyond the scope of this article.

Lower-extremity orthoses and shoes

This is a broad and complex topic, which focuses on common conditions and devices seen in the geriatric population. Orthoses should be durable, functional, and cosmetically acceptable to the patient for optimal efficacy [11]. They are commonly made from thermoplastic, carbon composites, leather, metal, or a combination of these materials. Orthotic devices can be classified by the joint crossed and the distal body segment where it attaches. An ankle-foot orthosis (AFO) crosses the ankle and attaches to the foot distally. There are also knee-ankle-foot orthoses and hip-knee-ankle-foot orthoses (Fig. 1).

Shoes

Often a well-chosen shoe can reduce the need for an orthotic device. Shoes are worn to support, protect, and distribute body weight to the feet during walking

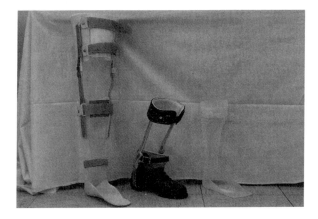

Fig. 1. (*left to right*) KAFO, metal AFO with t-strap attached to orthopedic shoe, molded AFO with posterior trim lines.

and standing. As such, they should be comfortable and conform to the shape of a patient's foot. Shoes should be about one index finger breadth longer than the longest toe to allow for movement of the foot during weight bearing and ambulation [12]. Loose shoes lead to increased friction over certain areas of the foot and can cause calluses, whereas tight shoes press on bony prominences and can cause ulcers or corns. Leather is a versatile material for most shoes because it is durable, breathable, warming, and conforms to a patient's shape over time. Leather shoes are suitable for most activities and can be easily modified.

Common shoe modifications

Once a shoe is appropriately fit to a patient, it can be modified for desired effect. Some factors to consider in shoe selection include skin sensation, skin integrity, lower-extremity edema, tone, and joint deformities. In patients with diabetes and peripheral neuropathy, shoes should have a high wide toe box to accommodate the toes and reduce pressure on any prominent areas. Patients with excessive tone around the ankle, chronic edema, or joint deformity should have shoes modified or be fit with custom orthopedic shoes that allow ease of donning and removal.

In general, shoes are modified to add stability, correct abnormal gait patterns, or to unload and redistribute forces encountered during ambulation and weight bearing. Excessive inversion and eversion at subtalar ankle joint can be compensated by a heel flare on either the medial or lateral heel depending on the motion being corrected. Lateral heel wedges promote eversion and can be used conservatively to treat medial compartment knee osteoarthritis. Lateral wedges distribute more force to the lateral knee compartment and unload the medial compartment of the knee. Medial heel wedges can be used in conjunction with medial sole wedges to promote supination, which corrects a flexible overly pronated foot. Whenever heel wedges are used the heel counter (posterior part of shoe upper) should be rigid enough to control the hind foot.

Severe metatarsal pain can be treated with a metatarsal bar on the external sole of the shoe to distribute the force to the metatarsal shafts rather than the metatarsal heads. Metatarsalgia can also be treated with a rocker bar, which is a convex bar on the external sole positioned posterior to the metatarsal heads to facilitate rollover and decrease pressure on the metatarsal heads. The increased height of the rocker bar requires an increase in heel height to facilitate rollover. In less severe cases an internal metatarsal pad can be placed inside the shoe posterior to the second through fourth metatarsal heads to distribute pressure; if this is not well tolerated by the patient, the metatarsal bar or rocker bar can be tried. Toe pain common in arthritis and gout, which is worse on ambulation, can be treated by decreasing flexibility of the shoe by adding extended shank with mild rocker sole thereby decreasing toe movement during ambulation.

Heel pain is commonly caused by plantar fasciitis, calcaneal spurs, and occasionally by tight heel cords. An external calcaneal bar analogous to the metatarsal bar can be used just posterior to the painful site to reduce symptoms during ambulation. Because overpronation can exacerbate plantar fasciitis, a Thomas heel with its medial anterior projection under the navicular bone can help push the foot into supination. Heel lifts or heel cushion relief (viscuelastic or gel cushion) pads within the shoe help cushion the heel and decrease Achilles tendon pain associated with excessive stretch on the tendon. Internal heel lifts can be used to correct a half-inch leg length discrepancy as measured from the tip of the anterior superior iliac spine to the medial malleolus. After correcting the first half-inch, additional discrepancy needs to be corrected with external heel pads. As the heel is built up, the sole also needs to be elevated with the addition of a rocker bottom to facilitate smooth transitions during ambulation.

Foot orthoses

Pronation and supination can also be controlled with foot orthoses. Soft foot orthoses are available over the counter; however, rigid and semirigid custom foot orthoses need to be fabricated by orthotists. Generally, soft foot orthoses provide some arch support and shock absorption. Fabricated foot orthoses are made to correct specific biomechanical abnormalities and are made from casts of patients' feet. Fabricated foot orthoses are semirigid and provide more arch support than soft orthoses and still have some shock absorption. In cases of severe pliable foot deformities a rigid foot orthosis is indicated.

As is the case with any rigid orthoses, it is important carefully to monitor patients' skin for any evidence of redness or breakdown. Semirigid foot orthoses can be used to treat flat and high-arched feet. They usually extend the length of the foot and provide arch support along the medial arch. In a high-arched foot they distribute some force along the arch in addition to functioning like an internal metatarsal pad. This supports the foot in gentle supination while pre-venting over supination. In a mildly flat foot, the medial build-up on the orthosis pushes the midfoot into slight supination. The medial build-up can be increased gradually so as not to overcorrect the deformity beyond the patient's tolerance. It is important that shoes be resized to accommodate foot orthoses, especially if they are used unilaterally.

Ankle foot orthoses

These are the most commonly used lower-extremity orthoses. They are commonly used to control motion at the ankle joint. Although they can provide static and dynamic control of ankle plantar flexion and dorsiflexion, they also afford mediolateral stability at the ankle. In addition, AFOs provide control of the knee during ambulation because of their effect on the ankle. Plantar flexion of the ankle helps to extend the knee and dorsiflexion of the ankle leads to flexion of the knee. During gait and weight bearing, AFOs exert effects on the knee, foot, and ankle, and have been shown to decrease the incidence of ankle contracture in patients with hemiparesis in upper motor neuron lesion (eg, acquired brain injury) [13]. AFOs are made from metal, leather, plastic, carbon composites, or some combination of these materials.

Thermoplastic AFOs are lightweight, durable, and compatible with most shoes; compact compared with metal AFOs; relatively inexpensive; and can provide control of the foot ankle and knee. Thermoplastic AFOs, also known as "molded AFOs" (MAFOs), can be custom made and cast to a patient's di-mensions, but they are also manufactured in various sizes that can be trialed on a patient. MAFOs are not pliable at room temperature and tend to be good for patients with sensate skin, stable lower-extremity edema, and good skin integrity.

The control of foot, ankle, and knee by MAFO depends on its trim line. The trim line refers to the anterior borders or edges at malleolar region of the MAFO. The width of ankle segment of MAFO determines the orthotic device's rigidity and its ability to control motion. Narrower MAFOs at the ankle joint exert less force to control motion during ambulation and weight bearing and are more flexible. Wider MAFOs are more rigid and can provide more mediolateral support; however, they can exert more force and tend to be worse at smooth energy transfer during ambulation. A hinge can be placed on a MAFO at the level of the malleoli to approximate the ankle joint. This facilitates energy transfer during gait and allows for control of plantar flexion or dorsiflexion during various phases of gait.

MAFOs have four basic components: (1) the calf shell, which encircles the calf; (2) the calf strap, which provides one proximal point of support; (3) the shoe insert, which goes into the shoe and helps control the foot; and (4) depending on the MAFO it may have a hinge at the level of the malleoli to simulate ankle movement. MAFOs shoe insert components should extend beyond metatarsal heads. MAFOs should provide enough dorsiflexion assist to clear the toes during ambulation. The MAFO calf shell should be about one inch below the fibular head to decrease the likelihood of peroneal nerve injuries. If the MAFO is to be worn unilaterally, the affected side's shoe should be about a half size bigger to accommodate the AFO. MAFOs can be modified using heat to deform the plastic in areas where there is too much pressure on a patient's skin.

Posterior leaf spring MAFOs have the narrowest trim line, and its calf shell encircles less than half the circumference. They function to aid weak ankle dorsiflexors during initial contact and swing phases of gait. They help to clear the foot during swing phase of gait. Posterior leaf spring MAFOs resist plantar flexion but do not prevent it. Because of their low narrow trim line, the posterior leaf spring is not considered when the ankle is unstable mediolaterally.

Solid AFOs restrict ankle dorsiflexion, ankle plantar flexion, and because of their anterior trim line in the foot can provide medial and lateral stability to the foot. They are useful to restrict motion at a painful ankle; help with plantar flexion spasticity after spastic hemiparesis (eg, acquired brain injury) [13]; and help treat foot drop in the setting of weak plantar flexors. It can be useful in minimizing motion at the ankle joint; however, because of its rigid nature and its lack of plantar flexion during stance, it can transmit forces proximally to destabilize the knee. Although it is important to monitor a patient's skin after use of any orthosis, because of its rigid nature it is necessary to re-evaluate the patient's skin in a solid AFO at each visit to monitor for evidence of breakdown.

A ground reaction AFO has a calf shell that wraps around the calf and takes advantage of the ground reaction force during ambulation to push the tibia posteriorly forcing the knee into extension while controlling motion at the ankle. This orthosis is useful in the setting of weak quadriceps with weak ankle dorsiflexors because it controls ankle motion and limits knee flexion. Hinged MAFOs can be used to control the ranges of plantar flexion and dorsiflexion, limited plantar flexion leads to more knee flexion, and limited dorsiflexion leads to more knee extension. Carbon composite AFOs are similar to MAFOs in function except that they cannot be modified once they have been manufactured. They come in various sizes and tend to be lighter and stronger that MAFOs.

Metal AFOs are also used to control motion at the ankle; however, their components and indications differ from those for MAFOs. The main components of a metal AFO include medial and lateral metal uprights attached to a shoe sole by a stirrup distally, with ankle joints in the metal uprights that allow for control of motion about the ankle joint. The metal AFO is attached proximally to the limb with a calf band. Metal AFOs are indicated for patients with insensate skin (eg, patients with neuropathy, fluctuating or excessive lower-extremity edema, or fragile skin as in the case of peripheral vascular disease) because there are fewer points of contact. Many older patients with metal AFOs who are candidates for plastic AFOs are hesitant to switch to MAFOs.

Padded resting ankle foot orthoses

Padded resting AFOs or multipodus boots are used to decrease pressure on a patient's heels during a period of being bed bound. They use a metal or carbon posterior upright to help attach the sheepskin-lined fasteners that distribute the weight of the patient's legs to reduce the likelihood of skin breakdown. In addition to distribution of weight, padded resting AFOs can be used for static positioning and correction of plantar flexion, eversion, and inversion deformity.

Unloading orthoses

These orthoses are total contact orthotic devices that use contact with soft tissues to unload distal segments of the lower extremities. Often called "patella tendon–bearing orthoses," these devices are used to support weight on the patella tendon and surrounding soft tissues to unload distal segments that may have healing skin ulcers, postoperative fusion, tibial fracture, or a more distal fracture that cannot take full weight bearing. They sometimes use a calf corset design to unload distal segments.

Knee-ankle-foot orthoses

Knee-ankle-foot orthoses provide mediolateral and anteroposterior stability to the knee, ankle, and foot through the combination of metal, leather, and plastic components. They usually involve an AFO with metal uprights, a metal knee joint, and thigh bands to anchor the device proximally. They can be used unilaterally in patients with polio and are often used bilaterally in patients with low thoracic or high lumbar spinal cord injuries. Knee-ankle-foot orthoses are often difficult to put on and remove; as such they tend to be used more for therapeutic walking and standing.

Knee orthoses

These devices only cross the knee and provide stabilization to the knee in various planes during ambulation. A knee unloader brace can be used to unload compartments of the knee affected by osteoarthritis. These braces apply external forces to the knee to decreased misalignment of the femur on the tibia to reduce the load on a particular compartment of the knee. Unloader braces are usually named medial or lateral for the knee compartment that is being unloaded. The Swedish knee cage is another example of an articulated knee orthosis, which is used for controlling hyperextension of the knee. It has mediolateral metal stays and a joint, which should approximate the femoral condyles. It uses a three-point system with one point above and one point below the knee as counter forces to the third point, which is behind the knee to help correct hyperextension during ambulation [14].

Lower-limb orthoses and shoes can be used to treat limb weakness, spasticity, pain, and joint deformities related to acquired brain injury, neuropathy, arthritis, or peripheral vascular disease in the geriatric population. Orthoses and shoes should be revaluated often to monitor for patient comfort, excessive wear, skin break down, and their effects on ambulation. Ideally, re-evaluation should occur through integrated communication with the patient, physical therapist, orthotist, and physician. Lower-extremity orthoses and appropriate footwear can reduce pain, decrease abnormal posture or tone, and can be used to correct abnormal gait patterns leading to increased efficiency during ambulation [11,14,15].

Physical therapy with prosthetics and orthoses

Therapy plays an integral role in preparing a patient for a lower-extremity orthotic or prosthetic device and training them with that device once it has been fabricated. A therapist is often asked to give their recommendation to a physician, orthotist, or prosthetist before a prescription is generated for an appropriate device. Once a patient receives a prosthetic or orthotic device, the therapist is then responsible for evaluating that patient with their device. After the initial evaluation has been completed, the therapist then designs goals with the physician, and their family taking into consideration their medical and social status and the results of their initial evaluation.

Goal setting for the authors' orthotic-prosthetic patients is very important because the goals become the foundation for treatment programs. The following are examples of common goals written for prosthetic and orthotic patients.

Independent home exercise program and patient-family education

Each patient or family member is issued a home exercise program once the initial evaluation has been completed. The patient and family are trained enabling them to perform the exercises at home independently. Home exercise programs may include flexibility exercises, strengthening exercises, and instructions on donning and doffing the prosthesis or orthotic device. Home exercise programs also include training on skin inspection and proper hygiene of their involved limb and device. Families are also trained in guarding techniques to assist their family member while performing all functional activities.

Independent preprosthetic-orthotic management

Before prosthetic training can begin all prosthetic candidates must be trained in residual limb wrapping. Residual limb wrapping controls edema, decreases pain, and increases circulation and healing. Wrapping is also important to obtain a conical-shaped residual limb to ease donning and doffing of the prosthesis. Residual limb shaping can be achieved with residual limb shrinker, ace wrap, or rigid or semirigid dressings [16]. Patients with orthotic devices may use compression stockings to help control edema of the lower extremity to prevent pressure sores. Prosthetic-orthotic patients are instructed on how properly to clean their residual limb or lower extremity and compressive socks or stockings on a daily basis.

Independent prosthetic-orthotic management

Prosthetic candidates and their families are trained on how to don and doff the prosthesis correctly. The patient and family are also trained on sock management, which includes instructing the patient and family on how properly to don and doff prosthetic socks and when to add or subtract prosthetic socks because of residual limb volume changes. Prosthetic training also includes skin inspection. Patients are trained how to inspect their skin for redness in pressure-sensitive areas, such as the crest of tibia on a transtibial amputee, on their residual limb that could lead to skin breakdown. Patients using orthotic devices are also trained how to don and doff the orthotic device correctly and inspect their skin once the orthosis has been taken off for redness as a result of pressure caused by improper orthotic fit or changes in lower-extremity edema.

Functional range of motion

Range-of-motion exercises are necessary to correct or prevent contractures. This can be accomplished by training the patient and family in proper positioning and range-of-motion exercises. Most commonly these patients develop hip or knee flexion contractures caused by poor positioning in bed and prolonged sitting in their wheelchair [16]. Patients using an orthotic device may also develop plantar flexion contractures because of loss of active movement. The patient and family are instructed on stretching exercises and proper positioning in bed or wheelchair to maintain flexibility, which enhances ambulation with a prosthetic-orthotic device. Maintaining or increasing trunk and upper extremity flexibility also allows for more efficient performance of functional activities.

Functional strength throughout

Energy expenditure for patients using an orthotic or prosthetic device is greater than an able-bodied individual [17]. Cardiovascular training is essential for these patients provided they are medically stable. Upper-extremity strengthening is also important to perform all transfers, bed mobility, donning and doffing of prosthetic-orthotic devices, and ambulation activities. Strengthening the trunk musculature helps to improve trunk stability, which enhances performance of all functional activities. Lower-extremity strengthening, with emphasis on the hip extensors, hip abductors, and knee flexors and extensors is very important in the patient with a an amputation. This enables a patient with a prosthetic device to accept weight through the prosthesis and allow them to ambulate efficiently [18]. Patients using orthotic devices are given exercise programs that include strengthening all of the lower-extremity musculature to help improve their gait pattern and allow them also to ambulate more efficiently.

Independent with desensitization activities

Prosthetic patients are also instructed on desensitization activities, which include massage and tapping to the residual limb and friction massage to the suture line to prepare the patient for weight bearing with the prosthesis [17].

Progressive weight bearing through the prosthesis also helps to desensitize the residual limb, improve strength around the hip and/or knee, and build up a tolerance to pressure on weight-bearing areas of their residual limb necessary for standing and ambulation activities (Fig. 2). Patients using orthotic devices are instructed on lower-extremity desensitization activities also to decrease hypersensitivity of the lower extremity to tolerate the pressure of the orthosis.

Improve balance to prevent falls and for independence of all functional activities

Patients requiring prosthesis or orthotic devices usually experience a loss of balance with functional activities. Amputees have been shown to have poorer static and dynamic balance than able-bodied individuals [19]. An amputee's balance can be challenged in different positions (ie, sitting, standing, quadriped, kneeling) with and without the prosthetic device. Patients are further challenged by placing them on soft or unstable surfaces, reaching for objects, picking objects up off the floor, obstacle courses, and accepting external forces while maintaining their balance. Objective measures are obtained on a patient's balance through use

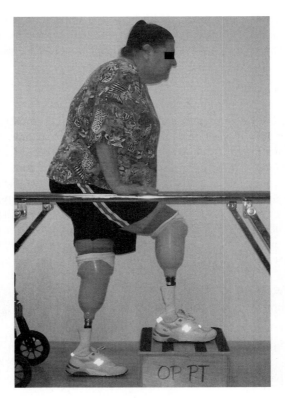

Fig. 2. Weight bearing activity.

of various balance tests. Loss of balance in standing or with ambulation activities caused by impaired motor control across the hip, knee, and ankle and diminished or absent sensation can be improved with the use of an orthotic device [20].

Independence with all activities of daily living

Dressing and hygiene

Patients are trained on proper cleaning and maintenance of their prosthetic-orthotic devices, residual limb socks, residual limb shrinkers, and footwear. Training is also given on proper care and cleaning of their affected and unaffected extremities. Patients are then trained on donning and doffing their lower body clothing while wearing a prosthetic-orthotic device.

Transfers

Patients perform various transfers with and without their prostheses or orthotic devices. They are trained to perform such transfers as wheelchair to bed, sit to stand with and without assistive device (Fig. 3), wheelchair or stand to toilet, wheelchair or stand to tub, wheelchair or stand to car, wheelchair to floor, and stand to floor (Fig. 4).

Ambulation

Initially, amputees are trained to ambulate safely with an appropriate assistive device without use of a prosthetic device for those occasions when they are unable to wear the prosthesis. Patients using prosthetic-orthotic devices are then

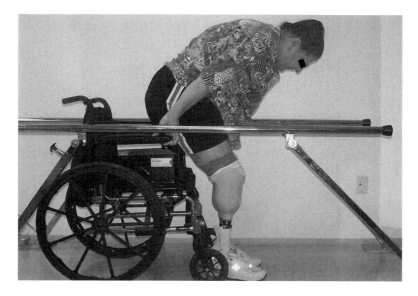

Fig. 3. Sit to stand transfer.

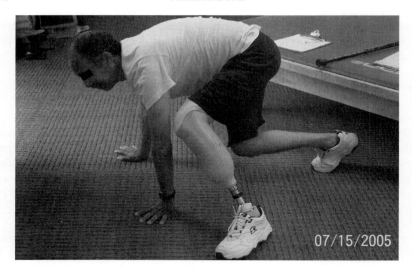

Fig. 4. Floor to stand transfer.

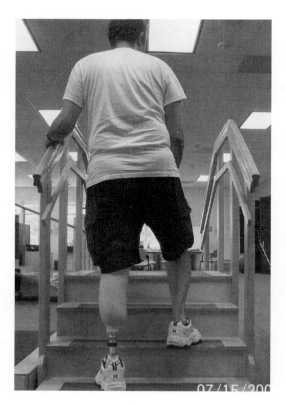

Fig. 5. Stair climbing.

trained to ambulate on even and uneven (ie, carpet, grass, sidewalks) surfaces with the appropriate assistive device. They are initially trained to ambulate household distances. If a patient is medically able, they are also trained to ambulate community distances.

Elevations

Ascending and descending elevations with a prosthetic-orthotic device includes 4-6-8 in stairs (Fig. 5) and 4-6-8 in curbs and inclines with and without the use of rail or assistive devices. Patients are also trained on bumping up and down stairs with or without their prosthetic-orthotic devices in case of an emergency.

Minimize gait deviations for safe and efficient ambulation on all surfaces

Once a patient receives the prosthetic-orthotic device the therapist performs a systematic check to determine if the device fits properly. The patient's gait pattern is then evaluated for deviations and asymmetry. Effective problem solving by the rehabilitation team helps to determine if the gait deviations are the result of a prosthetic-orthotic or a musculoskeletal issue.

Summary

Prosthetics and orthotics serve many purposes including optimizing function, joint protection, and reduction of pain. An individual might "get by" with a suboptimal prosthesis or orthosis or with inadequate therapy and rehabilitation. Proper prosthetic and orthotic selection, management, and patient education, however, contribute to a markedly enhanced quality of life for elderly and disabled individuals.

Acknowledgments

The authors acknowledge and thank Anna Paolino for her thorough and tireless assistance.

References

[1] Hiatt WR. Drug therapy: medical treatment of peripheral arterial disease and claudication. N Engl J Med 2001;344:1608–21.
[2] Hiatt WR. Atherosclerotic peripheral arterial diseases. In: Goldman L, Ausiello D, editors. Cecil textbook of medicine. 22nd edition. Philadelphia: WB Saunders; 2004. p. 465–71.
[3] Kay HW, Newman JD. Relative incidence of new amputations: statistical comparisons of 6,000 new amputees. Orthotics and Prosthetics 1975;29:3–16.

[4] Leonard JA, Meier RH. Upper and lower extremity prosthetics. In: DeLisa JA, Gans BM, editors. Rehabilitation medicine: principles and practice. 3rd edition. Philadelphia: Lippincott-Raven; 1998. p. 669–96.

[5] Wu Y, Krick H. Removable rigid dressing for below-knee amputees. Clinical Prosthetics and Orthotics 1987;11:33–44.

[6] Kavounoudias A, Tremblay C, Gravel D, et al. Bilateral changes in somatosensory sensibility after unilateral below-knee amputation. Arch Phys Med Rehabil 2005;86:633–40.

[7] Malone JM, Childer SJ, Underwood J, et al. Immediate postsurgical management of upper extremity amputation: conventional, electric and myoelectric prosthesis. Orthotics and Prosthetics 1981;35:1.

[8] Gitter A, Bosker G. Upper and lower extremity prosthetics. In: DeLisa JA, Gans BM, Walsh NE, editors. Rehabilitation medicine: principles and practice. 4th edition. Philadelphia: Lippincott Williams & Wilkins; 2005. p. 1325–54.

[9] Waters R, Mulroy S. The energy expenditure of normal and pathologic gait. Gait Posture 1999;9:207–31.

[10] Kirshblum SC, O'Connor KC, Benevento BT, et al. Spinal and upper extremity orthotics. In: DeLisa JA, Gans BM, editors. Rehabilitation medicine: principles and practice. 3rd edition. Philadelphia: Lippincott-Raven; 1998. p. 635–50.

[11] Braddom RL, Dumitru D, Johnson EW, et al. Lower limb orthoses. In: Branddom RL, editor. Physical medicine and rehabilitation. 2nd edition. Philadelphia: WB Saunders; 2000. p. 326–52.

[12] Xing Y, Alexander M. Lower limb orthotics. E Medicine topic 172 June 2002.

[13] Singer BJ, Dunne JW, Singer KP, et al. Non-surgical management of ankle contracture following acquired brain injury. Disabil Rehabil 2004;26:335–45.

[14] Molnar GE, Alexander MA. Orthotics and assistive devices. In: Molnar GE, editor. Pediatric rehabilitation, rehabilitation medicine library. Baltimore: Lippincott Williams & Wilkins; 1985. p. 157–77.

[15] Tan JC. Orthoses. In: Tan JC, editor. Practical manual of physical medicine and rehabilitation. 1st edition. Chicago: Mosby-Year Book; 1998. p. 178–228.

[16] May B. Amputations and prosthetics: a case study approach. Philadelphia: FA Davis; 1996.

[17] Seymour R. Prosthetics and orthotics: lower limb and spinal. Baltimore: Lippincott Williams & Williams; 2002.

[18] Nakollek H, Brauer S, Isles R. Outcomes after trans-tibial amputations: the relationship between quiet stance ability, strength of hip abductor muscles and gait. Physiotherapy Res Int 2002;7:203–14.

[19] Buckley JC, O'Driscoll D, Bennett SJ. Postural sway and active balance performance in highly active lower-limb amputees. Am J Phys Med Rehabil 2002;81:13–20.

[20] Wang R, Yen L, Wang M, et al. Effects of an ankle foot orthosis on balance performance in patients with hemiparesis of different durations. Clin Rehabil 2005;19:37–44.

ELSEVIER
SAUNDERS

CLINICS IN
GERIATRIC
MEDICINE

Clin Geriatr Med 22 (2006) 395–412

Balance in the Elderly

Brittany A. Matsumura, MD, Anne F. Ambrose, MD*

*Department of Rehabilitation Medicine, Mount Sinai School of Medicine, 1425 Madison Avenue,
New York, NY 10029–6574, USA*

Balance can be defined as the ability of an individual to successfully maintain the position of their body, or more specifically the center of gravity, within specific boundaries of space. Maintenance of balance may be either static (at rest) or dynamic (during motion). Balance is achieved by the complex integration between the sensory and musculoskeletal systems [1].

The functions of the balance system include

1. Correcting for inadvertent displacement of the center of gravity.
2. Providing perceptual information of body positioning.
3. Maintaining a clear image of the environment while the body is in motion.

With advancing age, changes related to normal aging, and those associated with diseases and their treatments, can affect the integrity and function of the musculoskeletal, vestibular, central, and peripheral nervous systems [2]. These effects are further compounded by a reduced capacity for plasticity and repair in the elderly.

Consequences of poor balance

One of the most serious outcomes of poor balance in the elderly is falls. More than one third of adults over the age of 75 fall each year [3]. In institutionalized patients, the fall rates are two to three times higher. Lipsitz and coworkers [4] found that 40% of 901 ambulatory nursing home patients fell two or more times

---

* Corresponding author.
E-mail address: anne.ambrose@mountsinai.org (A.F. Ambrose).

in the previous 6 months. One in 10 falls results in serious injury [3,5] and is the cause of mortality in 40% of injury- related deaths in adults over age 65 [6]. Serious injuries commonly resulting from falls include fractures of the femoral neck, limbs, and vertebrae, and subdural hematoma. Remaining on the ground for more than 1 hour after a fall is a marker of muscle weakness, illness, and social isolation in the elderly, and is associated with high mortality rates. Older adults who fall may experience decreased confidence in their physical capabilities and reduce their physical activities. This leads to sarcopenia (loss of muscle bulk), reduced physical endurance, and flexibility that may lead to further impairment of balance [1]. Fallers risk losing functional independence, becoming socially isolated, and developing depression [7,8]. Falls are often cited as a major contributing cause for nursing home admissions [9].

Expenses incurred by injury related to falls constitute a significant health care cost. Rice and MacKenzie [10] calculated in a report to the United States Congress in 1989 that falls in the elderly cost nearly $10 billion, or $4226 per injured person. Using Rice and Mackenzie's figures, Englander and coworkers [11] calculated that in 2020, expected cost of fall-related injuries in those over the age of 65 will total $43.8 billion.

Neuroanatomy of balance

Maintenance of balance relies on the harmonious integration and coordination of multiple body systems including the vestibular, visual, auditory, sensory, and autonomic systems [1]. The information from these different end organs is integrated in the central nervous system (CNS), an appropriate response is formulated, and the musculoskeletal system is directed to perform the appropriate head, eye, trunk, and limb movements to maintain posture [1].

Central nervous system pathways

Five pathways from the CNS to the periphery play crucial roles in maintaining balance. These pathways are the pyramidal, extrapyramidal, reticulospinal, medial vestibulospinal, and lateral vestibulospinal tracts. The pyramidal system (also called the corticospinal tract) begins in the pyramidal cells of the cerebral cortex, crosses over at the medullary pyramids, and extends the full length of the spinal cord. This tract controls voluntary movement.

The extrapyramidal system consists of the basal ganglia and four brainstem nuclei: (1) subthalamic nucleus, (2) substantia nigra, (3) red nucleus, and (4) reticular formation. The extrapyramidal system coordinates postural adjustments and reflexive movements. These two systems are the primary means of cortical influence over the peripheral motor centers [12].

The medial vestibulospinal tract is thought to play a role in coordinating eye movements and head position [12]. The lateral vestibulospinal tract relays information from the vestibular system and cerebellum to the lower motor neurons to maintain equilibrium by its influence over the extensor trunk and anti-gravity axial muscles. Originating in the pontine and brainstem medullary reticular formations, the reticulospinal tract indirectly receives input from the vestibular nuclei. It helps regulate muscle tone and inhibits reflex motor contractions [1].

Vestibular system

The paired vestibular system is housed in the petrous portion of the temporal bone. It consists of three semicircular canals and two otolithic organs, known as the "utricular maculae" and the "saccular maculae." The three pairs of semicircular canals (lateral, superior, and posterior) lie orthogonal to each other on either side of the head. Each canal is filled with a viscous fluid (endolymph), and contains neuroepithelial hair cells situated within a gelatinous structure called the cupola. Deflection of the neuroepithelial hair cells with rotational changes in head position informs the brain about angular acceleration, and the head's position in space [12]. The otolithic organs are more sensitive to linear accelerations. The utricle sends signals to the brain reporting forward and backward movement, whereas the saccule is primarily responsible for up and down motion. The vestibular system along with the visual system maintains visual focus during head movements. This ability to maintain a stable visual image during head movement is known as the "vestibulo-oculomotor reflex" [1,12].

The utricle and saccule project to the vestibular nuclei and on to the spinal cord by the medial longitudinal fasciculus and the lateral vestibulospinal tracts. Ascending tracts provide sensory information through the midbrain and thalamus to the vestibular cortex. The cerebellum is also involved in refining the response to balance challenge by mainly inhibitory synapses to the vestibular nuclei.

Peripheral afferent system

Mechanoreceptors located in muscles, joints, ligaments, and cutaneous tissues send sensory feedback to the CNS by afferent pathways to the cerebellum, brainstem, and cortex. These receptors are sensitive to the changes in shape, length, tension in muscle fibers, velocity, and direction of movement and transduce mechanical stimuli into neural signals. Sensory impulses are propagated toward the spinal cord by afferent nerve fibers with cell bodies located in the dorsal root ganglia. Within the spinal cord, sensory information is integrated by interneurons and filtered by descending information from the cortex and brainstem [13]. Proprioceptive information travels to the higher CNS centers in the cerebellum and cortex by the dorsal columns and the spinocerebellar tract. Signals traveling by the spinocerebellar tract are thought to relay nonconscious proprioceptive information (eg, muscle position and tone) [14], whereas dorsal columns relay conscious sensory information to the somatosensory cortex.

Cortical centers

The visual cortex (occipital lobe) receives information from the retina by the optic nerves and radiations. The visual cortex is connected to the frontal eye fields and the parietal cortex. Visual targeting is coordinated by connections with the superior colliculus, substantia nigra, and oculomotor nuclei to control smooth pursuit, saccadic, and optokinetic eye movements [12]. The vestibulo-ocular reflex maintains visual focus in response to fast head movements. The optokinetic and smooth pursuit reflexes maintain focus on objects during slow head movements. Saccadic eye movements rapidly change the orientation of the eyes to place a visual target on the center of the retina.

The balance system also includes the limbic system and the frontal cortex, which allows for learning complex experience-based postural and motor responses. These higher centers are important for development and adaptive purposes but also contribute to maladaptive behaviors, such as anxiety, avoidance, and phobia [1].

Vestibular compensatory mechanisms

Compensation is an adjustment process that progressively decreases symptoms of disequilibrium resulting from asymmetric peripheral vestibular afferent activity. It is a natural process that occurs after most vestibular insults, and involves neuronal changes in the brainstem and cerebellar nuclei in response to conflicting sensory information. Successful compensation leads to the ability to maintain stable gaze and upright posturing through secondary CNS processes [15]. Compensation is promoted by an active lifestyle and repeated exposure to specific stimuli. This process can be delayed by inactivity, or central vestibular dysfunction. Compensation after peripheral vestibular injury may be static or dynamic.

Static compensation

Static compensation occurs by modulating the resting activity of the vestibular nuclei to minimize side-to-side discrepancy provoked by changes in head position. This occurs within 24 to 72 hours after an acute vestibular disturbance, and is independent of head movement and visual input. The static compensation may help reduce symptoms of nausea and vertigo at rest seen with acute vestibular diseases [15]. The patient may continue, however, to experience motion-provoked disequilibrium and vertigo.

Dynamic compensation

Dynamic compensation takes place over days to weeks and involves reorganization of balance pathways in the cerebellum and brainstem. Dynamic compensation requires repeated exposure to motion stimuli to allow compensatory changes in posture and gaze response to head movement. Three important areas of dynamic compensation include adaptation, habituation, and sensory substitution [15].

Adaptation

Adaptation alters the vestibulo-ocular reflex to extinguish motion and visually provoked stimulation. Adaptation is context dependent for movement frequency, direction, eye position, and distance from the visual target; specific adjustments must be made for each scenario with alterations in the previously mentioned parameters [16].

Habituation

Attenuation or limitation of response to stimuli by repeated exposure to the stimulus is known as "habituation." Habituation requires consistent inputs to compensate appropriately and is not as effective in unstable vestibular lesions [15].

Substitution

In sensory substitution, the patient adopts alternate strategies relying on other sensory systems of posture and gaze control to replace the compromised sensory function. Although sensory substitution is helpful, it can be maladaptive for certain environments [15]. For example, a person who relies on visual input to compensate for sensory loss may have difficulty maintaining balance in the dark.

Causes of impaired balance in older adults

Normal aging is associated with decreased ability to maintain posture while standing in either unipedal or bipedal stance, when responding to unexpected perturbations, during normal or tandem walking, and when trying to avoid obstacles. The sensory, motor, and adaptive components of balance become vulnerable as they accumulate exposure to degenerative, infective, and injurious processes. Although mild changes in any one facet of the balance system may not result in significant perturbations, involvement of multiple components can lead to severe balance deficits [17].

Vestibular impairments

Aging has a significant effect on vestibular function. Hair cell loss occurs with aging, particularly in the ampulla [18]. It has been estimated that neuronal loss in the vestibular nuclei occurs at a rate of approximately 3% per decade from the age of 40 [2,19,20].

Elderly patients tend to show reductions in the gain of the vestibulo-ocular reflex and smooth pursuit and increases in saccade latencies [1]. The sensitivity of the semicircular canals for high-frequency sounds is reduced. Such age-related alterations might interfere with appropriate responses to fast head movements. Initially, reduction of the inhibitory system mediated through the cerebellum can compensate for decreased sensitivity. Over time, the combination of reduced peripheral sensitivity and central inhibition decreases the range in which the system can respond [21].

Vestibular failure also occurs in disease states (eg, vestibular neuronitis, cerebellar or brainstem hemorrhage). Patients with these conditions may present with symptoms of vertigo or dizziness because of discrepancies in information from both sides of the head.

Sensory impairments

Diseases commonly seen in the elderly including arthritis, diabetes, and atherosclerosis can impact balance [1,2]. Vessel occlusion by atherosclerosis can affect visual and somatosensory functions. Diabetic peripheral neuropathy and retinopathy can impair proprioception and vision. Peripheral neuropathy is commonly seen in elderly populations and can be caused by several etiologies including hereditary neuropathies; alcohol; lead; vitamin B_{12} deficiency; and medication use (eg, vincristine and dapsone) [22].

Visual impairments

Age-related changes in visual acuity, visual field, depth perception, contrast sensitivity, sensitivity to glare, and dark adaptation may also contribute to disequilibrium in the elderly because they affect overall visual input to the balance system. Some visual impairment may be reversible with corrective lenses or cataract surgery [23].

Musculoskeletal and neuromuscular impairments

Normal coordination of postural movement is dependent on appropriate timing relationships and sequence of muscle activation. Studies of coordinated muscle responses to balance perturbations have shown variability among activation timing relationships of muscles in the elderly when compared with their younger counterparts and increased response in muscles not generally active in the younger population [24,25].

Postural response latencies are increased in the healthy elderly compared with normal young subjects [24,25], which may result from slowing in stimulus encoding, central processing, and initiation of movement [26]. These deficits may lead to inadequate scaling of postural response to balance perturbation.

Approximately 30% of total body mass in a young healthy individual is muscle mass; however, by age 75 this percentage decreases to approximately 15% of body mass [27]. This muscle loss seen with aging is termed "sarco-

penia," and results from vascular, nutritional, hormonal, or metabolic disturbances. Sarcopenia is associated with poor structural parameters of bone and
impaired balance [28].

Joint mobility may be restricted in the elderly because of arthritis, which limits
postural readjustments. Reduced muscle strength and flexibility decrease the
body's ability to respond to balance perturbations [2]. In addition, spinal alignment abnormalities (ie, kyphosis and scoliosis) and leg length discrepancy can
alter the center of gravity. Deterioration of joint proprioception with older
subjects [29] has also been implicated in balance impairments.

Cardiovascular impairments

Advancing age is associated with decreased responsiveness to sympathetic
stimuli leading to blunting of exercise-induced heart rate and contractility, and
lowered cardiac output [30]. Studies suggest that baroreflex function is impaired
for both heart rate and sympathetic nerve activity in the elderly [31,32]. This may
lead to postural hypotension [33], a common cardiac cause of falls [34]. Many
diseases in older subjects are associated with postural hypotension, such as heart
failure, diabetes mellitus, and Parkinson's disease [35]. Drugs that can cause postural hypotension include antihypertensives, parkinsonian medications, antidepressants, antipsychotics, and diuretics [36].

Gait changes

Normal walking is dependent on several factors including the ability to
maintain upright stance, generate a rhythmic locomotor pattern, and control the
trajectory of the center of mass [37,38]. Control of dynamic balance in the elderly
can become increasingly challenging [39]. Gait patterns in the elderly may
exchange kinetic efficiency for increased postural stability [40,41] as seen by the
slowing of the gait cycle with prolonged stance and double support phases.

Many neurologic conditions, such as stroke, Parkinson's disease, myelopathy,
and cerebellar disorders, impair balance and gait. In older adults with strokes,
decreased lower-extremity strength can result in difficulty maintaining leg
extension and foot clearance during the swing phase of gait [42], which can lead
to difficulty in negotiating uneven terrain. The site of the lesion may affect
specific cognitive domains. Parietal lobe damage caused by strokes may impair
planning and execution of locomotor activities. Frontal lobe strokes may affect
judgment of safety. Brainstem and cerebellar strokes can affect balance by
interrupting critical pathways. In subjects with Parkinson's disease, falls are associated with rigid posture and inability to respond to external perturbations, with
attempts to overcome a "freezing episode" [43]. Cervical myelopathy results in
narrowing of the cervical canal and leads to loss of balance by compromising the
CNS pathways. Cerebellar lesions resulting from alcoholism, degeneration,

ischemia, or hemorrhages are associated with impaired balance. Wide-based gait and variability in step length in cerebellar lesions are associated with increased risk of falls [44].

Medications

Some common medications that have been implicated as major causes of falls in the elderly include sedatives, antidepressants, antiepileptics, cardiovascular drugs, and anti-inflammatory drugs [45]. Polypharmacy further increases this risk. Drug-induced mechanisms for poor balance include postural hypotension, cerebellar dysfunction, decreased attention, and arousal.

Evaluation of balance

History

Characteristics of the balance problem to be ascertained include onset of the symptoms, duration, frequency, exacerbating and relieving factors, severity, associated symptoms, and any past treatments and the treatment response. Enquire about the effect on overall functioning, activity level, and behavior [15]. Obtain a history of chronic medical illnesses, complications, and medications, both over the counter and prescription. The patient's living situation, physical environment, social support, and current and previous level of functioning can help guide management. In a patient with vestibular dysfunction, the history becomes a key component in determining whether the lesion is stable or unstable. A patient with incomplete vestibular compensation may complain of ongoing symptoms and it becomes imperative to determine if this is caused by an unstable lesion (lack of compensation because of frequently changing system) or an uncompensated stable lesion. Frequently, symptoms that are provoked by head or eye movements represent an uncompensated stable lesion, whereas symptoms that are more spontaneous in nature are caused by an unstable lesion [15]. In taking the history, it is important to try to elicit information as to why full compensation has not taken place. Such issues as avoidance of movement, concurrent medical conditions, and anxiety may contribute to deficits in compensation.

Physical examination

Physical examination of balance impairments includes evaluation of neurologic and sensory functions, posture, and gait. These assessments include evaluation of vision; eye movements; sensation; proprioception; reflexes; coordination (finger-to-nose testing); cerebellar function; and motor power. Balance assessment should be performed in the sitting and standing positions. Gait assessment tests dynamic balance and should include normal gait, tandem walking, dual task activities, and head movement during walking.

Performance-based assessments

Several performance-based assessments are available to test balance, gait, and falls in the elderly (Table 1). Table 2 summarizes commonly used specialized tests.

Table 1
Balance and gait assessment tools

Activities-Specific Balance Confidence Scale	Subjective 16-item questionnaire in which respondents rate their confidence that they will lose balance in the course of daily activities. Items rate from 0% (no confidence) to 100% (complete confidence).
Berg Functional Balance Scale	Objective 14-item functional balance performance assessment of daily activities including sitting, standing, and transitions. Items scored from 0 to 4 points with a maximum score of 56. A score less than 45 suggests increased risk of falling.
Gait assessment Rating Score	Predicts risk of falling among community-dwelling, frail older persons; 16-item rating scale to evaluate gait abnormalities, and movement in the trunk and upper and lower extremities. Rated from 0 to 3, 3 being the highest risk.
Tinetti Balance and Mobility Assessment	Predicts individuals who will fall at least once during the following year; 14-item balance and 10-item gait assessment. Maximum score is 40. Individuals scoring less than 36 are at greater risk of falling.
Dynamic Gait Index	Objectively assesses balance by evaluating response to changes in task demands during gait using eight functional tasks including walking, changing gait speed, walking with head turns in the vertical and horizontal directions, walking and turning, stepping over and around obstacles, and stair ascent and descent. Items scored on scale of 0 (severe impairment) to 3 (normal) with maximum total score of 24. A score less than 19 suggests increased risk for falling.
Timed up and go (TUG)	Objectively assesses level of functional mobility with three timed scenarios. (1) TUG Alone: from sitting in a chair, stand up, walk 3 m, turn around, walk back, and sit down. (2) TUG cognitive: complete the task while counting backwards from a randomly selected number between 20 and 100. (3) TUG manual: complete the task while carrying a cup of water. Participants taking longer than 13.5, 15, and 14.5 seconds to complete the TUG alone, TUG cognitive, and TUG manual, respectively, are at increased risk for falls.
One-leg stand	Predicts injurious fall in the elderly. Performed with eyes open and arms by the side of the trunk, the participant must stand unassisted on any one leg and is timed in seconds from the time one foot is lifted from the floor to the time when it touches the ground or the standing leg. Participants unable to perform the one-leg stand for at least 5 seconds are at increased risk for injurious fall.
Functional reach	Objectively assesses functional balance by measuring the maximal distance a person can reach beyond the length of their arm while maintaining a fixed base of support in the standing position. A reach less than or equal to 6 in predicts fall.

Treatment of balance impairment

Vestibular and balance rehabilitation

Vestibular rehabilitation is designed to restore homeostasis of the balance system. The goals of vestibular rehabilitation include decreasing dizziness, improving balance, and minimization the fall risk by improving vestibulo-ocular reflex accuracy, postural control, and oculomotor skills [46]. Various techniques used in vestibular and balance rehabilitation therapy include adaptation exercises, habituation exercises, substitution exercises, balance exercises, gait exercises, and general conditioning (Table 3) [15]. The prescribed program should be consistent with the patient's needs.

Recovery is improved when vestibular rehabilitation programs are initiated soon after the initial onset of symptoms. With age-related balance problems, customized programs may involve combinations of vestibular stimulation, gaze stabilization, ocular motor, dynamic balance, and gait exercises. Moderate-intensity exercise programs that include active stretching, endurance walking, muscle coordination, strengthening, and postural control have been shown to improve functional balance in community-dwelling elderly [47]. Recovery is influenced by the integrity of the patient's residual sensory systems and cerebellum, general physical health, cognitive processing, motivation, compliance, and motor skills. Age does not play a significant role in treatment outcomes of vestibular rehabilitation [48].

In addition to a vestibular rehabilitation exercise program, a patient may also require additional physical and occupational therapy services for supplemental physical conditioning. A home safety evaluation may help reduce fall risks by

Table 2
Specialty tests

Test	Use
Electro-oculography and Electronystagmography (ENG)	Measures important features of eye movements including saccades, pursuit, optokinetic nystagmus, and fixation. Useful in lesion localization.
Positional and positioning testing	Subset of ENG testing involving a battery of tests that include various head positions and movements and measurement of ocular and symptomatic responses. Useful in lesion localization.
Caloric testing	Subset of ENG testing involving irrigation of the external ear to affect changes in the movement of endolymph in the semicircular canal leading to alterations in afferent neural activity. Useful in lesion localization.
Rotational testing	Examination of the horizontal canal–ocular reflex involving rotation that stimulates the horizontal semicircular canal and recording of responsive horizontal eye movements. Useful in lesion localization.
Computerized dynamic posturography	Quantitative method for assessing balance functioning under various simulated tasks. Protocols are designed to test the sensory, motor, and biomechanical components of balance individually and in concert. May assist with lesion localization, identifying adaptive strategies and functional capabilities.

Table 3
Vestibular and balance rehabilitation exercises

Adaptation exercises	Goals to improve the VOR gain and gaze stability. Exercises include head movement with focus on a fixed target, progressively increasing the velocity of head movement repeating the cycle 20–30 times, and head movement with focus on a target moving in the opposite direction repeating the cycle 20–30 times. These exercises can be performed sitting and progressing to standing with increasingly sharpened stance (until one foot on top of the other).
Habituation exercises	Goal to extinguish pathologic positionally provoked responses. After evaluation, patients are instructed in an exercise program with repeated motions that provoke symptoms. These exercises are to be performed two to three times per day for several weeks until resolution of symptoms.
Substitution exercises	Goal to learn alternative strategies to compensate for deficits. Exercises teach patients to use cues from other components in the balance system and central preprogramming of movement (learned strategies for predictable or anticipated motions).
Postural control and gait exercises	Goal to improve postural control. Exercise focus on both static and dynamic balance. Gait exercises can include modifying walking surface or environmental conditions (ie, altered lighting or challenging surfaces, such as gravel) and adding performing concomitant tasks while walking (ie, throw and catch a ball).
Maintenance exercises	Goal to maintain active lifestyle. Exercises suited to patient's interests and abilities may include walking, jogging, cycling, golfing, tennis, bowling, or racquetball. Exercises should promote coordinated visual and body movements.

modifications of the home environment, such as proper lighting, handrails, walkways, and stairs.

Benign paroxysmal positional vertigo, a common cause of dizziness in the elderly, occurs when otoconia normally housed within the otolithic organs collects within the semicircular canals causing abnormal signaling from the vestibular system. For patients with benign paroxysmal positional vertigo, particle-repositioning maneuvers, such as the Epley maneuver, may resolve the symptoms (Fig. 1) [49–52]. The Epley maneuver consists of sequential movements of the head holding each position for approximately 30 seconds to remove debris from the semicircular canals. In most cases, balance retraining and gait exercises in addition to particle repositioning can significantly improve balance problems.

In several studies, a Tai Chi exercise has been shown to improve functional balance and decrease rates of falls in the elderly [53–57]. Visual and kinesthetic feedback programs can also be used in therapy to assist in balance rehabilitation [58].

Assistive devices

Assistive devices, including canes and walkers, can improve balance and mobility of patients with balance impairments by widening the base of support and improving somatosensory feedback.

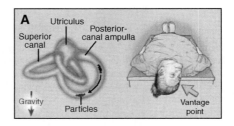

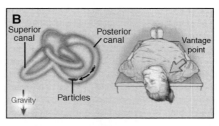

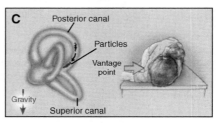

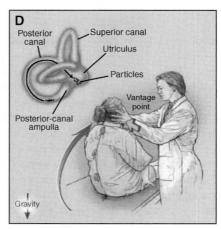

Fig. 1. (*A–D*) Performing the Epley maneuver for the right ear. Graphic also illustrates presumed position of debris. (*From* Furman JM, Cass SP. Benign paroxysmal positional vertigo. N Engl J Med 1999;341:1590–6: © 1999 Massachusetts Medical Society; with permission.)

Footwear

Redesigning footwear can improve stability in balance-impaired older adults. Heel elevation can reduce lumbar lordosis [59], increase pressure on forefoot [60], change toe-off [61], decrease stride length [62], increase energy consumption [63], and alter ankle-knee motion [64]. A study of low-resiliency sole material that retain compressed thickness during gait found improved stability with use of low-resiliency material compared with high-resiliency footwear [65]. The low-resiliency material may dissipate energy that might otherwise participate in reaction forces that alter posture. High heel collar is associated with greater ankle and subtalar stability in the frontal plane [66] and increased proprioceptive feedback [67]. Midsole flaring provides greater base of support and improves stability. Sensory contributions provided by footwear may also influence gait. In one study, the cutaneous sensory input provided by textured shoe inserts was found to alter gait patterns by changing muscle activity during walking [68]. Recent research also suggests low-level input mechanical or electrical noise (in the form of insoles or adhesive gel pads) may improve balance in the elderly by enhancing the sensitivity of the somatosensory system [69,70].

Medical therapy

The elderly are susceptible to injuries causing acute loss of vestibular function and intermittent vertigo, such as benign paroxysmal positional vertigo, Meniere's disease, and labrinthitis. In the acute phase, these disorders are frequently treated with vestibulosuppressive medications, such as meclizine or benzodiazepines, to reduce severity of symptoms including nausea and dizziness. It is important to use suppressive medications sparingly, especially in the elderly, and to minimize total treatment time because these medications can inhibit natural vestibular compensation. Symptoms of chronic disequilibrium are generally related to alteration of central neuronal functions or underlying vascular disease. In patients with constant disequilibrium of central origin, vestibulosuppressive medications can worsen their symptoms and should be avoided [1,15].

Surgical management

Surgical management of dizziness and vertigo is considered when conservative management fails to provide symptomatic relief. Individuals with unstable vestibular lesions, which progressively deteriorate or continuously fluctuate preventing adequate central compensation, are most suited for surgical intervention. History and auditory and vestibular testing should be performed to isolate the lesion to the peripheral vestibular system and identify the impaired side before surgical intervention. Surgical procedures for vertigo generally fall within one of two categories: preservation procedures and ablative procedures [71]. Vestibular preservation procedures (eg, posterior semicircular canal occlusion, endolymphatic sac surgery, microvascular decompression of the eighth nerve, perilymph fistula repair) are aimed to correct specific pathology and restore normal vestibular function but may be variable in their efficacy. Surgical interventions designed to ablate unilateral vestibular function (eg, vestibular neurectomy or labyrinthectomy) can be used to treat many vestibular pathologies, but can result in hearing loss [72]. Patients with poor central compensation tend to have less successful outcomes with surgical interventions.

Assessment of research and future areas of inquiry

Because of the complex nature of the balance system, the cause of balance dysfunction in individual patients is not easily defined. This may lead to variability among research outcomes depending on the stringency or lack thereof in the selection criteria. Additionally, there exists some inconsistency within the literature regarding what constitutes the normal process of aging and thereby the definition of a normal elderly individual. Although some argue that disease may be a natural process of aging, others support the notion that normal aging occurs in the absence of disease. As such, criteria in balance studies for the normal elderly individual vary widely and may limit the ability to generalize research outcomes in elderly populations. Large portions of the literature on balance rehabilitation define only short-term outcomes in small groups of patients. Further studies with larger study size concerning the long-term outcomes and appropriate time course for various balance interventions are warranted.

Advancing technology has expanded the possibilities in the diagnosis and treatment of balance disorders. Vestibular-evoked myogenic potentials are currently under investigation as a proposed supplement to the current vestibular testing battery [73–75]. Vestibular-evoked myogenic potentials are particularly useful in evaluating the saccular and inferior vestibular nerve function. One treatment of particular interest is neuroprosthetics [76,77]. Currently, investigations in prototype balance prostheses that transform information from inertial sensors for lateral head tilt into vibrotactile cutaneous display are underway [78].

Summary

Impairments in the sensory, musculoskeletal, and central and peripheral nervous systems commonly seen in the elderly can adversely affect the balance system, which requires a complex integration of many components. Balance dysfunction has serious implications on society because this is a major cause for falls, injury, and loss of functional independence in the elderly population. A thorough investigation into the cause of balance dysfunction in an elderly patient is essential to the implementation of appropriate treatment. Balance problems in the older adult are often multifactorial and require a multidisciplinary approach. Several treatment options including a variety of rehabilitation therapy approaches, assistive devices and equipment, medication for symptomatic relief, and surgical interventions are available and can have positive effects with appropriate referral.

References

[1] Konrad HR, Girardi M, Helfert R. Balance and aging. Laryngoscope 1999;109:1454–60.

[2] Girardi M, Konrad HR. Imbalance and falls in the elderly. In: Cummings CW, Flint PW, Haughey BH, et al, editors. Otolaryngology: head & neck surgery. 4th edition. St. Louis: Elsevier-Mosby; 2005. p. 3319–20.

[3] Tinetti ME, Speechley M, Ginter SF. Risk factors for falls among elderly persons living in the community. N Engl J Med 1988;319:1701–7.

[4] Lipsitz LA, Jonsson PV, Kelley MM, et al. Causes and correlates of recurrent falls in ambulatory frail elderly. J Gerontol 1991;46:M114–22.

[5] Nevitt MC, Cummings SR, Hudes ES. Risk factors for injurious falls: a prospective study. J Gerontol 1991;46:M164–70.

[6] New South Wales Health Department. The epidemiology of falls in older in NSW. Sydney, Australia: New South Wales Health Department; 1994.

[7] Murphy J, Isaacs B. The post-fall syndrome: a study of 36 elderly patients. Gerontology 1982;28:265–70.

[8] Howland J, Lachman ME, Peterson EW, et al. Covariates of fear of falling and associated activity curtailment. Gerontologist 1998;38:549–55.

[9] Tinetti ME, Liu WL, Claus EB. Predictors and prognosis of inability to get up after falls among elderly persons. JAMA 1993;269:65–70.

[10] Rice DP, MacKenzie EJ. Cost of injury in the United States: a report to Congress. San Francisco: Institute for Health and Aging, University of California; 1989.

[11] Englander F, Hodson TJ, Terregrossa RA. Economic dimensions of slip and fall injuries. J Forensic Sci 1996;41:733–46.

[12] Shepard NT, Telian SA. Balance disorder patient. San Diego: Singular Publishing Group; 1996.

[13] Leonard CT. The neuroscience of human movement. St Louis: Mosby-Year Book; 1998.

[14] Warren S, Yezierski RP, Capra NF. The somatosensory system. I: Discriminative touch and position sense. In: Haines DE, Ard MD, editors. Fundamental neuroscience. New York: Churchill Livingstone; 1997. p. 220–35.

[15] Shepard NT, Telian SA. Vestibular and balance rehabilitation: program essentials. In: Cummings CW, Flint PW, Haughey BH, et al, editors. Otolaryngology: head & neck surgery. 4th edition. St. Louis: Elsevier-Mosby; 2005. p. 3310–7.

[16] Shelhamer M, Robinson DA, Tan HS. Context-specific adaptation of the gain of the vestibule-ocular reflex in humans. J Vestib Res 1992;2:89–96.

[17] Tinetti ME, Williams CS, Gill TM. Dizziness among older adults: a possible geriatric syndrome. Ann Intern Med 2000;132:337–44.

[18] Rosenhall U. Degenerative patterns in the aging human vestibular neuro-epithelia. Acta Otolaryngol 1973;76:208–20.

[19] Tang Y, Lopez I, Baloh RW. Age-related change of the neuronal number in the human medial vestibular nucleus: a stereological investigation. J Vestib Res 2001–2002;11:357–63.

[20] Lopez I, Honrubia V, Baloh RW. Aging and the human vestibular nucleus. J Vestib Res 1997; 7:77–85.

[21] Nakayama M, Helfert RH, Konrad HR, et al. Scanning electron microscopic evaluation of age-related changes in the rat vestibular epithelium. Otolaryngol Head Neck Surg 1994;111: 799–806.

[22] Verghese J, Bieri PL, Gellido C, et al. Peripheral neuropathy in young-old and old-old patients. Muscle Nerve 2001;24:1476–81.

[23] Harwood RH. Visual problems and falls. Age Ageing 2001;30(Suppl 4):13–8.

[24] Woollacott MH. Gait and postural control in the aging adult. In: Bles WI, Brandt T, editors. Disorders in posture and gait. Amsterdam: Elsevier Science Publishers; 1986. p. 325–35.

[25] Woollacott M, Inglin B, Manchester D. Response preparation and posture control: neuro-muscular changes in the older adult. Ann N Y Acad Sci 1988;515:42–53.

[26] Stelmach GE, Worringham CJ. Sensorimotor deficits related to postural stability: implications for falling in the elderly. Clin Geriatr Med 1985;1:679–94.

[27] Manolagas S. Aging and the musculoskeletal system. In: Beers MH, Berkow R, editors. The Merck manual of geriatrics. Whitehouse Station (NJ): Merck Research Laboratories; 2000. p. 467–71.

[28] Szulc P, Beck TJ, Marchand F, et al. Low skeletal muscle mass is associated with poor structural parameters of bone and impaired balance in elderly men–the MINOS study. J Bone Miner Res 2005;20:721–9.

[29] Skinner HB, Barrack RL, Cook SD. Age-related decline in proprioception. Clin Orthop Relat Res 1984;184:208–11.

[30] Fleg JL, O'Connor FC, Gerstenblith G, et al. Impact of age on the cardiovascular response to dynamic upright exercise in healthy men and women. J Appl Physiol 1995;78:890–900.

[31] Ferrari AU, Grassi G, Mancia G. Alterations in reflex control of the circulation associated with aging. In: Amery A, Staessen J, editors. Handbook of hypertension: hypertension in the elderly, vol. 12. Amsterdam: Elsevier Science; 1989. p. 39–50.

[32] Matsukawa T, Sugiyama Y, Watanabe T, et al. Baroreflex control of muscle sympathetic nerve activity is attenuated in the elderly. J Auton Nerv Syst 1998;73:182–5.

[33] Ferrari AU, Radaelli A, Centola M. Invited review: aging and the cardiovascular system. J Appl Physiol 2003;95:2591–7.

[34] Kario K, Tobin JN, Wolfson LI, et al. Lower standing systolic blood pressure as a predictor of falls in the elderly: a community-based prospective study. J Am Coll Cardiol 2001;38:246–52.

[35] Tilvis RS, Hakala SM, Valvanne J, et al. Postural hypotension and dizziness in a general aged population: a four-year follow-up of the Helsinki Aging Study. J Am Geriatr Soc 1996;44: 809–14.

[36] Mets TF. Drug-induced orthostatic hypotension in older patients. Drugs Aging 1995;6:219–28.

[37] Winter DA, Frank JS, Patla AE. Assessment of balance control in humans. Med Prog Technol 1990;16:31–53.

[38] Winter DA. Human balance and posture control during standing and walking. Gait Posture 1995;3:193–214.

[39] Winter DA, Frank JS, Patla AE, et al. Biomechanical walking pattern changes in the fit and healthy elderly. Phys Ther 1990;70:340–6.

[40] Shkuratova N, Morris ME, Huxham F. Effects of age on balance control during walking. Arch Phys Med Rehabil 2004;85:582–8.

[41] Guimaraes RM, Isaacs B. Characteristics of the gait in old people who fall. Int Rehabil Med 1980;2:177–80.

[42] Tideiskar R. Falling in old age: its prevention and treatment. New York: Springer-Verlag; 1989.

[43] Paulson GW, Schafer K, Hallum B. Avoiding mental changes and falls in older Parkinson's patients. Geriatrics 1986;41:59–62, 67.

[44] Hausdorff JM, Edelberg HK, Mitchell SL, et al. Increased gait unsteadiness in community-dwelling elderly fallers. Arch Phys Med Rehabil 1997;78:278–83.

[45] Cumming RG. Epidemiology of medication-related falls and fractures in the elderly. Drugs Aging 1998;12:43–53.

[46] Herdman SJ, Schubert MC, Tusa RJ. Strategies for balance rehabilitation: fall risk and treatment. Ann N Y Acad Sci 2001;942:394–412.

[47] Means KM, Rodell DE, O'Sullivan PS. Balance, mobility, and falls among community-dwelling elderly persons: effects of a rehabilitation exercise program. Am J Phys Med Rehabil 2005;84: 238–50.

[48] Whitney SL, Wrisley DM, Marchetti GF, et al. The effect of age on vestibular rehabilitation outcomes. Laryngoscope 2002;112:1785–90.

[49] Richard W, Bruintjes TD, Oostenbrink P, et al. Efficacy of the Epley maneuver for posterior canal BPPV: a long-term, controlled study of 81 patients. Ear Nose Throat J 2005;84:22–5.

[50] Chang AK, Schoeman G, Hill M. A randomized clinical trial to assess the efficacy of the Epley maneuver in the treatment of acute benign positional vertigo. Acad Emerg Med 2004;11: 918–24.

[51] Ruckenstein MJ. Therapeutic efficacy of the Epley canalith repositioning maneuver. Laryngo-scope 2001;111:940–5.

[52] Furman JM, Cass SP. Benign paroxysmal positional vertigo. N Engl J Med 1999;341:1590–6.

[53] Li F, Harmer P, Fisher KJ, et al. Tai Chi and fall reductions in older adults: a randomized controlled trial. J Gerontol A Biol Sci Med Sci 2005;60:187–94.

[54] McGibbon CA, Krebs DE, Parker SW, et al. Tai Chi and vestibular rehabilitation improve vestibulopathic gait via different neuromuscular mechanisms: preliminary report. BMC Neurol 2005;5:3.

[55] Wang C, Collet JP, Lau J. The effect of Tai Chi on health outcomes in patients with chronic conditions: a systematic review. Arch Intern Med 2004;164:493–501.

[56] Wu G. Evaluation of the effectiveness of Tai Chi for improving balance and preventing falls in the older population: a review. J Am Geriatr Soc 2002;50:746–54.

[57] Wolf SL, Barnhart HX, Kutner NG, et al. Reducing frailty and falls in older persons: an investigation of Tai Chi and computerized balance training. Atlanta FICSIT Group. Frailty and Injuries: Cooperative Studies of Intervention Techniques. J Am Geriatr Soc 1996;44: 489–97.

[58] Hamman RG, Mekjavic I, Mallinson AI, et al. Training effects during repeated therapy sessions of balance training using visual feedback. Arch Phys Med Rehabil 1992;73:738–44.

[59] Bendix T, Sorensen SS, Klausen K. Lumbar curve, trunk muscles, and line of gravity with different heel heights. Spine 1984;9:223–7.

[60] Corrigan JP, Moore DP, Stephens MM. Effect of heel height on forefoot loading. Foot Ankle 1993;14:148–52.

[61] McBride ID, Wyss UP, Cooke TD, et al. First metatarsophalangeal joint reaction forces during high-heel gait. Foot Ankle 1991;11:282–8.

[62] Merrifield HH. Female gait patterns in shoes with different heel heights. Ergonomics 1971; 14:411–7.

[63] Ebbeling CJ, Hamill J, Crussemeyer JA. Lower extremity mechanics and energy cost of walking in high-heeled shoes. J Orthop Sports Phys Ther 1994;19:190–6.

[64] Gollnick PD, Tipton CM, Karpovich PV. Electrogoniometric study of walking on high heels. Res Q 1964;35:370–8.

[65] Robbins S, Waked E, Krouglicof N. Improving balance. J Am Geriatr Soc 1998;46:1363–70.

[66] Johnson GR, Dowson D, Wright V. A biomechanical approach to the design of football boots. J Biomech 1976;9:581–5.

[67] Petrov O, Blocher K, Bradbury RL, et al. Footwear and ankle stability in the basketball player. Clin Podiatr Med Surg 1988;5:275–90.

[68] Nurse MA, Hulliger M, Wakeling JM, et al. Changing the texture of footwear can alter gait patterns. J Electromyogr Kinesiol 2005;15:496–506.

[69] Priplata AA, Niemi JB, Harry JD, et al. Vibrating insoles and balance control in elderly people. Lancet 2003;362:1123–4.

[70] Gravelle DC, Laughton CA, Dhruv NT, et al. Noise-enhanced balance control in older adults. Neuroreport 2002;13:1853–6.

[71] LaRouere MJ, Seidman MD, Kartush JM. Medical and surgical treatment of vertigo. In: Jacobson GP, Newman CW, Kartush JM, editors. Handbook of balance function testing. St. Louis: Mosby-Year Book; 1993. p. 337–57.

[72] Telian SA. Surgery for vestibular disorders. In: Cummings CW, Flint PW, Haughey BH, et al, editors. Otolaryngology: head & neck surgery. 4th edition. St. Louis: Elsevier-Mosby; 2005. p. 3290–308.

[73] Akin FW, Murnane OD, Panus PC, et al. The influence of voluntary tonic EMG level on the vestibular-evoked myogenic potential. J Rehabil Res Dev 2004;41(3B):473–80.

[74] Welgampola MS, Colebatch JG. Characteristics and clinical applications of vestibular-evoked myogenic potentials. Neurology 2005;64:1682–8.
[75] Rauch SD, Silveira MB, Zhou G, et al. Vestibular evoked myogenic potentials versus vestibular test battery in patients with Meniere's disease. Otol Neurotol 2004;25:981–6.
[76] Kentala E, Vivas J, Wall III C. Reduction of postural sway by use of a vibrotactile balance prosthesis prototype in subjects with vestibular deficits. Ann Otol Rhinol Laryngol 2003;112: 404–9.
[77] Wall III C, Merfeld DM, Rauch SD, et al. Vestibular prostheses: the engineering and biomedical issues. J Vestib Res 2002–2003;12:95–113.
[78] Wall III C, Weinberg MS, Schmidt PB, et al. Balance prostheses based on micromechanical sensors using vibrotactile feedback of tilt. IEEE Trans Biomed Eng 2001;48:1153–61.

CLINICS IN
GERIATRIC
MEDICINE

Clin Geriatr Med 22 (2006) 413–434

ELSEVIER
SAUNDERS

Principles of Geriatric Dentistry and Their Application to the Older Adult with a Physical Disability

Daniel E. MacDonald, DMD, MSD[a,b,c,d,*]

[a]Division of Periodontology, Columbia University College of Dental medicine, 630 West 168th Street,
PH-7-E-110, New York, NY 10032, USA
[b]Langmuir Center for Colloids & Interfaces, Fu School of Graduate Engineering,
Columbia University, 500 West 120th Street, Mail Code 4711, New York, NY 10027, USA
[c]Division of Mineralized Tissue Research, Hospital for Special Surgery, 535 East 70th Street,
New York, NY 10021, USA
[d]James J. Peters VA Medical Center, 130 West Kingsbridge Road Bronx, NY 10468, USA

Dental disease, such as caries, gingivitis, and periodontal disease, has been linked with a variety of neurologic impairments including stroke [1,2], Parkinson's disease [3], and spinal cord injury [4]. Rheumatologic diseases, such as rheumatoid arthritis, systemic lupus erythematosus, and systemic scleroderma, have also been linked to a higher incidence of caries, believed to be related to impaired salivary gland function [5]. Marton [6] described reduction of mouth opening caused by temporomandibular joint dysfunction in rheumatoid arthritis and systemic sclerosis, and deceased salivary gland output in Sjögren's syndrome.

This article provides to clinicians caring for older adults with physical or cognitive impairments an understanding of age-related changes in dentition, common pathology of the oral cavity, and special concerns as they apply to this population.

* Division of Periodontology, Columbia University School of Dental and Oral Surgery, New York, NY.
   E-mail address: dem14@columbia.edu

0749-0690/06/$ – see front matter © 2006 Elsevier Inc. All rights reserved.
doi:10.1016/j.cger.2005.12.009   geriatric.theclinics.com

Age-related changes in the oral cavity

Tooth changes

It is difficult to distinguish between normal physiologic changes and pathologic changes that affect the teeth. Teeth change in shape and color with increasing age. Attrition and wear can both result in loss of tooth length and altered
enamel thickness. As a result, the underlying dentin become more prominent and
contributes to the observed increased yellow appearance of the teeth and reduced
translucency because of the loss of the overlying enamel. Teeth may also demonstrate attrition, abrasion, erosion, and caries, all of which alter the appearance
and shape of the tooth.

Dentin formation continues even beyond full eruption of the tooth. The con-
tinuation of dentin mineralization results in a reduction in the size of the pulp
chamber [6,7]. This diffuse mineralization can be visualized clinically; dental
radiographs show narrowing of the pulp chamber by further dentin deposition
on the ceiling and floor or along the walls of the pulp chamber.

Aside from narrowing of the pulp chamber [8], the degree of pulpal vas-
cularity is also markedly reduced with age [9]. These changes reduce the success
the tooth has to be able to recuperate after the insult from caries has occurred.

Changes of oral mucous membranes and periodontium

The oral mucosa may be classified into a masticatory mucosa found on
the gingiva around teeth and hard palate, the lining mucosa of the cheek, soft
palate, floor of the mouth, and lateral surface of the tongue, and a specialized
mucosa found on the dorsum of the tongue and lips [10]. Variation of the various
tissue types seems to be related to cell density, degree of keratinization, variation in the density of collagen, organization of collagen bundles, and quantity of
elastic fibers [11]. The diameters of elastic fibers increase regularly with age.
Aging does not result in changes in the appearance of the oral mucosa [12].
Nevertheless, the oral mucosa becomes increasingly more thin and dry. These
changes have been described histologically with diminished keratinization
[13] and thinning of the epithelial structure [14]; however, there is no evidence
for a change in the morphology of the human oral epithelial cells as a result
of aging [15]. It is important to note, however, that some of the human mucosal alteration with age may be caused by factors other than aging alone, such
as dietary deficiencies of certain vitamins, reduced estrogen levels, or other systemic influences [16,17]. Studies evaluating an association between age and
the rate of oral mucosal cell renewal are inconclusive [18–20]. It is possible that
aging may reduce the homeostasis of epithelial cell development, resulting in
a greater variation of tissue quality. Histologic evaluation of the periodontal
ligament, fibers that attach the root surface to surrounding alveolar bone, as
a function of age has revealed a decrease in fiber content and increase in interstitial
compartments with vasculature, but no change seems to occur in the fiber bundle

orientation [21]. Gingival recession is common in geriatric individuals. This results in exposure of the dental root to the oral environment [22].

Oral bone changes

Evaluation of bone for men and women between the ages of 35 and 70 shows that the bones become increasingly more brittle [23]. Age-related changes in the microscopic structure of the bone matrix and chemical composition affect the strength of bone. In the oral cavity, bone loss manifests itself as increased tooth loss in the dentate individual [24] or resorption of the residual ridges in the edentulous patient [25]. Studies in women of 50 years or older showed a decrease in alveolar bone height relative to root length when compared with younger age groups [24]. Part of this associated bone loss is caused by the loss of periodontal attachment, which is more prevalent in the elderly. This chronic inflammatory disease accelerates the loss of alveolar bone secondary to any bone loss from aging. Continual loss of the residual ridges in the edentulous patient is manifested by the need to have removable dental prosthetic appliances either relined or refabricated.

Age-related changes of the salivary glands

Diminished salivary flow has been associated with aging [26]. Studies on the submandibular gland have reported the loss of approximately 40% of acinar cells with aging [27,28]. Similar morphologic changes have been reported in the parotid gland [29] and labial salivary glands [30]. Because acinar cells are salivary elements capable of fluid production, this may explain such a reduction in salivary sections. Studies vary as to whether there is a decrease [31] or no difference [32,33] in salivary flow output between elderly and young adults. No changes have been observed between parotid and submandibular salivary secretions from individuals of different ages [34,35], but differences in minor labial glands have been described [36]. It is reasonable to suggest that salivary flow reduction may be different for each gland type.

Clinically, a reduction in saliva resulting in oral dryness (xerostomia) and elderly patient complaints about dry mouth, difficulty chewing, and loss of taste, should not be considered simply a consequence of aging [37]. Other factors, most notably medications, may directly affect salivary gland output. A number of these drugs with secondary salivary side effects have been listed elsewhere [38]. Radiation and chemotherapy may also result in salivary impairment. Ionizing radiation used in the management of head and neck cancers damages and destroys acinar cells of the salivary glands [39]. Lastly, any autoimmune disease may also impair salivary function. One example is Sjögren's syndrome, which either affects the salivary or lacrimal glands alone or may be associated with a rheumatoid disease (ie, rheumatoid arthritis or lupus) [40].

Age may act as a contributing factor in making the salivary gland more vulnerable to disease, but age alone does not result in salivary compromise [41,42].

Dental caries and periodontal disease

Dental caries and periodontal disease are common among the elderly. The following sections outline each separately.

Dental caries

Today's older adult population has a very different oral profile than earlier generations. Individuals are keeping their teeth longer. The prevalence of decayed and missing teeth in the United States has decreased approximately 50% since 1962 [43,44]. This suggests a noticeable decline in the number of edentulous persons in the United States. By contrast, the annual coronal caries increment per year in older adults was greater than that of children [45]. The clinician should be aware that older individuals, despite different dietary habits from children, are prone to dental caries.

Coronal dental caries is a destructive infection in which certain oral bacteria cavitate and penetrate through the enamel into the dentin of a tooth. The carious lesion can be confined to one or more tooth surfaces. The cavitation of the tooth structure is caused by certain species of oral microorganisms.

Three essential requirements are necessary for caries to occur: (1) the predominance of cariogenic bacteria, (2) a food source, and (3) an acidic environment within which to replicate on a substrate. Caries that affects the crown portion of the tooth, composed of enamel, is referred to as "coronal." Caries that affects the root surface is referred to as "root caries." The three most common bacteria associated with both lesions are (1) *Streptococcus mutans*, (2) *Lactobacillus*, and (3) *Actinomyces* [46,47]. Some elderly are predisposed to dental caries because of a diet high in fermentable carbohydrates because of limited finances or their inability to chew harder foods. Such softer diets are also more cariogenic [48].

Root caries

Root caries affects the surface of the tooth roots. Epidemiologic studies on root caries suggest an increase in the percentage of individuals with root caries who are from older populations [49]. The prevalence of root caries is double for individuals of 60 years of age compared with 30 year olds [49]. The mandibular facial surfaces of premolar and molar teeth, typically those showing gingival recession, exhibit the greatest prevalence of root caries [50,51]. The prevalence of root caries in the senior population may range as high as 60% [44]. Low socioeconomic status, infrequent dental care, nursing home residence, nonfluoridated water supply, and poor oral hygiene are all factors associated with the increased prevalence of root caries [52–54]. Other local factors include previous history

of coronal and root caries, high plaque presence, and low salivary flow rate
[53,55,56].

Incidence of root caries with clinical dental treatment

In studies involving overdenture abutments and the incidence of root caries,
most root caries occurred within the first year of prosthetic placement. Thereafter, the incidence is reduced by more than 50% [57,58]. Restorative procedures for root caries eliminated the incidence of recurrent root caries up to 1 year
follow-up [59]. Fixed prosthetics had a lower incidence of root caries when
compared with removable partial dentures over a 5-year period.

Periodontal surgery and incidence of root caries

Patients receiving periodontal surgery are not at increased risk of developing
root caries compared with those treated nonsurgically provided preventive maintenance schedules are implemented [60,61].

Nursing home versus community residents and root caries

The prevalence of root caries is higher in nursing homes than elderly individuals residing in the community [53,62]. The incidence of root caries increases
almost eightfold when residents are afflicted with a neurodegenerative disease,
such as Alzheimer's disease, when compared with elderly living within the same
community [63].

Topical fluoride and root caries

Several clinical studies have shown the value of topical fluoride application on
root caries. A 2-year clinical study evaluating the use of topical fluoride showed
that 100% of shallow lesions were reversible when lightly disked followed by
fluoride application [64]. Eighty percent of root carious lesions were arrested
simply by applying topical fluoride. An 18-month investigation on root caries
reversibility reported 100% success through the use of topical fluoride treatments
and fluoridate toothpaste used twice daily [65].

A 4-year study of root caries in older adults dwelling in a fluoridated community showed that sodium fluoride rinse daily or acidulated phosphofluoride (APF)
gel reduced the number of new lesions [66]. Further, sodium fluoride or APF
use also resulted in a greater number of reversed lesions than the placebo group.

Periodontal disease in the elderly population

The periodontium are those supporting structures of the teeth in the jaw-
bone and include the gingiva, cementum, the periodontal ligament, and bone.
Cementum is a mineralized tissue that is present on the surface of the root into
which the periodontal ligament attaches. The periodontal ligament is composed
of collagenous fibers that serve to attach the root cementum to the alveolar bone.

Bacterial plaque has been shown experimentally to produce gingivitis (gingival inflammation) in humans [67]. Other risk factors include oral hygiene, age,

type of bacteria, gender, and tobacco use [68,69]. Gingivitis is an inflammatory disease with bacterial plaque being the primary risk factor. It is characterized by erythematous, edematous gingival tissue with bleeding on gentle tissue manipulation. The cause of gingivitis is bacterial plaque associated with poor oral hygiene. Gingivitis develops rapidly in the aging population, but reversal of the process occurs readily with treatment and healing is not affected by age [70].

Periodontal disease occurs when the inflammation of the attachment tissue results in loss of bony support of the teeth. It is believed to be a progression from gingivitis. The proportion of individuals with periodontal disease increases in the elderly population [71]. This is also associated with an increase in attachment loss, recession [43], and decrease in oral cleanliness with increasing age [72]. The incidence of periodontitis is higher among all age groups for those with poor oral hygiene versus those with good oral hygiene [73]. There are at least two microorganisms associated with progressive periodontal disease: *Actinobacillus actinomycetemcomitans* and *Porphyromonas gingivalis* [74]. Although age is a good predictor of periodontitis, its effect is negligible when oral hygiene is maintained [73]. A number of epidemiologic studies of institutionalized individuals suggest that the severity and percentage of individuals with advanced periodontal disease is greater in this population than noninstitutionalized populations [75–77]; however, the exact cause of this difference requires further study.

Periodontitis is the destruction of the underlying supporting alveolar bone. Bone loss eventually results in loosening of teeth and their loss. Periodontitis in the elderly population is referred to as "chronic periodontitis," characterized by episodic periods of quiescence followed by short bursts of bony destruction.

Age is not a risk factor for periodontal disease [78]; however, certain habits or nutritional deficiencies may play a contributing role. Smoking has been shown to be an important contributor to periodontal disease facilitating the formation of calculus and reducing gingival healing [79]. Smokeless tobacco is an important risk factor for severe periodontal disease [80]. Diet may also play an important role in the susceptibility of the disease [81].

A relationship between the diabetic patient and the risk for more severe periodontal disease compared with a healthy population has been observed [82]. Other studies have shown a possible association between periodontal disease and coronary arthrosclerosis, because both maladies share similar inflammatory mediators and embolus formation from oral plaque microorganisms. It is not yet clear whether there exists an association between periodontal disease and coronary heart disease [83,84].

It is important for the clinician to understand that the effect of age alone does not cause tooth loss. Further, the presence of severe periodontal disease in an elderly individual should not be considered a normal occurrence in the aging process. Regardless of age, plaque accumulation leads to gingival inflammation [85]. Apart from any systemic risk factors, this process is reversible through proper oral hygiene and professional dental maintenance. Plaque, gingivitis, and loss of attachment remain significantly reduced in an elderly population maintained on a 2- to 3-month dental recall program consisting of oral hygiene instruction and prophylaxis [86,87]. This population group should be carefully monitored and maintained by a systematic regiment of professional recall visits.

Oral cancer in the elderly population

Over 375,000 new cases of oral cancer were diagnosed worldwide in 1980 [88]. It is estimated that one American dies every hour from oral cancer [89]. Oral cancer is found on the lip, oral cavity, tongue, and pharynx. The appearance of these and other oral lesions are nicely depicted in several oral pathology textbooks [90–92].

Lip cancer

Lip cancer is generally a squamous cell carcinoma on the vermilion border of the lower lip in fair-skinned individuals [93]. The 5-year survival rates for lip cancer for men and women are 91% and 84%, respectively. A combination of sunlight with other factors, such as cold and wind, may be important in the etiology of this cancer [94].

Cancer of the oral cavity, tongue, and pharynx

Cancer of the oral cavity, tongue, and pharynx is generally a squamous cell carcinoma and occurs more frequently in the elderly. Oral leukoplakia, erythroplakia, and erythroleukoplakia are considered premalignant [95]. Smoking remains a major risk factor for oral and pharyngeal cancer [96]. Smokeless tobacco and alcohol are also risk factors [96,97].

Oral cancer is primarily squamous cell carcinoma and frequently presents itself as an asymptomatic red or white lesion that does not heal. Pain or paresthesia suggests a more invasive form of the disease. It is most commonly found under the tongue in the floor of the mouth and the area behind the last molar teeth in the mandible. For base of the tongue squamous cell carcinoma the survival rates are low when diagnosed in advanced stages most perish within 2 years following detection [98]. Other areas can include the soft palate and lateral borders of the tongue. Any suspicious lesion that has not resolved within 1 to 2 weeks should be biopsied to rule out oral cancer.

Preventive dentistry

Development of dental oral health services for the elderly is still limited in many health institutions. Certainly prevention is a better approach than management through costly emergency treatment alone. Dental treatment needs to go simultaneously with a program of preventive management.

Because periodontal disease and dental caries are both of bacterial plaque origin, their treatment and prevention are important in the maintenance and dental well-being of the patient. Limited manipulative skills by the elderly coupled with a history of missing teeth, defective restorations, and faulty prosthesis all contribute to plaque accumulation [99]. Neurologic diseases, such as stroke, Parkinson's disease, or Alzheimer's disease, all limit the individual's manipulative skills, predisposing this population to dental disease. The geriatric dental patient requires a set of oral hygiene appliances that facilitate oral hygiene procedures despite their limited manual dexterity.

For elderly individuals with grasping difficulties, one might consider providing a toothbrush with a wider handle. An electric toothbrush not only provides a wider handle, but also removes the necessity for the individual to navigate the brush. The electric toothbrush itself provides the mechanical work. This is particularly important in individuals with limited neuromuscular activity or severe arthritis. Because cleaning between teeth (interproximal cleaning) is so important, dental floss is the implement of choice. Dental floss is used with both hands and passed between the teeth. For individuals with manipulative problems, the use of a floss holder or dental toothpick may be a good substitute.

As an adjunct to mechanical oral hygiene, elderly patients may also use an antimicrobial mouth rinse that helps reduce supragingival plaque. Chlorhexidine has been found to reduce these microbiota. Unfortunately, rinsing does not reduce pathogenic microorganisms situated subgingivally. Even with subgingival irrigation, these microbiota eventually recolonize the area if not professionally monitored [100].

Professional mechanical debridement of periodontal pockets removes the subgingival bacterial accumulations and significantly reduces plaque-induced diseases. It is important that family members and professional staff assist with the debilitated elderly individual's oral hygiene and the schedule of professional maintenance visits. Both family members and staff need to increase their dental awareness through education. This can be accomplished by imparting information to the family member and having professional health providers attend periodic seminars on dental issues related to the geriatric patient.

It is important for the professional to understand that there is a difference in patient-perceived need for dental treatment. A comparison examining the dental prosthetic treatment needs of an elderly population showed that the clinician-assessed need was approximately 25% higher than the perceived need on the part of the geriatric patient [101,102]. Further, variation in the degree of dental care use seems to be related to socioeconomic and cultural factors [103]. Those individuals of lower socioeconomic status had a higher propensity for not seeking dental care than those of middle or higher social class [104].

Oral health

The epidemiologic literature shows that both root and coronal caries are prevalent in the older individual because of social and behavioral factors. Poor oral hygiene leads to increasing amounts of plaque and calculus, resulting in the increased incidence of gingivitis and periodontitis [105]. The lack of proper oral hygiene has been observed to increase with age [106].

The most common oral lesion in the elderly is denture stomatitis, caused by poor denture hygiene and ill-fitting dentures [107]. This can be reduced by proper hygiene measures, including proper brushing and soaking of the prosthesis, by the elderly patient or caregiver. A number of over-the-counter denture cleansers are available. Finally, removable partial and full denture prosthetics should not be worn at night when saliva is reduced and bacterial counts increase.

In developing a program for the elderly, it is important to note that the traditional barrier to cost for services influences use only slightly [108]. More importantly, the lack of perceived need by the patient seems to be the major reason why individuals do not seek dental services [109]. Aside from providing high-quality dental services, the clinician must shape the patient's attitudes and perceived needs related to oral health needs.

Behavioral changes are difficult to accomplish. It is difficult to encourage a patient with a lifelong history of poor hygiene to evolve into one with meticulously oral home care. A major part of any oral hygiene regimen involves primarily education of both the patient and caregiver. It is equally important that the caregiver be educated in oral hygiene techniques and the importance thereof. Research has shown that the knowledge of the attendant transgresses that of the patient [4]. Caregivers with a higher prevalence of dental disease of their own and low dental knowledge had patients exhibiting similar attributes [4].

Providing oral health information both verbally combined with individual demonstrations on dental cleaning techniques is most effective for a geriatric population when compared with verbal alone [110]. Repetition is also essential to avoid memory regression. This can be reinforced through individual discussions, group slide presentations, group meetings, and directly at each follow-up dental visit [111].

A second group of individuals who require exposure to information on dental health care issues are the health care workers directly involved with residential homes. Often the amount of dental care knowledge of health care staff is very limited [112]. Very often caregivers perceive that oral hygiene is of low priority, not linked to health risks, and noncurative [113]. Further, many health care workers believe the act of handling the teeth or dentures of an individual is unpleasant and jeopardizes the patient's privacy. Courses in oral hygiene issues are often not sought out by health care staff [114]. Changes of such attitudes can only be brought about through a comprehensive dental education program targeting the staff within the hospital ward or elderly facility. Only through health-promoting programs can health care providers acquire the necessary skills and knowledge to aid in the early detection and prevention of geriatric-related oral health problems.

Role of physicians in oral health

Physicians should recognize the benefits of oral health to the overall health of the elderly patient. Aside from the functional aspect of the mouth in masticating food, it is also important in speaking, facial expression, affection, and self-esteem [115].

Oral maladies can affect one or more of these important activities, which can have both physiologic and psychologic consequences. Because the face and mouth are important for daily communication, any facial disfigurement makes the individual self-conscious and depressed. Further, oral ailments can make food mastication difficult resulting in the potential for nutritional impairment. It has been reported that the intake of nutrients was lower in edentate than dentate older individuals [116]. More aggressive oral diseases, such as malignancies or abscesses (and attendant bacteriemia and septicemia), can potentially be life-threatening particularly in the medically compromised elderly individual. The importance of geriatric medicine has been growing steadily with the increasing demands from a heterogeneous aging population. Acquisition of specialized knowledge in this area should also include aspects of oral health. Most medical programs do not presently devote sufficient time toward geriatric dental issues for their residents.

Pertinent medical history

To define a particular oral problem, it is important to elicit information about the symptoms of which the geriatric patient complains. Medical work-up by the physician is crucial for the evaluation of nondental causes of nutritional and medical contributors to the ailment.

The first criterion is to determine if there is any confusion or if the individual is cognizant and providing reliable responses to questioning. Responses to critical questions are essential if the cause of the chief complaint is to be elucidated. Elderly individuals underreport orofacial pain compared to younger adults [117]. Adult men are less likely than women to seek urgent dental care [118]. Location, duration, and degree of discomfort are important information to aid in finding a potential cause of the ailment. Even discussing dental ailments with the spouse or significant other may elicit additional information.

Tooth loss is a common finding in most elderly individuals. Fortunately, the number of edentulous adults decreased from the 1960s (49%) to the 1990s (25%) [44,45,119], caused in part by better public education and a change in the dental school philosophy to preserve the dentition. Fortunately, most oral diseases are treatable or preventable.

Other oral conditions

Oral candidiasis

Aside from hosting a number of microorganisms, the oral cavity also has a low count of yeast. The major pathogenic yeast is *Candida albicans*. This yeast can proliferate, infiltrate the oral mucosal layers, and result in an inflection known as "oral candidiasis."

Oral candidiasis can occur in individuals with altered immunity, such as HIV, diabetes mellitus, or head and neck radiation. Chronic use of antibiotics, chemotherapeutic agents, and steroid therapy can also predispose to candidiasis. Candidiasis can also be present under poorly fitting maxillary dentures characterized as an erythematous area under the prosthesis. Xerostomia can also predispose the individual to this condition.

Oral candidiasis can present itself in an acute or chronic form. The acute form can appear as a pseudomembranous or atrophic form. Chronic candidiasis presents itself as atrophic or hyperplastic. The two most common forms found in the elderly individual are acute pseudomembranous or chronic atrophic. The pseudomembranous form, or thrush, appears as a curdlike elevation and is generally associated with a burning mouth. It can be present anywhere on the soft tissue of the oral cavity including the pharynx and tongue. The lesion can be removed with a gauze and a definitive diagnosis made microscopically by the presence of yeast and hyphae.

Angular cheilitis is chronic atrophic candidiasis that presents itself along the commissures of the lips. This occurs when saliva is allowed to pool around the corners of the mouth and presents itself as an erythematous lesion in the commissures on either one or both sides.

Treatment for oral candidiasis

Treatment of oral candidiasis consists of using oral antifungal agents. Nystatin oral suspension (100,000 U/mL) is rinsed four times daily after meals and at bedtime. If nystatin is available in powder form (1 billion units) one can mix one eighth teaspoon into half a cup of water and have the patient swish for 1 minute. Both treatments should be performed over a 2-week period and the patient should be NPO one-half hour after giving the medication. In situations of denture stomatitis or angular cheilitis, application of a nystatin ointment or cream is useful (100,000 U/g), applied to the inner denture or the corner of the mouth four times daily for a 2-week period. For a systemic approach, ketoconazole, 200 mg, can be given once per day over a 2-week period. Fluconazole, 100 mg, is a good alternative because of the one dosage per day regiment, namely two tablets on the first day followed by one tablet for the remaining 13 days. It is recommended that the patient's denture be soaked in a solution of half a cup of 0.12% chlorhexidine gluconate to water or 1 teaspoon sodium hypochlorite in one cup of water during the treatment phase.

Xerostomia

Saliva is important in the digestive process by furnishing lubrication during the masticatory process. It also provides for oral pH balance, maintains a high level of calcium and phosphate, and has both antimicrobial and antifungal properties. For a variety of reasons the quantity of saliva may be reduced, a condition referred to as "xerostomia." Several reasons can contribute to this condition including medications used, alcoholism, autoimmune disorders, glandular blockage, Parkinson's disease, and radiation therapy of the salivary glands. The most common reason for xerostomia is the use of medications [120,121]. It is important to note that drug-induced xerostomia is reversible when the medication is changed. This is not the case with xerostomia caused by glandular damage from disease or radiation therapy.

Management of xerostomia

Treatment depends very much on the cause. For drug-induced xerostomia, changing the causative medication may reverse the condition. Alternatively, providing the medication at night, when the mouth is normally dry, or during meal time when saliva is most stimulated are additional strategies to help ease the situation. The use of sugarless chewing gum or candies may provide additional relief. The patient should be advised to have an adequate intake of water to avoid dehydration and avoid alcohol-containing mouthwashes and salty foods, which tend to desiccate the oral tissues. Caffeine-containing beverages should be limited because caffeine can also contribute to oral dryness.

Although there are salivary substitutes available on the market, such as Oralbalance Gel (Laclede, Garden, California), Optimoist (Colgate Oral Pharmaceuticals, Canton, Massachusetts), Xerolube (Scherer Laboratories, Dallas, Texas), and Moi-Stir (Kingswood Lab, Indianapolis, Indiana), these may only provide temporary relief and need to be applied regularly. In this population, a more serious issue is the potential for tooth decay. Proper oral hygiene is important in this regard. If the aged individual cannot perform the task effectively, then a trained health care provider should provide assistance. In addition to fluoridated toothpaste, it is recommended that an additional home fluoride gel (5000 pmm F^-) be prescribed as a supplement. The patient can swish this in the mouth or it can be applied with an oral mouth guard that the patient wears for 1 to 2 minutes. This should be accomplished after normal oral homecare procedures once or twice a day, particularly before sleep when salivary flow rate is reduced.

Oral ulcerations

Ulcerations are most commonly caused by oral trauma and may be present on the lips, mucosa, gingiva, and tongue [122]. Improperly fitting removable partial or denture prosthesis is the most common etiology. The trauma induced by fractured teeth may also contribute to oral ulcerations. Dental restorative and prosthetic treatment should resolve these areas of ulceration. Nevertheless, lesions of no apparent traumatic origin, which fail to heal after 1 to 2 weeks, should be suspect of being oral cancer.

Another oral ulcerative condition includes recurrent aphthous lesions that are generally present on the movable, nonkeratinized oral mucosa. These lesions are painful and resolve within a 1- to 2-week period. The cause is not known, but precipitating factors include local trauma; stress; food sensitivity; hormone imbalance; and smoking cessation [123]. Treatment is only palliative and rarely are systemic steroids required [124].

Lichen planus also presents as an erosive ulceration. It is believed to be an autoimmune condition and is characterized as an ulcerative region circumscribed by a lacelike white pattern. It is found primarily on the tongue, gingiva, and cheek mucosa and may be initiated by stress, drug allergy, infection, or genetic predisposition [125]. Lichen planus is painful and episodic. Treatment consists of the application of either clobetasol propionate ointment 0.05%, fluocinonide gel 0.05%, or trimcinolon acetonide in gel base 0.1% topical medications [126]. These are applied to the lesions four times daily. For lesions not responsive to oral applications, systemic steroids should be considered [127]. It is important to note that approximately 1% of oral cancers may appear with the same clinical morphology and distribution as erosive or erythematous lichen planus [128]. These lesions should be followed-up periodically to exclude malignant transformation.

Hyperkeratotic lesions

Hyperkeratotic lesions are most often the result of chronic trauma, seen associated with dentures or on the lateral border of the tongue. These lesions appear as a white plaque referred to as "leukoplakia." In the event the traumatic etiology cannot be ascertained, the lesion should be biopsied to rule out the potential of cancer. Detection of oral cancer in early asymptomatic stages is possible, a period when curative therapy is most effective. A simple screening method uses a computer-assisted brush biopsy technique (OralCDx, CDx Laboratories, Suffern, New York) that is very effective in screening unexplained red, white, mixed, ulcerative, or hyperkeratotic lesions for the possibility of cancer [129]. This minimally invasive technique serves as an adjunct to the oral examination and determines whether an innocuous clinical lesion requires surgical biopsy. With this transepithelial biopsy technique, a biopsy brush is moistened with the patient's saliva, pressed firmly on the surface of the lesion until the tissue becomes reddened or slight bleeding is observed, and rotated several times. The brush is then removed and the specimen from the brush transferred onto a glass slide. The cellular material on the slide is treated with a fixative solution, dried, fixed, and stored in a special slide holder. The brush is then placed into a second transport vial containing fixative and sealed. Both items are then delivered to CDx Laboratories for pathologic interpretation. All oral lesions with abnormal brush biopsy findings of dysplasia should be subjected to incisional scalpel biopsy.

Lesions of dental prosthetic origin

Aged patients most likely have lost some of their teeth. Either a full denture replacing all the teeth in an arch, or a partial denture or bridge in which localized areas of missing teeth are substituted, replace their lost teeth. With the extraction of teeth there are changes in the level of the osseous ridge that continues over time. As a result, both full and partial dentures become ill-fitting resulting in episodic mechanical trauma to the underlying gingival tissues, particularly during mastication. This trauma results in an overgrowth of gingival connective tissue evident along the borders of the prosthesis. Treatment involves adjusting the prosthesis or fabricating a new one. In more severe cases of gingival outgrowth, oral surgery is required to remove this excess tissue.

Painful, burning mouth

The primary symptom is a generalized painful, burning sensation of the oral cavity. This can affect the entire mouth or be localized to the tongue alone. The primary cause to consider is oral *Candida* infection [130]. Other possible causes include vitamin B deficiency, xerostomia, iron deficiency, diabetes mellitus, allergies, nonfunctional oral habits, and menopause [131,132].

Treatment depends on the etiology. These treatments include antifungal medication in the case of *Candida* infection. For xerostomia, finding the causative drug and providing helpful procedures to stimulate salivary flow and using salivary substitutes may be helpful. In some cases, vitamin or iron supplementation may be indicated. Treatment may also involve determining the reason for a nonfunctional oral habit, such as a sharp tooth or broken denture. Simply smoothing the tooth or denture may provide some patient relief. Oral hygiene should always be considered, because particles of food also serve as an irritant to the soft tissues. Treatment involves proper brushing and interdental cleaning by the patient or health caregiver. In the case of an oral denture prosthesis, treatment involves having the patient remove the prosthesis at least 6 hours a day (generally while sleeping); brushing the prosthesis and underlying soft tissue; and soaking the prosthesis overnight in a solution of denture cleaner.

Systemic disease affecting the oral condition

Any systemic disease that limits a patient's ability to masticate and ingest food and perform proper oral hygiene impacts the oral condition. Some conditions in this category include arthritis, stroke, dementia, and cancer.

Arthritis

Arthritis results in the deformation of the individual's fingers making oral hygiene more difficult. Thickening of the handle of a manual toothbrush facilitates manipulation. An electric or sonic toothbrush with a wider handle is a good substitute for the conventional toothbrush and requires less hand motion. If gripping continues to be a problem, using an elastic or Velcro band or cloth helps retain the toothbrush within the hand. In patients with a limited range of motion because of arthritic shoulders, the handle of a toothbrush can be lengthened by using a piece of wood or plastic. For cleaning between the teeth, a Y-shaped floss holder is particularly useful. Floss is threaded between the ends to the holder and passed between the teeth while holding the handle. Several designs are available on the market (Flossaid, Santa Clara, California; Butler, Chicago, Illinois). The Proxabrush (Butler) is a small brush mounted on a handle that can be used between teeth with larger spaces. A limitation is that some dexterity is required and the brushes must be replaced periodically. The use of a thin wooden interdental toothpick made of orangewood (Stimudents, Johnson and Johnson, New Brunswick, New Jersey) is also a good substitute requiring less manipulative skills.

Osteoarthritis and rheumatoid arthritis may affect the temporomandibular joint [133,134] and fall under the general category of "temporomandibular disorders," which is a collection of problems that affect the muscles of mastication and the temporomandibular joint itself. The temporomandibular joint, or jaw joint, is the hinge that connects the mandible to the temporal bone of the skull. The symptoms are numerous ranging from discomfort in the face or head region, tinnitus, paresthesia, discomfort while masticating, headaches, and hearing problems [135]. These individuals are best managed with a multidisciplinary team of a dentist, physical therapist, rheumatologist, and neurologist. During periods of discomfort, these patients are advised to limit jaw activity and switch to a softer diet.

Stroke

Stroke is characterized by paresis or paralysis of the extremities and difficulty with speech. Survivors frequently are left with compromised motor ability, numbness, and difficulty swallowing. Their compromised motor ability results in poor oral hygiene. A spouse or caregiver needs to assist the patient with brushing and ensure that all food has been removed from the oral cavity. Oral numbness further complicates the situation, because the patient is unaware that portions of food may still be in the mouth. Aspiration is always a concern because many of these individuals have a swallowing disorder. Every effort should be made by the caregiver to ensure good oral care to avoid aspiration of oral microbiota. Fabrication of any dental prosthesis for the semidentate or edentulous stroke patient should be delayed until the individual demonstrates enough rehabilitation and progress that they can properly function with a new prosthesis.

Dementia

This population is characterized by a loss of cognitive function. The spouse and caregiver should include oral hygiene into the dementia patient's daily routine. With advanced dementia, the patient may require increasing assistance with oral hygiene coupled with a high-level fluoride gel or toothpaste (5000 ppm). This patient group may also be less cognizant of sensory stimulation and unable appropriately to relay pain. Because of the progressive nature of the disease, dental restorative procedures should be completed during the early onset of the disease, avoiding a more difficult situation if dental services are required during the terminal stages of the disease.

Radiation and cancer

Radiation used to treat cancers of the head and neck can cause several acute and chronic oral problems. When the salivary glands are placed within the field of radiation, the result is radiation-induced xerostomia or hyposalivation [136]. Along with a decrease in salivary flow is a decrease in taste, smell acuity, and trouble masticating food [132]. Patients need to function with the compromised amounts of saliva. Some patients experience some benefit using pilocarpine hydrochloride, a drug that stimulates salivary gland secretion, before and after radiation therapy (5 mg three times a day) [137]. Use of sugar-free lozenges or sugar-free chewing gum, sweetened with xylitol, also helps increase salivation. Further, a specially designed Biotene Dry Mouth Gum is available on the market (Laclede, Rancho Dominguez, California) to stimulate salivary flow.

To reduce the incidence of caries, placement of oral custom-fabricated trays around the teeth containing a high-level fluoride gel (5000 ppm) for 5 minutes per day at bedtime is recommended. Frequency of application can be increased in more severe cases of dental caries. As an alternative to the tray, high-fluoride application can be delivered by toothpaste. Some brands of high-fluoride toothpaste include PreviDent 5000 Plus (Colgate Oral Pharmaceutics, Canton, Massachusetts); Fluoridex 5000 ppm Neutral Sodium Fluoride Toothpaste (Discus Dental, Culver City, California); and ControlRx (Omnii Oral Pharmaceuticals, West Palm Beach, Florida). All dental work and a thorough oral prophylaxis should be completed before radiation therapy. Teeth of hopeless prognosis should be extracted before the radiation therapy is started. This avoids the increased risk of osteoradionecrosis of the surrounding bone in the event extractions become necessary post–radiation therapy.

Cancer patients receiving radiation or chemotherapy experience other oral complications. One such manifestation is mucositis, an inflammation of the oral mucous membranes. It is characterized by a reddened, inflamed, and painful oral mucosa. Although generally not life-threatening, many cancer patients who develop this complication may experience difficultly eating and swallowing. A 0.12% chlorhexidine gluconate rinse provided during chemotherapy can reduce the severity of mucositis [138]. Patients may find additional relief from the new drug palifermin recently approved by the US Food and Drug Administration. Palifermin is recombinant human keratinocyte growth factor, which stimulates the growth and repair of cells in skin, oral mucosa, stomach, and colon [139]. A study of palifermin on 212 cancer patients showed that 63% of the patients taking the drug developed mucositis and that the condition lasted for an average of 3 days. In contrast, 98% of the patients who were not on the drug developed mucositis and the condition lasted for an average of 9 days [139]. Palifermin reduces both the duration and severity of the oral mucositis. This drug is administered intravenously 3 days before radiation or chemotherapy and for 3 days following chemotherapy, but not on the same day as radiation or chemotherapy. Finally, to avoid oral trauma to the sensitive oral mucosa in the patient with mucositis, premoistened sponges on handles (Toothette, SAGE Products, Cary, Illinois) are available to clean and maintain the oral cavity. These are nonabrasive and reduce the chance of traumatizing the inflamed tissues.

Summary

By 2010, almost 40 million Americans will be 65 years old or older. The increase in life expectancy and numbers of elderly has magnified the need for research and focus on geriatric dentistry. This population is more at risk of systemic diseases with oral manifestations, which need to be recognized and managed. It is incumbent on the health care provider to understand the etio-pathogenesis, clinical presentation, and management of oral diseases in an aging population. Additional Online information can be found at the following sites: American Dental Association, www.ada.org; American Academy of Periodontology, www.perio.org; and National Center for Chronic Disease Prevention and Health Promotion, www.cdc.gov/aging/health_issues.htm.

Acknowledgments

The author would like to thank Christopher Cardozo, MD, Associate Professor of Medicine and Pharmacology and Biological Chemistry, Mount Sinai School of Medicine and George Dietrick, MD, Assistant Professor of Surgery, Mount Sinai School of Medicine for their insightful suggestions and reviewing the manuscript.

References

[1] Maupone G, Gullion CM, White BA, et al. Oral disorders and chronic systemic diseases in very old adults living in institutions. Spec Care Dentist 2003;23:199–208.
[2] Grau AJ, Becher H, Ziegler CM, et al. Periodontal disease as a risk factor for ischemic stroke. Stroke 2004;35:496–501.
[3] Anastassiadou V, Katsarou Z, Naka O, et al. Evaluating dental status and prosthetic need in relation to medical findings in Greek patients suffering from idiopathic Parkinson's disease. Eur J Prosthodont Restor Dent 2002;10:63–8.
[4] Stiefel DJ, Truelove EL, Persson RS, et al. A comparison of oral health in spinal cord injury and other disability groups. Spec Care Dentist 1993;13:229–35.
[5] Simonova MV, Grinin VM, Nasonova VA, et al. Clinical factors essential for dental caries intensity in rheumatic patients. Stomatologiia (Mosk) 2002;81:15–9.
[6] Marton K. Oral symptoms of immunologic disorders. Part 1. Systemic autoimmune diseases. Fogorv Sz 2003;96:9–15.
[7] Nitzan DW, Michaeli Y, Weinreb M, et al. The effect on aging on tooth morphology: a study of impacted teeth. Oral Surg Oral Med Oral Pathol 1986;61:54–60.

[8] Oi T, Saka H, Ide Y. Three-dimensional observation of pulp cavities in the maxillary first premolar tooth using micro-CT. Int Endod J 2004;37:46–51.

[9] Bennet CG, Kelln EE, Biddington WR. Age changes of the vascular pattern of the human dental pulp. Arch Oral Biol 1965;10:995–8.

[10] Schroeder HE. Differentiation of human oral epithelia. Basel: Karger; 1981.

[11] Gogly B, Godeau G, Gilbert S, et al. Morphometric analysis of collagen and elastic fibers in normal skin and gingiva in relation to age. Clin Oral Investig 1997;1:147–52.

[12] Wolff A, Ship JA, Tylenda CA, et al. Oral mucosal appearance is unchanged in healthy, different-aged persons. Oral Surg Oral Med Oral Pathol 1991;71:569–72.

[13] Shklar G. The effects of aging upon oral mucosa. J Invest Dermatol 1966;47:115–20.

[14] Löe H, Karring T. The three dimensional morphology of the epithelium connective tissue interface of the gingiva as related to age and sex. Scand J Dent Res 1971;79:315–26.

[15] Plewig G. Regional differences of cell sizes in the human stratum cornium II. Effects of sex and age. J Invest Dermatol 1970;54:19–23.

[16] Bottomly WK. Physiology of the oral mucosa. Otolaryngol Clin North Am 1979;12:15–20.

[17] Belding JH, Tade WH. Evaluation of epithelial maturity in hormonally related stomatitis. J Oral Med 1978;33:17–9.

[18] Ryan EJ, Toto PD, Garguilo AW. Aging in human attached gingival epithelium. J Dent Res 1974;53:74–6.

[19] Maidhof R, Hornstein OP. Autoradiographic study of some proliferative properties of human buccal mucosa. Arch Dermatol Res 1979;265:165–72.

[20] Thomson PJ, Potten CS, Appleton DR. In vitro labelling studies and the measurement of epithelial cell proliferative activity in the human oral cavity. Arch Oral Biol 2001;46:1157–64.

[21] Severson JA, Moffett BC, Kokich V, et al. A histological study of age changes in the adult human periodontal joint (ligament). J Periodontol 1978;49:189–200.

[22] Furseth R, Tolo K, Mjör I. Periodontium. In: Mjör I, editor. Reaction patterns in human teeth. Boca Raton (FL): CRC Press; 1983. p. 157–219.

[23] Martin B. Aging and strength of bone as a structural material. Calcif Tissue Int 1993; 53(Suppl 1):S34–40.

[24] Salonen L, Frithiof L, Wouters F, et al. Marginal alveolar bone height in an adult Swedish population: a radiographic cross-sectional epidemiologic study. J Clin Periodontol 1991;18: 223–32.

[25] Hirai T, Ishijima T, Hashikawa Y, et al. Osteoporosis and reduction in residual ridge in edentulous patients. J Prosthet Dent 1993;69:49–56.

[26] Langer A. Oral signs of aging and their clinical significance. Geriatrics 1976;31:63–9.

[27] Waterhouse JP, Chisholm DM, Winter RB, et al. Replacement of functional parenchymal cells by fat and connective tissue in human salivary glands: an age-related change. J Oral Pathol 1973;2:16–27.

[28] Scott J. Degenerative changes in the histology of the human submandibular gland occurring with age. J Biol Buccale 1977;5:311–9.

[29] Scott J, Flower EA, Burns J. A quantitative study of histological changes in the human parotid gland occurring with adult age. J Oral Pathol 1987;16:505–10.

[30] Drummond JR, Chisholm DM. A qualitative and quantitative study of the aging human labial salivary glands. Arch Oral Biol 1984;29:151–5.

[31] Ben-Aryeh H, Miron D, Szargel R, et al. Whole saliva secretion rates in old and young healthy subjects. J Dent Res 1984;63:1147–8.

[32] Parvinen T, Larmas M. Age dependency of stimulated salivary flow rate, pH, and lactobacillus and yeast concentrations. J Dent Res 1982;61:1052–5.

[33] Ship JA, Baum BJ. Is reduced salivary flow normal in old people? Lancet 1990;336:1507.

[34] Heft MW, Baum BJ. Unstimulated and stimulated parotid salivary flow rates in individuals of different ages. J Dent Res 1984;63:1182–5.

[35] Tylenda CA, Ship JA, Fox PC, et al. Evaluation of submandibular salivary flow rate in different age groups. J Dent Res 1988;67:1891–4.

[36] Smith DJ, Joshipura K, Kent R, et al. Effect of age on immunoglobulin content and volume of human labial gland saliva. J Dent Res 1992;71:1891–4.

[37] Wu AJ, Ship JA. A characterization of major salivary gland flow rates in the presence of medications and systemic diseases. Oral Surg Oral Med Oral Pathol 1993;76:301–6.

[38] Sreebny LM, Schwartz SS. A reference guide to drugs and dry mouth. Gerodontology 1986;5: 75–99.

[39] Silverman Jr S. Precancerous lesions and oral cancer in the elderly. Clin Geriatr Med 1992;8: 529–41.

[40] Talal N. Overview of Sjögren's syndrome. J Dent Res 1987;66:672–4.

[41] Baum BJ, Ship JA, Wu AJ. Salivary gland function and aging: a model for studying the interaction of aging and systemic disease. Crit Rev Oral Biol Med 1992;4:53–64.

[42] Baum BJ. Evaluation of stimulated parotid saliva flow rate in different age groups. J Dent Res 1981;60:1292–6.

[43] Johnson ES, Kelly JE, Van Kirk LE. Selected dental findings in adults by age, race, and sex, United States, 1960–1962. Vital Health Stat 11 1965;11:1–35.

[44] Miller AJ, Brunelle JH, Carlos JP, et al. Oral health of United States adults: the national survey of oral health in US employed adults and seniors, 1985–1986: National findings. Epidemiology and oral disease prevention program: National Institute of Dental Research. Bethesda: US Department of Health and Human Services, Public Health Service, National Institutes of Health; 1987. NIH publication no. 87–2868.

[45] Katz RV, Neely AL, Morse DE. The epidemiology of oral diseases in older adults. In: Holm-Pedersen P, Löe H, editors. Textbook of geriatric dentistry. Copenhagen: Munksgaard; 1996. p. 263–301.

[46] vanHoute J. Bacterial specificity in the etiology of dental caries. Int Dent J 1980;30:305–26.

[47] Bowden GHW. Microbiology of root surface caries in humans. J Dent Res 1990;69:1205–10.

[48] Gordon SR, Kelley SL, Sybyl JR, et al. Relationship in very elderly veterans of nutritional status, self-perceived chewing ability, dental status and social isolation. J Am Geriatr Soc 1985; 33:334–9.

[49] Katz RV. Assessing root caries in populations: the evaluation of the root caries index. J Public Health Dent 1980;40:7–16.

[50] Wallace MC, Retief DH, Bradley EL. Prevalence of root caries in a population of older adults. Gerodontics 1988;4:84–9.

[51] Katz RV, Hazen SP, Chilton NW, et al. Prevalence and intraoral distribution of root caries in an adult population. Caries Res 1982;16:265–71.

[52] Galan D, Lynch E. Epidemiology of root caries. Gerodontology 1993;10:59–71.

[53] MacEntee MI, Clark DC, Glick N. Prediction of caries in old age. Gerodontology 1993;10: 90–7.

[54] Stamm JW, Banting DW, Imrey PB. Adult root caries survey of two similar communities with contrasting natural water fluoride levels. J Am Dent Assoc 1990;120:143–9.

[55] Graves RC, Beck JD, Disney JA, et al. Root caries prevalence in black and white North Carolina adults over age 65. J Public Health Dent 1992;52:94–101.

[56] Powell LV, Mancl LA, Senft GD. Exploration of prediction models for caries risk assessment of the geriatric population. Community Dent Oral Epidemiol 1991;19:291–5.

[57] Toolson LB, Smith DE. A 2-year longitudinal study of overdenture patients. I. Incidence and control of caries on overdenture abutments. J Prosthet Dent 1978;40:486–91.

[58] Ettinger RL, Jakobsen J. Caries: a problem in an overdenture population. Community Dent Oral Epidemiol 1990;18:42–5.

[59] Levy SM, Jensen ME, Doering JV, et al. Evaluation of a glass ionomer cement and a microfilled composite resin in the treatment of root surface caries. Gen Dent 1989;37:468–72.

[60] Keltjens H, Schaeken T, van der Hoeven H, et al. Epidemiology of root surface caries in patients treated for periodontal diseases. Community Dent Oral Epidemiol 1988;16:171–4.

[61] Ravald N, Hamp SE, Birkhed D. Long-term evaluation of root surface caries in periodontally treated patients. J Clin Periodontol 1986;13:758–67.

[62] Kitamura M, Kiyak HA, Mulligan K. Predictors of root caries in the elderly. Community Dent Oral Epidemiol 1986;14:34–8.

[63] Jones JA, Lavalee N, Alman J, et al. Caries incidence in patients with dementia. Gerodontology 1993;10:76–82.

[64] Billings RJ, Brown LR, Kaster AG. Contemporary treatment strategies for root surface dental caries. Gerodontics 1985;1:20–7.

[65] Nyvad B, Fejerskov O. Active root surface caries converted into inactive caries as a response to oral hygiene. Scand J Dent Res 1986;94:281–4.

[66] Wallace MC, Retief DH, Bradley EL. The 48-month increment of root caries in an urban population of older adults participating in a preventive dental program. J Public Health Dent 1993; 53:133–7.

[67] Theilade E, Wright WH, Jensen SB, et al. Experimental gingivitis in man, II. A longitudinal clinical and bacteriological investigation. J Periodontal Res 1966;1:1–13.

[68] Jette AM, Feldman HA, Tennstedt SL. Tobacco use: a modifiable risk factor for dental disease among the elderly. Am J Public Health 1993;83:1271–6.

[69] Beck JD, Koch GG, Rozier RG, et al. Prevalence and risk indicators for periodontal attachment loss in a population of older community-dwelling blacks and whites. J Periodontol 1990; 61:521–8.

[70] Holm-Pederson P, Agerbaek N, Theilade E. Experimental gingivitis in young and elderly individuals. J Clin Periodontol 1975;2:14–24.

[71] Albandar JM. Epidemiology and risk factors of periodontal diseases. Dent Clin North Am 2005;49:517–32.

[72] Sheiham A. The prevalence and severity of periodontal disease in a British population. Dental surveys of employed populations in Great Britain. Br Dent J 1969;726:115–22.

[73] Abdellatif HM, Burt BA. An epidemiological investigation into the relative importance of age and oral hygiene status as determinants of periodontitis. J Dent Res 1987;66:13–8.

[74] Genco RJ. Current view of risk factors for periodontal diseases. J Periodontol 1996;67:1041–9.

[75] Vigild M. Oral hygiene and periodontal conditions among 201 dentate institutionalized elderly. Gerodontics 1988;4:140–5.

[76] Miyazaki H, Shirahama R, Ohtani I, et al. CPITN assessments in institutionalized elderly people in Kitakyushu, Japan. Community Dent Health 1991;8:239–43.

[77] Jenkins WMM, Kinane DF. The high risk group in periodontitis. Br Dent J 1989;167:168–72.

[78] Suzuki J, Niessen L, Fedele D. Periodontal diseases in the older adult. In: Papas A, Niessen L, Chauncey H, editors. Geriatric dentistry: aging and oral health. St. Louis: Mosby Yearbook; 1991. p. 189–201.

[79] Fenesy KE. Periodontal disease: an overview for physicians. Mt Sinai J Med 1998;65:362–9.

[80] Fisher MA, Taylor GW, Tilashalski KR. Smokeless tobacco and severe active periodontal disease, NHANES III. J Dent Res 2005;84:705–10.

[81] Al-Zahrani MS, Bissada NF, Borawski EA. Diet and periodontitis. J Int Acad Periodontol 2005; 7:21–6.

[82] Grossi SC, Genco RJ. Periodontal disease and diabetes mellitus: a two-way relationship. Ann Periodontol 1998;3:51–61.

[83] Geerts SO, Legrand V, Charpentier J, et al. Further evidence of the association between periodontal conditions and coronary artery disease. J Peridontol 2004;75:1274–80.

[84] Hujoel PP, Drangsholt M, Spiekerman C, et al. Periodontal disease and coronary heart disease risk. JAMA 2000;284:1406–10.

[85] Holm-Pedersen P, Agerbaek N, Theilade E. Experimental gingivitis in young and elderly individuals. J Clin Periodontol 1975;2:14–24.

[86] Axelsson P, Lindhe J. Effect of controlled oral hygiene procedures on caries and periodontal disease in adults. J Clin Periodontol 1978;5:133–51.

[87] Axelsson P, Lindhe J, Nystrom B. On the prevention of caries and periodontal disease: results of a 15-year longitudinal study in adults. J Clin Periodontol 1991;18:182–9.

[88] Parkin DM, Läärä E, Muir CS. Estimates of the worldwide frequency of sixteen major cancers in 1980. Int J Cancer 1988;41:184–97.

[89] Slavkin HC. Clinical dentistry in the 21st century. Compend Contin Educ Dent 1997;18:212-8.

[90] Neville BW, Damm DD, White DK. Color Atlas of Clinical Oral Pathology. Baltimore: Williams & Wilkins; 1999.

[91] Laskaris G. Color Atlas of Oral Diseases. New York: Theime; 2003.

[92] Field A, Longman L. Tyldesley's Oral Medicine. Oxford: Oxford University Press; 2003.

[93] Keller AZ. Cellular types, survival, race, nativity, occupations, habits and associated diseases in the pathogenesis of lip cancers. Am J Epidemiol 1970;91:486-99.

[94] Prestin-Martin S, Henderson BE, Pike MC. Descriptive epidemiology of cancers of the upper respiratory tract in Los Angeles. Cancer 1982;49:2201-7.

[95] Silverman SJ, Gorsky M, Lozada F. Oral leukoplakia and malignant transformation: a follow-up study of 257 patients. Cancer 1984;53:563-8.

[96] Blot WJ, McLaughlin JK, Winn DM, et al. Smoking and drinking in relation to oral and pharyngeal cancer. Cancer Res 1988;48:3282-7.

[97] Rosenquist K, Wennerberg J, Schildt EB, et al. Use of Swedish moist snuff, smoking and alcohol consumption in the aetiology of oral and orophoryngeal squamous cell carcinoma. A population-based case-control study in southern Sweden. Acta Otolaryngol 2005;125:991-8.

[98] Zhen W, Karnell LH, Hoffman HT, et al. The National Cancer Data Base report on squamous cell carcinoma of the base of tongue. Head Neck 2004;26:660-74.

[99] Addy M, Bates JF. Plaque accumulation following the wearing of different types of removable partial dentures. J Oral Rehabil 1979;6:111-7.

[100] Westling M, Tynelius-Bratthall G. Microbiological and clinical short-term effects of repeated intracrevicular chlorhexidine rinsings. J Periodontal Res 1984;19:202-9.

[101] Vigild M. Denture status and need for prosthodontic treatment among institutionalized elderly in Denmark. Community Dent Oral Epidemiol 1987;15:128-33.

[102] Mojon P, MacEntee MI. Discrepancy between need for prosthodontic treatment and complaints in an elderly edentulous population. Community Dent Oral Epidemiol 1992;20:48-52.

[103] Manski RJ, Magder LS. Demographic and socioeconomic predictors of dental care utilization. J Am Dent Assoc 1998;129:195-200.

[104] Chattopadhyay A, Kumar JV, Green EL. The New York State minority health survey: determinants of oral health care utilization. J Public Health Dent 2003;63:158-65.

[105] Ambjørnsen E. Remaining teeth, periodontal condition, oral hygiene and tooth cleaning habits in dentate old age subjects. J Clin Periodontol 1986;13:583-9.

[106] Johnson NW. Detection of high risk groups and individuals for periodontal diseases. Int Dent J 1989;39:33-47.

[107] Budtz-Jørgensen E, Bertram U. Denture stomatitis. I. The etiology in relations to trauma and infection. Acta Odontol Scand 1970;28:71-92.

[108] Kiyak HA. Recent advances in behavioral research in geriatric dentistry. Gerodontology 1988; 7:27-36.

[109] Mann J, Mersel A, Ernest M, et al. Dental behavioral aspect of a non-institutionalized elderly population. Gerodontology 1990;9:83-7.

[110] Ambjørnsen E, Rise J. The effect of verbal information and demonstration on denture hygiene in elderly people. Acta Odontol Scand 1985;43:19-24.

[111] Reynolds MW. Education for geriatric oral health promotion. Spec Care Dentist 1997;17: 33-6.

[112] Rak OS, Warren K. An assessment of the level of dental and mouth care knowledge amongst nurses working with elderly patients. Community Dent Health 1990;7:295-301.

[113] Eadie DR, Schou L. An exploratory study of barriers to promoting oral hygiene through carers of elderly people. Community Dent Health 1992;9:343-8.

[114] Fiske J, Gelbier S, Watson RM. Barriers to dental care in an elderly population resident in an inner city area. J Dent 1990;18:236-42.

[115] Berkey DB, Shay K. General dental care for the elderly. Clin Geriatr Med 1992;8:579-97.

[116] Sheiham A, Steele JG, Marcenes W, et al. The relationship among dental status, nutrient intake, and nutritional status in older people. J Dent Res 2001;80:408-13.

[117] Lipton JA, Ship JA, Larach-Robinson D. Estimated prevalence and distribution of reported orofacial pain in the United States. J Am Dent Assoc 1993;124:115–21.

[118] Riley III JL, Gilbert GH, Heft MW. Orofacial pain: patient satisfaction and delay of urgent care. Public Health Rep 2005;120:140–9.

[119] Kelly JE, Harvey CR. Basic data of dental examination findings of persons 1–74 years, United States, 1971–74. Vital Health Stat 11 1979;214:1–33.

[120] Navazesh M, Brightman VJ, Pogoda JM. Relationship of medical status, medications, and salivary flow rates in adults of different ages. Oral Surg Oral Med Oral Pathol Oral Radiol Endod 1996;81:172–6.

[121] Bergdahl M, Bergdahl J. Low unstimulated salivary flow and subjective oral dryness: association with medication, anxiety, depression, and stress. J Dent Res 2000;79:1652–8.

[122] Greer RO. A problem oriented approach to evaluation of common mucosal lesions in the geriatric patient. Gerodontics 1985;1:68–74.

[123] Scully C, Gorsky M, Lozada-Nur F. The diagnosis and management of recurrent aphthous stomatitis: a consensus approach. J Am Dent Assoc 2003;134:200–7.

[124] Sarmadi M, Ship JA. Refractory major aphthous stomatitis managed with systemic immunosuppressants: a case report. Quintessence Int 2004;35:39–48.

[125] Regezi JA, Sciubba JJ. Oral pathology: Clinical Pathologic Correlations. Philadelphia: Saunders; 1999.

[126] Gibson G, Niessen LC. Aging and the oral cavity. In: Cassel CK, Leipzig RM, Cohen HJ, et al, editors. Geriatric medicine, an evidence-based approach. New York: Springer; 2003. p. 901–17.

[127] Chainani-Wu N, Silverman Jr S, Lozada-Nur F, et al. Oral lichen planus: patient profile, disease progression and treatment responses. J Am Dent Assoc 2001;132:901–9.

[128] Eisen D. The clinical features, malignant potential, and systemic associations of oral lichen planus: a study of 723 patients. J Am Acad Dermatol 2002;46:207–14.

[129] Sciubba JJ. Improving detection of precancerous and cancerous oral lesions. J Am Dent Assoc 1999;130:1445–57.

[130] Terai H, Shimahara M. Atropic tongue associated with Candida. J Oral Pathol Med 2005; 34:397–400.

[131] Pinto A, Stoopler ET, DeRossi SS, et al. Burning mouth syndrome: a guide for the general practioner. Gen Dent 2003;51:458–61.

[132] Scala A, Checci L, Montevecchi M, et al. Update on burning mouthy syndrome: overview and patient management. Crit Rev Oral Biol Med 2003;14:275–91.

[133] Koh ET, Yap AU, Koh CK, et al. Temporomandibular disorders in rheumatoid arthritis. J Rheumatol 1999;26:1918–22.

[134] Emshoff R, Innerhofer K, Rudisch A, et al. The biological concept of internal derangement and osteoarthrosis: a diagnostic approach in patients with temporomandibular joint pain? Oral Surg Oral Med Oral Pathol Oral Radiol Endod 2002;93:39–44.

[135] Iacopino AM, Wathen WF. Craniomandibular disorders in the geriatric patient. J Orofac Pain 1993;7:38–53.

[136] Fox PC. Acquired salivary dysfunction: drugs and radiation. Ann N Y Acad Sci 1998;842: 132–7.

[137] Johnson JT, Ferretti GA, Nethery WJ, et al. Oral pilocarpine for post-irradiation xerostomia in patients with head and neck cancer. N Engl J Med 1993;329:390–5.

[138] Ferretti GA, Raybould TP, Brown AT, et al. Chlorhexidine prophylaxis for chemotherapy and radiotherapy induced stomatitis: a randomized double-blind trial. Oral Surg Oral Med Oral Pathol 1990;69:331–8.

[139] Spielberger R, Stiff P, Bensinger W, et al. Palifermin for oral mucositis after intensive therapy for hematologic cancers. N Engl J Med 2004;351:2590–8.

CLINICS IN
GERIATRIC
MEDICINE

Clin Geriatr Med 22 (2006) 435–447

Rehabilitation of the Older Adult with an Osteoporosis-Related Fracture

Julie T. Lin, MD[a,b,*], Joseph M. Lane, MD[a,c]

[a]Hospital for Special Surgery, 535 East 70th Street, New York, NY 10021, USA
[b]Department of Rehabilitation Medicine, Weill Medical College of Cornell University,
1300 York Avenue, New York, NY 10021, USA
[c]Department of Orthopedic Surgery, Weill Medical College of Cornell University,
1300 York Avenue, New York, NY 10021, USA

Fractures can result in significant disability and dysfunction. Osteoporosis is the leading cause of fracture in the elderly and is the most common metabolic bone disease in the world. It is a condition in which there is decreased bone mass; less advantageous distribution of the bone mass; altered microarchitecture with decreased interconnectivity; and poor quality of bone, related to altered mineralization or collagen. As a result there is increased bone fragility, leading to enhanced fracture risk. Fractures classically take place in the setting of no or minimal trauma.

Etiology

The leading cause of fracture in many cases is preceding fall. This is particularly true in hip fractures, in which more than 90% of fractures are related to fall. Other factors include direct impact to the hip following fall, energy absorption in soft tissue, and bone strength [1]. Falls are multifactorial and can result from intrinsic factors, or factors that are inherent to an individual, and extrinsic factors, such as environmental issues including cluttered surroundings.

Insufficiency or fragility fractures are a type of stress fracture in which there is normal stress applied to abnormal bone, such as osteoporotic bone. Insuffi-

* Corresponding author. Hospital for Special Surgery, 535 East 70th Street, New York, NY 10021.
E-mail address: linj@hss.edu (J.T. Lin).

0749-0690/06/$ – see front matter © 2006 Elsevier Inc. All rights reserved.
doi:10.1016/j.cger.2005.12.010

ciency fractures typically occur in the absence of significant trauma. Instead, they typically result from either no trauma, or minimal trauma, such as fall from a standing position. Insufficiency or fragility fractures are the hallmark of osteoporosis.

Consequences of fracture

Osteoporotic fractures can result in both increased morbidity and mortality. Kado and coworkers [2] demonstrated that there was increased mortality in women with radiographically documented vertebral fracture. Hip fractures in particular are worrisome because they dramatically increase morbidity and mortality and are projected to continue to grow in incidence [3].

Types of fracture

Most osteoporotic fractures involve the vertebral bodies, hips, and distal radius, with the remainder of fractures occurring throughout the body. Each year in the United States there are over 1.5 million osteoporotic fractures, of which 700,000 are vertebral fractures, 300,000 are hip fractures, and 200,000 are distal radius fractures. Estimated lifetime risk of developing hip fracture is approximately 14% in postmenopausal women and 6% in men [4].

Identification of the older patient at risk

Risk factors for osteoporosis can be divided into modifiable and nonmodifiable risk factors as outlined by the National Osteoporosis Foundation (NOF). According to the NOF guidelines, major risk factors for osteoporosis include family history of fragility fracture in a first-degree relative; personal history of fracture as an adult; current smoking; less than 127 lb (based on a 5-ft, 5-in height); and use of oral corticosteroids for more than 3 months. Additional risk factors include overall poor health and frailty, lifelong low calcium intake, dementia, estrogen deficiency at a young age, impaired vision, recent falls, low physical activity, and more than two alcoholic drinks per day. Increased age is a significant risk factor for fractures, and is an independent risk factor for fracture in osteoporotic fractures [5]. Secondary osteoporosis can increase the fracture risk from either the disease or the therapy.

Recurrent falls and poor balance represent major risk factors for osteoporosis. Patients with history of recurrent falls or history of significant balance dysfunction should be screened for potentially reversible or modifiable conditions, such as diabetic peripheral neuropathy. In addition, patients at risk should receive appropriate balance training and risk factor prevention with minimization or elimination of fall risks.

Bone mineral density (BMD) testing should be performed in patients with history of insufficiency fracture; those with multiple risk factors (other than being female and white); and in any patients considering treatment for osteoporosis. The gold standard for BMD testing is dual-energy x-ray absorptiometry. Dual-energy vertebral assessment, one system of imaging the lateral spine to determine the presence of vertebral fractures, can provide clinicians with a comprehensive fracture risk assessment [6].

The fracture index is one tool that has been proposed to be a 5-year assessment of hip and other osteoporotic fractures [7]. This index considers age; BMD T-score; fracture after age 50 years; maternal hip fracture after age 50; weight ≤125 lb (57 kg); smoking status; and ability to stand up from a chair without the use of arms. Although this tool has not been widely adopted for use by many clinicians, its use in the future may help clinicians screen for those patients most at risk for osteoporotic fracture who would benefit from further evaluation and treatment.

Patients with prior fractures are at significantly increased risk of sustaining refracture [8]. Refracture risk seems to be highest immediately following fracture [9]. Presence of one or more vertebral fractures at baseline increases the risk of sustaining a vertebral fracture by fivefold during the year following fracture [10].

Radiographs are not considered a sensitive indicator of osteoporosis. Osteopenia may be appreciated on radiographs; however, a considerable amount of bone loss has to take place before osteopenia is seen. Radiographs are, however, extremely helpful in detecting fracture.

Diagnosis of fracture

Diagnostic imaging helps to confirm clinical suspicion for osteoporotic fracture. Radiographs may demonstrate fracture, although they are notoriously insensitive for certain types of fractures, such as sacral fractures [11,12]. MRI is an extremely sensitive modality that can be useful in detecting subtle fractures. Bone scan may also be used to detect fractures, and can be useful in detecting the presence of multiple fractures. CT is one of the best methods to image bone and is often used to complement bone scan findings. Its major drawback, however, is its radiation dosage.

Undertreatment of osteoporotic patients

Osteoporosis unfortunately remains a medical condition that is underdiagnosed and undertreated. This is likely caused by myriad reasons. Like silent diseases, such as hypertension, osteoporosis is silent until it manifests late in the course of the disease. In the case of osteoporosis, manifestations are often devastating consequences, such as fracture and deformity. Because osteoporosis is silent, it is often overlooked by health care providers. In addition, it is likely that limited training or exposure to the condition by health care providers limits appropriate treatment. Furthermore, patients may often not understand the condition and its relationship to fracture and deformity. This may be true even in patients who have sustained multiple osteoporotic fractures.

Several studies have shown that patients at highest risk for fracture (those with hip fracture) routinely are not treated appropriately with antiosteoporotic medication. One study demonstrated that in patients with nontraumatic hip fracture, only 13% of participants were receiving adequate treatment for osteoporosis as defined by the NOF guidelines for osteoporosis, 47% reported partial treatment that did not meet NOF guidelines, and 40% were receiving no treatment for osteoporosis [13].

Who is responsible for screening and treating patients?

Part of the problem may be that both physicians and patients do not recognize the potentially deleterious effects of the disease. In addition, it is likely that lack of time or appropriate training limits the attention given to the disease. In addition, it is often unclear under whose domain osteoporosis falls. For example, does the internist, orthopedist, or physiatrist accept the most responsibility for the appropriate treatment of this disease? Whatever the right answer, it is encouraging that the rate of treatment of osteoporosis has been gradually improving over the past several years [14]. A retrospective study was conducted in patients with hip fracture, who are typically the patients with the most advanced disease and at the highest risk for refracture. The study found that between the years 1997 and 2000, 11%, 13%, 24%, and 29%, respectively, of hip fracture patients were discharged from the hospital with a prescription for some medication targeting osteopenia, either supplemental calcium or an antiosteoporotic medication (estrogen, calcitonin, a bisphosphonate, or raloxifene).

A recent double-blind, randomized trial demonstrated that heightened awareness of osteoporosis results in improved treatment for osteoporosis. In this study, patients in the control group were given a list of questions to review with their primary physician, asking them about osteoporosis and their treatment, whereas patients in the control group received a brochure on fall prevention. At 6-month follow-up, 42% of patients in the study group compared with 19% of patients in the control group had their osteoporosis addressed by their primary physician [15]. This study demonstrates that improved attention to osteoporosis and treatment can affect higher rates of osteoporotic treatment.

Such studies are encouraging and demonstrate that as physicians and the public become more aware of osteoporosis and its potential consequences, improved treatment for the condition can be attained. Both physicians and patients must advocate a comprehensive treatment program for osteoporosis that includes both medical and nonmedical management.

Treatment

Appropriate treatment of osteoporotic fracture involves both pharmacologic and nonpharmacologic management. A comprehensive program incorporates all aspects of treatment, preferable to focusing only on medication management.

Pharmacologic management

Pharmacologic treatment should be initiated for anyone with a T score of less than −2 on hip BMD, anyone with a T score of less than −1.5 on hip BMD with one or more risk fracture, and anyone with prior hip or vertebral fracture. Medications including calcium and vitamin D, oral and intravenous bisphosphonates, calcitonin, selective estrogen receptor modulators, and the anabolic agent teriparatide are available in the treatment of osteoporotic fracture.

Daily dosages of 1200 to 1500 mg calcium and 800 IU of vitamin D are recommended, with the higher dosages recommended in most cases. Calcium is primarily available in the forms of calcium citrate and calcium carbonate. Calcium citrate is typically preferred because it is more reliably absorbed by most individuals than calcium carbonate. In addition, calcium carbonate is relatively contraindicated in individuals who are taking antacids, because they require an acidic environment to be activated.

The bisphosphonates include the oral bisphosphonates risedronate, alendronate, and the newly released ibandronate and the intravenous bisphosophonates pamidronate and zoledronate. The oral bisphosphonates are considered first-line agents; however, in those individuals who cannot tolerate the oral bisphosphonates secondary to side effects, such as gastrointestinal complaints, the intravenous bisphosphonates represent good alternatives. Numerous studies have substantiated the efficacy of the oral bisphosphonates to improve both bone density and reduce fracture risk. They are available in daily, weekly, and now monthly doses (ibandronate). The intravenous bisphosphonates have not been approved by the Food and Drug Administration for use in osteoporosis, and are used off-label. Preliminary studies suggest that the intravenous bisphosphonates offer similar increases in bone density and reductions in fracture risk as the oral bisphosphonates [16]. Side effects of the intravenous bisphosphonates include flulike syndromes, such as fevers, chills, and myalgias, and bony pain. In addition, these medications pose an increased risk of renal insufficiency and, rarely, avascular necrosis of the jaw [17,18].

Another medication that may be useful in treatment of fracture is calcitonin, which the authors primarily use for its analgesic effect [19]. Calcitonin has been shown to be effective in its 200 IU daily dose in reducing the risk of vertebral fractures [20] but similar findings have not been shown in nonvertebral fractures [19]. Calcitonin is often used as a second-line agent or only for analgesia.

Selective estrogen receptor modulators, such as raloxifene, an antiresorptive agent, have been found to reduce the risk of vertebral fracture, but have no effect on nonvertebral fractures [21]. In addition, drawbacks to its use include risks of venous thromboembolism, hot flashes, and leg cramps.

Intermittent parathyroid hormone or teriparatide is the only anabolic agent approved for use in osteoporosis by the Food and Drug Administration. It is available as a 20-µg subcutaneous daily injection and has been found to decrease both vertebral and nonvertebral fracture risk and increase BMD [22]. There is some evidence that teriparatide alone is more efficacious than both teriparatide used in combination with bisphosphonate medication, such as alendronate, and more efficacious than alendronate alone [23].

Nonpharmacologic management

Nonpharmacologic management involves rehabilitation and exercise programs, hip protectors, and orthoses. In addition, the procedures vertebroplasty and kyphoplasty and surgical stabilization may be appropriate.

An appropriate comprehensive treatment program for osteoporotic patients with fracture includes education and skill building to increase knowledge about fall risk factors; exercise to improve strength and balance; home modifications to reduce fall hazards; medication assessment to minimize side effects, such as dizziness and grogginess [24]; hip protectors; and orthoses.

Physical therapy programs should emphasize back extensor strengthening exercises, balance training, and body mechanics. In particular, resistive exercises for the spine and proprioceptive re-education are useful, with the latter useful in improving balance and posture [25]. Exercise programs range from Tai Chi, a Chinese martial art form especially efficacious in improving balance, to osteoporosis fitness classes, which provide further reinforcement of appropriate exercises and body mechanics in a group setting. Studies have demonstrated that Tai Chi is the most effective exercise to reduce fall risk, with reductions in fall risk of 47.5% [26].

Exercise in combination with appropriate oral medication has been shown to result in larger gains than the use of oral medication alone. One study in heart transplant recipients demonstrated that resistance exercise plus alendronate was more efficacious than alendronate alone in restoring BMD [27].

Home modifications

Environmental modifications in the home can help to diminish fall risk. Modifications include the use of grab bars, nonslip mats, and removal of throw rugs. One study demonstrated that some common recommendations made by occupational therapists include removal of mats and throw rugs (48%); changes of footwear (24%); and use of nonslip bathmats (21%). In this study, only 52% of recommendations were made with partial adherence [28]. A major reason why these recommendations were not followed was that patients did not believe that making these changes would diminish their fall risk. Another study demonstrated that home visits to patients with history of falls resulted in diminished falls [29]. In this randomized controlled trial, patients in both groups received a geriatric assessment, with the intervention group receiving a home visit and home interventions, whereas controls received recommendations and usual care at home. Home interventions in the intervention group included a diagnostic home visit, with assessment of the home for environmental hazards, advice about possible changes, offer of facilities for any necessary home modifications, and training in the use of technical and mobility aids. At 3-month follow-up, an additional visit was made to reinforce the recommendations. The study found that there were 31% fewer falls in the intervention group than in the control group, with the interventions most effective in the highest-risk patients (ie, patients with history of two or more falls).

Hip protectors

Hip protectors are orthoses that typically consist of undergarments with pads placed over the hips. The goal of hip protectors is to diminish fall risk by absorbing the impact of fall. A randomized, controlled trial involving 1801 participants [30] demonstrated that the use of an external hip protector can result in reductions in hip fracture in frail elderly adults. In this study, 13 and 67 subjects sustained hip fracture in the hip-protector and control groups, respectively. A recent meta-analysis found that hip protectors are particularly useful for those living in institutional care at highest risk for hip fracture [31]. The major drawback, however, has been low rates of acceptability by users of the protectors because of discomfort and practicality. Other reviews have found hip protectors effective clinically and from a cost-effectiveness standpoint, particularly in the institutionalized elderly. Some controversies have existed in the literature regarding the efficacy of hip protectors, with one meta-analysis stating that hip protectors are only effective in the nursing home setting, and even there, their use requires further confirmation [32].

Compliance clearly remains one of the major drawbacks to the use of hip protectors. In one study, leading concerns raised by patients with respect to hip protectors include effectiveness (83%); fit (82%); comfort (78%); laundering (66%); cost (57%); not showing (55%); and looking well (54%) [33]. One study demonstrated that in institutionalized patients, an interdisciplinary approach is necessary to help effect compliance [34]. Constant reinforcement to the patient by physicians and by caregivers is paramount to help maximize rates of compliance.

Hip protectors are simple, relatively inexpensive orthoses that require little from patients except for compliance. Patients should be continually encouraged to wear hip protectors as much as tolerated, because the risks of developing hip fractures certainly outweigh any inconveniences related to the hip protectors. Patients should be encouraged to wear the protectors especially during high-risk situations, such as during the night for those patients who frequently get up in the middle of the night to urinate.

Bracing

Orthoses, such as various thoracolumbar braces, can help to improve back extensor strength and provide proprioceptive reminders to the spine, especially the thoracolumbar spine. Some orthoses include the Jewett and Cruciform Anterior Spinal Hyperextension brace, which are both hyperextension braces. In addition, the posture training support brace is now available in the form of a weighted backpack and in the form of a vest with weights. Prior studies have found the posture training support may be effective in improving back extensor strength [35]. Another study found that the posture training support resulted in diminished pain in patients with vertebral fractures and may be better tolerated than other thoracolumbar braces [36]. One study demonstrated that wearing another thoracolumbar brace for 6 months resulted in improvements in back extensor strength, abdominal flexor strength, decreased kyphosis, decreased body sway, increased vital capacity, decrease in pain, increase in well-being, and decrease in limitations [37].

Surgical interventions and vertebroplasty or kyphoplasty

Surgical fixation may be required to stabilize fractures, such as hip fractures and distal radius fractures. The exact surgical fixation used depends on several factors, such as the exact location of the fracture and the age and activity level of the patient. In impacted and valgus femoral neck fractures, a cannulated screw is used to stabilize the fracture. In displaced fractures, if the individual is young or active, reduction must take place urgently, followed by either placement of a cannulated screw or a total hip replacement. Nonactive individuals with displaced femoral neck fractures should undergo a unipolar or bipolar hemiarthroplasty. Patients with stable intertrochanteric fractures undergo fixation with a dynamic hip screw, which is a sliding hip screw, whereas patients with unstable intertrochanteric fractures undergo fixation with an intramedullary nail.

Vertebroplasty and kyphoplasty are two new minimally invasive interventions that are used in patients with painful vertebral compression fractures. Both procedures involve the infiltration of cement into fractured vertebral bodies, but kyphoplasty includes the use of an inflatable bone tamp resembling a balloon to create a cavity into which polymethyl methacrylate is infiltrated. Kyphoplasty specifically addresses kyphosis in addition to stabilization and pain reduction, whereas vertebroplasty does not reduce the kyphosis beyond positioning. Both procedures have been shown to be effective in reducing pain from vertebral fractures. Some authors suggest that kyphoplasty may be a safer procedure because it involves the construction of a cavity into which the bone cement is injected, rather than the cement being forced into the vertebral body under high pressure in the absence of a cavity, such as in vertebroplasty.

Indications for vertebroplasty and kyphoplasty include intractable pain from vertebral fracture, which has not responded to conservative management including analgesic medication, bracing, and rehabilitation. In addition, kyphoplasty is used to help improve severe kyphosis, particularly in situations where extreme kyphosis results in functional limitations. These limitations include compromised pulmonary function and decreased tolerance for oral intake secondary to severe compromise of the thoracic cavity. Risks of kyphoplasty include extravasation of cement into adjacent disk spaces, along nerve roots, and into the spinal canal, and embolization of cement to the lungs.

Some authors have reported conflicting results with respect to the reduction in kyphosis that may be achieved with vertebroplasty versus kyphoplasty. One study demonstrated that vertebroplasty improved the pretreatment height of compression fractures in one third of patients (in those that reduce with position) by a mean of 47.6% ($P < .001$), with only 15% showing no improvement. In addition, the authors reported a mean improvement in kyphosis angle of 6 degrees and an improvement in the wedge angle of 3.5 degrees [38]. Other studies have reported reductions in kyphosis in kyphoplasty but not vertebroplasty [39].

Relative contraindications to vertebroplasty and kyphoplasty include an older (ie, greater than 6 months) vertebral fracture and a vertebral fracture that is so severely compressed (ie, less than 25% of its normal vertebral body height) that proper placement of the instruments into the vertebral bodies is unlikely. In addition, cases involving patients with suspected metastatic disease involving the vertebral bodies from solid tumors should be approached with extreme caution.

Case studies

Hip fracture

AG is a 78-year-old woman with a history of vertebral compression fracture who presents status post fall in her bathroom. She arrives in the emergency room with complaints of severe pain and inability to ambulate on her right lower extremity. Radiographs demonstrate right femoral neck fracture, Garden classification III. She has been on alendronate for 1 year, but has not been taking calcium and vitamin D.

The patient underwent surgical fixation of her femur with open reduction and internal fixation. She was also placed on a minimum of 1500 mg of calcium and 800 IU of vitamin D and continues taking her alendronate. The patient participated in a rehabilitation program with emphasis on strengthening exercises of the hip muscles, especially the hip abductors.

Garden [40–43] developed a classification system of femoral fracture. Garden I are incomplete or impacted fractures. In these fractures, the trabeculae of the inferior neck are still intact. Garden II are complete fractures without displacement. Radiographs demonstrated that the weight-bearing trabeculae are interrupted by a fracture line across the entire neck of the femur. Garden III fractures are complete fracture with partial displacement. In this fracture, there is frequently shortening and external rotation of the distal fragment. The trabecular pattern of the femoral head does not line up with that of the acetabulum, demonstrating incomplete displacement between the femoral fracture fragments. Garden IV fractures are complete fractures with total displacement of the fracture fragments. In this fracture all continuity between the proximal distal fragments is disrupted.

Vertebral fracture

TR is an 86-year-old woman with history of emphysema and multiple compression fractures who presents with complaints of sharp lower back pain following a fall onto her right side. Since the development of this back pain, she reports occasional dyspnea, which has limited her ability to ambulate for more than two blocks. On physical examination, she has significant percussion and palpation tenderness over her T10 and T11 vertebral bodies. MRI of the thoracic spine demonstrates edema in the T10 and T11 vertebral bodies, with losses of 60% and 70% height, respectively. The clinical and MRI findings are consistent with acute compression fractures. Initially, the patient is prescribed analgesic medication, prescribed physical therapy, and fitted for a thoracolumbar brace. She reports discomfort with the brace, however, and reports no improvement in her pulmonary symptoms after 4 weeks. On return examination, she is noted to have labored breathing and now reports increasing difficulty with tolerating oral intake. She notes continued severe, constant pain that has not responded adequately to oral medications or to physical therapy modalities. She continues to have palpation and percussion tenderness over her lower thoracic spine and reports a 5- to 7-lb weight loss.

The decision is made to have the patient undergo kyphoplasty, a procedure that augments the fractured vertebral bodies, reduces kyphosis, and results in pain reduction. It is hoped that the kyphoplasty will alleviate the patient's dyspnea. Vertebral fractures are known to have deleterious effects on pulmonary function, with compromises in vital capacity for each compression fracture noted [44]. The patient will receive an infusion of intravenous zoledronic acid during her overnight stay at the hospital following kyphoplasty. The patient will continue to perform gentle thoracic back extensor strengthening exercises. Precautions include avoidance of excessive flexion biased exercises; abdominal crunches; and heavy weights (greater than 5 lb).

Distal radius fractures

Patient JM is a 63-year-old woman who presents with right forearm pain following a fall in her apartment. She is found to have a minimally displaced distal radius fracture. She has never undergone an evaluation for osteoporosis and is not taking any osteoporotic medications, including calcium and vitamin D. She does not have a history of prior fracture.

The patient was referred to a hand and elbow surgeon who placed the patient in a light, short-arm fiberglass cast. She was advised to take calcium and vitamin D and is to undergo an osteoporosis evaluation, including BMD study. She was placed on appropriate antiosteoporotic medication accordingly. Six-week follow-up demonstrated fracture healing and the patient was given a splint. The patient started a hand rehabilitation program consisting of hand exercises, such as extension and abduction-adduction of digits, grasp exercises, and claw exercises with the metacarpophalangeal joint of the fingers extended but the interphalangeal joint flexed.

Future areas of inquiry

Future areas of inquiry include the use of additional substances into fractured vertebral bodies. Currently, polymethyl methacrylate is injected in vertebroplasty and kyphoplasty. It has been suggested that increased fractures may occur in the areas adjacent to the levels treated with vertebroplasty or kyphoplasty secondary to the properties of the bone cement. It would be interesting to consider the use of a more biologic agent to mimic the properties of normal bone, with the goal of reducing fracture rate. Important educational websites include the National Osteoporosis Foundation, www.nof.org, and Arthritis Foundation, www.arthritis. org. Commercial websites with product information on orthoses, hip protectors, and kyphoplasty include www.camphealthcare.com, www.epill.com, www. hipprotectors.com, and www.kyphon.com. Educational lectures and articles can be found on www.osteo.org and www.hss.edu.

References

[1] Lauritzen JB, McNair PA, Lund B. Risk factors for hip fractures. A review. Dan Med Bull 1993; 40:479–85.
[2] Kado DM, Browner WS, Palermo L, et al. Vertebral fractures and mortality in older women: a prospective study. Study of Osteoporotic Fractures Research Group. Arch Intern Med 1999; 159:1215–20.
[3] Kannus P, Parkkari J, Sievanen H, et al. Epidemiology of hip fractures. Bone 1996;18(1 Suppl): 57S–63S.
[4] Lauritzen JB. Hip fractures: epidemiology, risk factors, falls, energy absorption, hip protectors, and prevention. Dan Med Bull 1997;44:155–68.
[5] Kanis JA, Johnell O, Oden A, et al. Ten year probabilities of osteoporotic fractures according to BMD and diagnostic thresholds. Osteoporos Int 2001;12:989–95.
[6] Vokes TJ, Dixon LB, Favus MJ. Clinical utility of dual-energy vertebral assessment (DVA). Osteoporos Int 2003;14:871–8.
[7] Black DM, Steinbuch M, Palermo L, et al. An assessment tool for predicting fracture risk in postmenopausal women. Osteoporos Int 2001;12:519–28.
[8] Gunnes M, Mellstrom D, Johnell O. How well can a previous fracture indicate a new fracture? A questionnaire study of 29,802 postmenopausal women. Acta Orthop Scand 1998;69:508–12.
[9] Johnell O, Kanis JA, Oden A, et al. Fracture risk following an osteoporotic fracture. Osteoporos Int 2004;15:175–9.
[10] Lindsay R, Silverman SL, Cooper C, et al. Risk of new vertebral fracture in the year following a fracture. JAMA 2001;285:320–3.

[11] Lin J, Lachmann E, Nagler W. Sacral insufficiency fractures: a report of two cases and a review of the literature. J Womens Health Gend Based Med 2001;10:699–705.
[12] Lin JT, Lane JM. Sacral stress fractures. J Womens Health (Larchmt) 2003;12:879–88.
[13] Bellantonio S, Fortinsky R, Prestwood K. How well are community-living women treated for osteoporosis after hip fracture? J Am Geriatr Soc 2001;49:1197–204.
[14] Gardner MJ, Flik KR, Mooar P, et al. Improvement in the undertreatment of osteoporosis following hip fracture. J Bone Joint Surg Am 2002;84:1342–8.
[15] Gardner MJ, Brophy RH, Demetrakopoulos D, et al. Interventions to improve osteoporosis treatment following hip fracture: a prospective, randomized trial. J Bone Joint Surg Am 2005; 87:3–7.
[16] Heijckmann AC, Juttmann JR, Wolffenbuttel BH. Intravenous pamidronate compared with oral alendronate for the treatment of postmenopausal osteoporosis. Neth J Med 2002;60:315–9.
[17] Marx RE. Pamidronate (Aredia) and zoledronate (Zometa) induced avascular necrosis of the jaws: a growing epidemic. J Oral Maxillofac Surg 2003;61:1115–7.
[18] Tarassoff P, Csermak K. Avascular necrosis of the jaws: risk factors in metastatic cancer patients. J Oral Maxillofac Surg 2003;61:1238–9.
[19] Munoz-Torres M, Alonso G, Raya MP. Calcitonin therapy in osteoporosis. Treat Endocrinol 2004;3:117–32.
[20] Chesnut III CH, Silverman S, Andriano K, et al. A randomized trial of nasal spray salmon calcitonin in postmenopausal women with established osteoporosis: the prevent recurrence of osteoporotic fractures study. PROOF Study Group. Am J Med 2000;109:267–76.
[21] Cranney A, Adachi JD. Benefit-risk assessment of raloxifene in postmenopausal osteoporosis. Drug Saf 2005;28:721–30.
[22] Neer RM, Arnaud CD, Zanchetta JR, et al. Effect of parathyroid hormone (1–34) on fractures and bone mineral density in postmenopausal women with osteoporosis. N Engl J Med 2001; 344:1434–41.
[23] Finkelstein JS, Hayes A, Hunzelman JL, et al. The effects of parathyroid hormone, alendronate, or both in men with osteoporosis. N Engl J Med 2003;349:1216–26.
[24] Stevens JA, Olson S. Reducing falls and resulting hip fractures among older women. MMWR Recomm Rep 2000;49(RR-2):3–12.
[25] Sinaki M. Critical appraisal of physical rehabilitation measures after osteoporotic vertebral fracture. Osteoporos Int 2003;14:773–9.
[26] Wolf SL, Barnhart HX, Kutner NG, et al. Selected as the best paper in the 1990s: reducing frailty and falls in older persons. An investigation of tai chi and computerized balance training. J Am Geriatr Soc 2003;51:1794–803.
[27] Braith RW, Magyari PM, Fulton MN, et al. Resistance exercise training and alendronate reverse glucocorticoid-induced osteoporosis in heart transplant recipients. J Heart Lung Transplant 2003;22:1082–90.
[28] Cumming RG, Thomas M, Szonyi G, et al. Adherence to occupational therapist recommendations for home modifications for falls prevention. Am J Occup Ther 2001;55:641–8.
[29] Nikolaus T, Bach M. Preventing falls in community-dwelling frail older people using a home intervention team (HIT): results from the randomized Falls-HIT trial. J Am Geriatr Soc 2003; 51:300–5.
[30] Kannus P, Parkkari J, Niemi S, et al. Prevention of hip fracture in elderly people with use of a hip protector. N Engl J Med 2000;343:1506–13.
[31] Parker MJ, Gillespie LD, Gillespie WJ. Hip protectors for preventing hip fractures in the elderly. Cochrane Database Syst Rev 2004;3:CD001255.
[32] Sawka AM, Boulos P, Beattie K, et al. Do hip protectors decrease the risk of hip fracture in institutional and community-dwelling elderly? A systematic review and meta-analysis of randomized controlled trials. Osteoporosis Int 2005;16(12):1461–74.
[33] Myers AH, Michelson JD, Van NM, et al. Prevention of hip fractures in the elderly: receptivity to protective garments. Arch Gerontol Geriatr 1995;21:179–89.
[34] Burl JB, Centola J, Bonner A, et al. Hip protector compliance: a 13-month study on factors and cost in a long-term care facility. J Am Med Dir Assoc 2003;4:245–50.

[35] Kaplan RS, Sinaki M, Hameister MD. Effect of back supports on back strength in patients with osteoporosis: a pilot study. Mayo Clin Proc 1996;71(3):235–41.

[36] Kaplan RS, Sinaki M. Posture training support: preliminary report on a series of patients with diminished symptomatic complications of osteoporosis. Mayo Clin Proc 1993;68:1171–6.

[37] Pfeifer M, Begerow B, Minne HW. Effects of a new spinal orthosis on posture, trunk strength, and quality of life in women with postmenopausal osteoporosis: a randomized trial. Am J Phys Med Rehabil 2004;83:177–86.

[38] Dublin AB, Hartman J, Latchaw RE, et al. The vertebral body fracture in osteoporosis: restoration of height using percutaneous vertebroplasty. AJNR Am J Neuroradiol 2005;26:489–92.

[39] Grohs JG, Matzner M, Trieb K, et al. Minimal invasive stabilization of osteoporotic vertebral fractures: a prospective nonrandomized comparison of vertebroplasty and balloon kyphoplasty. J Spinal Disord Tech 2005;18:238–42.

[40] Garden RS. Stability and union in subcapital fractures of the femur. J Bone Joint Surg Br 1964;46:630–47.

[41] Garden RS. The significance of good reduction in medial fractures of the femoral neck. Proc R Soc Med 1970;63(11 Part 1):1122.

[42] Garden RS. Malreduction and avascular necrosis in subcapital fractures of the femur. J Bone Joint Surg Br 1971;53:183–97.

[43] Garden RS. Reduction and fixation of subcapital fractures of the femur. Orthop Clin North Am 1974;5:683–712.

[44] Leech JA, Dulberg C, Kellie S, et al. Relationship of lung function to severity of osteoporosis in women. Am Rev Respir Dis 1990;141:68–71.

ELSEVIER
SAUNDERS

CLINICS IN
GERIATRIC
MEDICINE

Clin Geriatr Med 22 (2006) 449–468

Traumatic Brain Injury in the Elderly: Diagnostic and Treatment Challenges

Steven R. Flanagan, MD*, Mary R. Hibbard, PhD,
Brian Riordan, MD, Wayne A. Gordon, PhD

*Rehabilitation Medicine, Mount Sinai School of Medicine, 1 Gustave L. Levy Place, Box 1240,
New York, NY 10029, USA*

The purpose of this review is to introduce geriatric practitioners to issues and challenges presented in the elderly after onset of traumatic brain injury (TBI). Issues discussed include the magnitude of TBI in the elderly, mechanisms of onset, issues specific to both acute and rehabilitation care for the elderly with TBI, and specific physical and behavioral manifestations of TBI that may need to be addressed on an inpatient or outpatient basis. General guidelines are provided for the diagnosis and treatment of older individuals who have TBI, with specific clinical scenarios illustrating key points.

Scope of the problem

In 2000, the United States Census estimated the population of individuals over the age of 65 to be 35 million, with an anticipated growth to more than 86 million by the year 2050. Among elderly Americans, the largest growth in population will occur in the number of those older than 85 years, projected to reach 20 million by 2050 [1]. Although the population most at risk for TBI is young adults, a second peak incidence occurs in those aged 65 years or older [2]. This trend in population growth and distribution, indicating a large expansion of the geriatric population, suggests that geriatric TBI will become a significant health care issue in the coming decades, presenting health care providers and government officials with substantial challenges.

---

* Corresponding author.
E-mail address: steve.flanagan@mssm.edu (S.R. Flanagan).

The consequences of TBI are staggering, although they are poorly recognized and appreciated by the health care industry. TBI is far more widespread than most clinicians realize, accounting for 20 times more hospitalizations than traumatic spinal cord injury [3] and representing one of the most common disabling conditions in the United States. Each year, TBI afflicts at least 1.4 million individuals and accounts for 50,000 deaths and 235,000 hospitalizations [4]. The prevalence of individuals living with a TBI-related condition is 5.3 million [5], although this figure most likely underestimates the true scope of the problem, because only 15% of individuals are known to the medical system [6]. Individuals who have milder injuries typically do not seek medical attention; thus their TBIs remain undiagnosed. Other individuals who have TBI are misdiagnosed with psychiatric disorders, because the consequences of TBI frequently manifest as cognitive or behavioral impairments, rather than the more obvious physical impairments associated with neurologic injury. The cost of misdiagnosis or nondiagnosis of TBI is high in that the cognitive and behavioral disorders related to TBI frequently prevent successful community reintegration, even in the presence of good physical recovery. Failure correctly to identify the TBI may also lead to inappropriate or ineffective treatments. This problem is compounded in the elderly, because behavioral and cognitive manifestations of TBI may be misinterpreted as signs of dementia, erroneously leading clinicians toward inaccurate prognoses and limiting implementation of appropriate treatment.

The overall leading cause of TBI is falls, particularly in the elderly population; falls account for more than half of all TBIs in those aged 65 years or older [1], whereas young adults are more likely to sustain a TBI in a motor vehicle–related collision. As individuals age, they become more likely to fall and sustain a TBI. Compared with adults aged 65 years or less, people aged 65 to 74 are three times as likely to be hospitalized with a TBI-related fall, with the relative risk increasing to 7.6 and 16.4 for those aged 75 to 84 and 85 or older, respectively. The yearly cost associated with elderly fall-related TBI in California alone was estimated to be $50 million [7], underscoring the need for preventive measures to decrease fall rates in the elderly.

Mortality of TBI varies by age at onset. The overall TBI-related mortality decreased during the 1990s, most likely owing to a combination of several factors, including advances in emergency care, greater enforcement of seat belt laws, and a reduction in assault-related TBIs. However, this reduction was not realized for those aged 75 years or older, who experienced a surprising increase in mortality as a group and had the highest overall mortality [8]. It is unclear whether this reported increase is the result of better coding, of enhanced detection of TBI in the elderly, or of more frequent or severe comorbid conditions that may predispose the elderly to higher death rates following trauma [9–12]. The increased mortality is unrelated to injury severity, because mortality is greater among the elderly across all injury severities, including mild TBI [13]. Older individuals who have TBI also have lower long-term survival rates than their age-matched noninjured peers [14], indicating that TBI predisposes the elderly to premature death.

Understanding the pathophysiology of traumatic brain injury in the elderly

Pathologic changes after TBI may be divided into two broad categories: focal versus diffuse and primary versus secondary. Focal injuries involve an injury to a localized area of the brain, whereas diffuse injuries involve a wider region. Primary injuries occur at the time of impact, whereas secondary injuries occur at some point in time after the initial blow to the head and may be avoided or minimized by treatment.

Focal injuries include cerebral contusions, lacerations, localized hemorrhages, and focal ischemic lesions. Contusions occur when the brain strikes the hard, rough inner surface of the skull during trauma. Although contusions may occur anywhere in the cerebral cortex, the configuration of the skull and brain predisposes the inferior frontal lobes and anterior portion of the temporal lobes to contusions. Additionally, contusions may manifest as coup-contrecoup lesions, which occur when the brain strikes the skull, causing it to rebound and strike the opposite side of the skull. Lacerations occur at points where the dura is lacerated, either by a depressed skull fracture or a penetrating object. Focal regions of ischemia result from interruption of blood flow caused by either vasospasm following a traumatic subarachnoid hemorrhage or physical compression of arteries, resulting in a focal region of cerebral infarction. Deep penetrating arteries are at risk for shearing during trauma, which may cause small hemorrhages in the deeper regions of the brain.

Extra-axial hemorrhages occur frequently after TBI and include epidural, subdural, and subarachnoid hemorrhages. Epidural hemorrhages typically occur in association with a skull fracture that lacerates the middle meningeal artery. The hemorrhage is situated between the skull and the dura, which often limits the extent of bleeding because of the tight adherence of the dura to the skull at the bony sutures. Subarachnoid hemorrhages are located between the pia mater and the arachnoid, predisposing cerebral arteries to vasospasm and poorer outcomes following TBI [15].

Subdural hemorrhages arise from shearing of the bridging veins, resulting in bleeding within the space defined by the dura mater and arachnoid. Elderly individuals are particularly vulnerable to subdural hemorrhages (SDH) because bridging veins become more susceptible to shearing forces as the brain naturally atrophies with advancing age. A large acute SDH manifests as a rapid deterioration of arousal or development of focal neurologic impairments. However, an SDH may not be clinically evident during the acute stages in older adults, because of the enlargement of the subdural space that naturally occurs with aging. This state permits a larger volume of blood to accumulate before the development of clinically significant cerebral compression. An SDH may also slowly expand in the elderly as a result of abnormalities of blood vessels [16,17], increased fibrinolysis, and abnormal coagulation [18], which partially account for the late deterioration of mental abilities often observed in elderly people who have SDH.

SDH frequently occurs in older adults after apparently trivial trauma and often is related to a fall in which there was no direct trauma to the head [19,20]. Not surprisingly, many older individuals are unable to recall the inciting event leading to the hemorrhage.

Widespread cerebral injury results from diffuse axonal injury (DAI), systemic hypoxia, and poor cerebral circulation. DAI occurs when the brain is exposed to stretch and torque forces, typically in an acceleration/deceleration event such as a motor vehicle collision, resulting in axonal stretch. This event alters the cytoskeleton structure of the neurons, resulting in abnormal axonal transport and electrolyte disturbances that cause the neuron to malfunction. When immediate loss of consciousness occurs after TBI, it is most likely the result of DAI. Depending on the extent of stretch, this process may ultimately lead to complete axonal disruption, which is believed to result in significant impairments in both cognition and behavior post-TBI [21]. DAI is a microscopic process, and its structural sequelae are typically not seen on standard CT and MRI scans. Therefore, individuals with significant cognitive and behavioral problems post-TBI may have normal-appearing neuroimaging studies [22,23], which often complicates the process of making a correct diagnosis.

Treatment course after traumatic brain injury in the elderly

Acute care management

In elderly persons who experience a severe TBI, the primary focus of acute care management is on preventing secondary brain injury that may arise as a result of diffuse cerebral ischemia. Increased intracerebral pressure, resulting from intracranial hemorrhages or brain swelling, often impedes cerebral blood flow, particularly in instances of systemic hypotension. The trauma team must diligently monitor intracerebral pressure and lower it if it is elevated, using such measures as evacuation of extra-axial hemorrhages, osmotic diuresis, and pharmacologic induction of coma. Mechanical hyperventilation is not routinely used, because it lowers cerebral pressure by inhibiting blood flow. Mean arterial pressure is also closely monitored to ensure adequate cerebral perfusion. Likewise, continuous assessment of systemic oxygenation is crucial to avert additional cerebral injury. Individuals who have severe TBI may be placed on mechanical ventilation to prevent hypoxemia [24].

Rehabilitation following TBI is ideally initiated shortly after hospitalization, often while the patient resides in an intensive care setting. The immediate goal of rehabilitation is to prevent the complications associated with a prolonged period of immobilization, such as joint contracture, skin breakdown, venous stasis, and pulmonary compromise. After reviewing the medical records and noting the nature and extent of the injury, the rehabilitation consultant completes a full physical and mental state examination of the patient, which includes a thorough assessment of his or her neurologic and functional condition.

A prescription for rehabilitation intervention is generated, which ideally includes initiation of neuropsychologic, physical, occupational, and speech therapies, as well as specific recommendations for the primary trauma team. An important initial goal is to preserve joint mobility of paralyzed limbs; this is achieved by ranging all limbs through a full range of motion several times daily. Common orthotic devices or splints that properly position a paralyzed limb are particularly useful during this period of immobilization but are not an adequate substitute for the routine passive range-of-motion exercises that should be performed by therapists, nurses, physicians, family members, and, when feasible, by the patient. During this early stage, speech therapists will assess swallowing safety and communication problems and, when dysphagia is present, determine which food and liquid consistencies are safe to consume orally. When oral feeding is deemed unsafe, nutritional support by means of gastrostomy or jejunostomy tube is generally preferred to nasogastric tube feedings, particularly when a prolonged period of dysphagia is predicted. Communication boards may be useful soon after TBI for patients who have lost their ability to verbalize because of aphasia, mechanical ventilation, or tracheotomy. Neuropsychologists assess the extent of cognitive and behavioral impairments and make recommendations for decreasing post-TBI agitation and enhancing cognitive recovery.

Inpatient rehabilitation

Older individuals who manifest persistent physical or cognitive impairments beyond the acute phase after TBI should be considered candidates for intensive inpatient rehabilitation in a specialized brain injury rehabilitation service.

Criteria for admission of an elderly person who has a new TBI are identical to those for other candidates for rehabilitation: namely, the patient is medically stable, has the physical ability to participate in at least 3 hours of daily therapy, demonstrates the need for an interdisciplinary treatment approach that cannot adequately be provided in a less intensive setting, and has the potential to improve functional skills in response to treatment in a reasonable amount of time. Once an individual has been determined to meet these criteria, transfer to inpatient rehabilitation should be commenced as early as possible. Less intensive settings for rehabilitation, such as subacute facilities and home-based treatment, should be considered when acute inpatient rehabilitation is not appropriate or is too taxing for the individual. Subacute services provide a similar range of services to those provided in acute facilities, but with less intensity.

The rehabilitation team is composed of numerous professionals, the patient, and the patient's loved ones. The team is best described as interdisciplinary, meaning that all members have commonly shared responsibilities in addition to their specific roles. Team members and their roles are summarized in Table 1.

Intensive inpatient rehabilitation should continue as long as services cannot be provided safely and appropriately in a less intensive setting and the patient is demonstrating reasonable improvement on a regular basis. Such improvement is typically determined by weekly updates. The elderly person often achieves significant functional recovery following TBI in response to intensive rehabilitation interventions, although improvements are realized over a longer period of time.

Table 1
Roles of the rehabilitation team

Physiatrist	A physician with specialized training in physical medicine and rehabilitation
	Serves as the team leader and is responsible for directing the rehabilitation process
	Provides medical care of the patient
	Coordinates treatment rendered by all members of the team
	Coordinates treatment by other medical consultants.
Rehabilitation nurse	Provides patient care 24 hours a day
	Plans nursing care directed toward elderly patients with TBI
	Assesses and manages many TBI-related behavioral and medical problems
Physical therapist	Maximizes muscle strength, endurance, balance, and mobility through exercises and adaptive equipment
Occupational therapist	Maximizes upper limb strength and ADL skills through exercises and adaptive equipment
Speech language pathologist	Addresses language, speech, and swallowing impairments
Neurophysiologist	Assesses cognition and behavior
	Makes recommendations to rehabilitation team to maximize cognitive skills and minimize maladaptive behaviors
	Provides supportive counseling to patients and loved ones
	Provides cognitive intervention in groups or individually
Recreational therapist	Complements therapy provided by other team members through recreational activities
Social workers/Case managers	Determine extent and availability of financial resources and plan for potential long-term disability

Abbreviation: ADL, activities of daily living.

In fact, most older individuals who sustain a TBI are ultimately capable of returning to their communities after intense inpatient rehabilitation [25]. Unfortunately, reimbursement to rehabilitation facilities is a factor that may determine the financial viability of providing inpatient services to the elderly. The Center for Medicare and Medicaid Services (CMS) recently established the Prospective Payment System (PPS) for Medicare beneficiaries. Under this system, CMS provides a specific predetermined reimbursement to rehabilitation facilities for Medicare beneficiaries based on diagnosis and extent of disability. A recent analysis indicated that PPS may reimburse rehabilitation facilities significantly less than their actual costs for treating individuals who have TBI. This problem may have a tremendously adverse impact on how long and where elderly patients with TBI receive needed rehabilitation services [26], with many centers potentially viewing aggressive rehabilitation as too costly to provide. In part, the CMS decisions may have been based on limited research into older adults' ability to profit from intensive rehabilitation efforts over time.

Specifically, older individuals are less likely than their younger counterparts to care for themselves independently after TBI and have poorer functional outcomes than younger individuals with the condition [13,27–29]; these appear to persist long after the injury occurred [30]. However, with few exceptions, most studies examining functional skills of older individuals after TBI use measures that insensitively assess changes in functional skill, minimizing improvements that typically result in enhanced quality of life. Additionally, outcomes are usually assessed within several months of the injury and therefore do not account for functional improvements that typically take longer in older adults.

Finally, these studies rarely control for comorbid conditions. Together, these considerations suggest that the studies need to be interpreted cautiously. Superficial review of these reports may suggest that rehabilitation interventions for older individuals who have TBI are impractical, based on the presumption that meaningful recovery is unlikely.

Preparation for discharge from rehabilitation

When discharge to the community is planned, appropriate arrangements are made to continue rehabilitation services in either the home or the outpatient setting. Considerable planning is often required to ensure that adequate assistance is provided, because many older individuals require continued help with mobility and activities of daily living after hospital discharge. These needs frequently present a problem for elderly patients who live alone or with a physically or cognitively disabled spouse. When feasible, a combination of extended family members, visiting nursing services, and privately reimbursed companions may be necessary to assist with physical care or supervision to provide a safe home environment. Therapists, social workers, and nurses ensure that all needed durable medical equipment is available at the time of discharge and that the persons responsible for providing home care have been properly trained. In the event that a discharge home is impractical, alternatives are discussed with the patient and his or her loved ones. These may include continued rehabilitation treatment in a subacute facility, where supervision and assistance are continuously available while rehabilitation interventions continue at a lower intensity. Assisted living facilities provide another option for individuals who require less intense supervision but who cannot return to their homes. Finally, long-term care facilities may be necessary for some older individuals following TBI.

Specific physical changes after traumatic brain injury

Several physical changes specific to TBI necessitate focused rehabilitation.

Paralysis

Paralysis secondary to TBI is common and often manifests as hemiplegia, which may be bilateral. Both physical and occupational therapists work to enhance motor recovery using a variety of methods, such as neurodevelopmental techniques, focused exercises, and electrical stimulation. Although maximizing motor recovery is an important goal, the extent of motor return varies from person to person. Therefore, various orthotic and assistive devices are used by hemiplegic patients to enhance their function. Braces may be fitted on the distal end of the leg to align the foot and ankle properly during standing and walking activities. Similarly, braces are often used to position the upper limb to prevent joint contracture. Many devices are available to assist patients who have hemiplegia in their progress toward independent ambulation, including parallel bars and various types of walkers and canes.

Orthostatic hypotension

A frequent obstacle to full participation in an aggressive rehabilitation program is orthostatic hypotension, typically resulting from periods of prolonged bed rest following trauma, particularly in elderly individuals with multiple comorbid conditions that require treatment with multiple drugs. Physiatrists need closely to monitor patients' cardiovascular response to exercise as well as when shifting from the supine to upright position.

When orthostatic hypotension is present, drug regimens may need to be altered to permit full participation in the rehabilitation process. Additional steps may be required, including using pressure stockings for the lower limbs and abdominal binders to support blood pressure while the patient is standing or sitting upright. Other physiologic responses to exercise may need to be assessed during physical activity, including oxygen saturation and pulse rate, with modifications made to the rehabilitation process to prevent further injury.

Hydrocephalus

Hydrocephalus may follow TBI as a result of traumatic subarachnoid hemorrhage or infection that scars the arachnoid, preventing absorption of cerebral spinal fluid into the general circulation. Clinical manifestations of hydrocephalus often include failing cognitive skills, worsening gait, and urinary incontinence. However, during the rehabilitation process, it may also manifest as a failure of the patient to demonstrate improved function. Clinicians need to be on the alert for signs of hydrocephalus and order appropriate tests to confirm the diagnosis. These typically include neuroimaging studies, which in the presence of hydrocephalus reveal enlarged ventricles out of proportion to the sulci. However, neuroimaging results are often inconclusive. In this scenario, a cerebral spinal fluid (CSF) tap test may be indicated: a large volume of CSF is removed during a lumbar puncture, and evidence of clinical improvement is sought by all members of the rehabilitation team. Timely treatment of hydrocephalus is indicated to speed resumption of the rehabilitation process.

Neuropsychologic testing should also be considered to evaluate changes in cognitive abilities due to hydrocephalus and extent of cognitive recovery once hydrocephalus has been treated.

Spasticity

Abnormal muscle tone, referred to as dystonia, frequently accompanies paralysis following injury to the central nervous system. It is manifested by either flaccidity (ie, complete paralysis without resistance to passive stretch) or various degrees of abnormal resistance to passive stretch of a limb across a joint. Spasticity, one of many forms of dystonia, is characterized by a velocity-dependent increase in resistance to passive stretch. It often complicates the disabling effects of paralysis by contributing to pain and development of joint contractures and pressure sores and by making hygiene and mobility more difficult. However, some patients may actually receive functional benefits from spasticity. For example, hypertonia of leg extensor muscles may provide a splinting effect in an otherwise weak limb, enabling an individual to ambulate or transfer with greater ease.

Goals of spasticity treatment include facilitating hygiene, positioning, and mobility as well as pain reduction. Treatment initially begins with range-of-motion exercises and proper patient positioning to maximize joint flexibility. Prolonged stretching of joints reduces the likelihood of contractures; this may be achieved either by using splints or by applying a series of plaster casts across a spastic limb. Several medications are available to reduce spasticity, such as tiza-nidine, diazepam, and baclofen, which do so by inhibiting muscle stretch reflexes in the central nervous system.

Alternatively, dantrolene sodium inhibits spasticity by inhibiting muscle contraction. However, all these medications frequently cause adverse effects on cognition and arousal. This problem limits their usefulness following TBI, particularly in the elderly, who are typically taking many other pharmacologic agents and are more susceptible to medication effects.

Intrathecal baclofen (ITB) is a new treatment method that delivers baclofen directly to the intrathecal space. The primary advantage of ITB is its capacity to place high doses of baclofen near its site of action, largely avoiding the sedating and cognitively impairing effects associated with oral administration. ITB more effectively reduces spasticity in lower limbs than in upper limbs, an important consideration when choosing potential patients for treatment.

Often spasticity of a single muscle or muscle group is troublesome to patients. In these circumstances, when generalized muscle tone reduction is neither indicated nor desirable, focal nerve blocks or muscle injections provide a means of decreasing spasticity at specified sites. Phenol is an inexpensive means of inhibiting the muscle stretch reflex by denervating motor points within a spastic muscle. However, when it is injected in close proximity to sensory nerves, painful dysesthesia may develop. Currently, most motor point blocks are achieved through targeted injections of botulinum toxin. Unlike phenol, botulinum toxin has activity only against motor nerves, eliminating the risk for sensory nerve injury. Like that of phenol, its effect on spasticity reduction is time-limited to several months, necessitating repeated injections for many patients.

Limited doses of botulinum toxin may be provided at any one time, making injections of many muscles impractical. Significant and clinically meaningful reduction in muscle is achievable using motor point blocks [31–33].

Specific cognitive and behavioral changes after traumatic brain injury

Cognition impairments in traumatic brain injury

Following moderate to severe TBI, the diagnosis of brain injury is typically straightforward regardless of age, with cognitive and physical sequelae obvious at the time of injury or shortly thereafter. However, older adults who experience an apparently trivial event in which there has been a minor trauma to the head, with either a brief loss of consciousness or a period of altered mental state, often present with more insidious and delayed symptom onset of an undiagnosed TBI. These delayed symptoms reflect the unique pathophysiology of the older brain [34], which places these individuals at greater risk for slowly expanding SDH [35]. In situations where DAI occurs without other trauma-related lesions, neuroimaging tests typically add little to the diagnostic process. As a result, geriatricians should maintain an "index of suspicion of TBI" [36] when older adults present with cognitive or physical decline occurring over a period of several weeks or months. Because of the overlap in clinical presentations of TBI, dementia, and early-onset Alzheimer's disease (AD), correct diagnosis is key; prognostic implications will vary with the selected diagnosis based on anticipated ability to profit from specific interventions.

Individuals who have TBI or AD present with cognitive impairments in the areas of memory [37], attention [38], language [39], and executive functioning [40–43]. Similarly, the presence of comorbid psychiatric disabilities (eg, major depression and anxiety disorders) is observed following TBI [44,45] but is also noted during the early stages of dementia [46] and AD [47–49]. Hence these psychiatric comorbidities add little to clarification of the diagnosis. Finally, a history of a prior brain injury has been related to the subsequent development of AD [50–52]. Indeed, the presence of a prior TBI appears to increase the risk for onset of AD in later life [53–56], with this risk proportionately increased when select genetic risk markers are present [57].

To diagnose a TBI accurately, clinicians should conduct clinical interviews with both patients and their families. The goal of these interviews is to establish a prior history of falls or other events leading to possible head trauma, a timeline of cognitive and physical decline after the identified event or events, and the adequacy of the older adult's cognitive functioning before the identified event. Timely procurement of neuroimaging studies and referral for neuropsychologic testing should be implemented to help confirm a correct diagnosis. As noted previously, many individuals who have mild TBI, including older adults, have normal-appearing neuroimaging studies, which do not rule out the diagnosis of

TBI. In such cases, neuropsychologic evaluation will provide validation of a TBI and help differentiate TBI from dementia or normal aging.

Normal age-related declines in memory are characterized by a fairly narrow range of impaired performance in acquisition and retrieval of new information [58,59] and by decreased processing speed when multiple tasks are involved [60]. In contrast, cognitive deficits in TBI are more pervasive and thus are easily differentiated from normal aging.

Testing profiles differ in TBI from those observed in AD, in that individuals who have TBI demonstrate an ability to learn and retain newly learned information over time (albeit at a reduced level), whereas no such learning is noted in individuals who have AD [61]. Beyond validation of the diagnosis of TBI, a neuropsychologic evaluation will pinpoint an older adult's preserved cognitive strengths, as well as current cognitive deficits, and dictate recommendations regarding cognitive remediation interventions needed to maximize learning abilities and community functioning. Thus, by maintaining an "index of suspicion of TBI," geriatricians may effectively spare older adults who have TBI the erroneous diagnosis of dementia or AD and direct these individuals toward focused rehabilitation interventions that may enhance their cognitive and functional abilities in the community.

Behavioral disturbances

Behavioral disturbances manifested by individuals after TBI are frequently the most challenging problems faced by health care professionals and loved ones. Maladaptive behaviors often impede both the rehabilitation process and reintegration into the patient's community. Apathy, restlessness, irritability, and aggression are common TBI-related problems that manifest throughout the rehabilitation process and may become chronic, requiring ongoing assessments, interventions, and understanding from the rehabilitation team, loved ones, and key members of the community. Treatment interventions are geared toward specific behaviors and use a combination of supportive or cognitive therapies, behavioral modification techniques, and medications.

Agitation can be a significant behavioral challenge in the elderly following TBI. Manifestations of agitation following TBI range from mild irritability to frank physical or verbal aggression. Successful interventions to mitigate agitation begin with identification of the inciting causes, such as noxious or excessive sensory stimulation, problems that commonly occur during the acute phase of recovery. If the undesirable behavior persists after the inciting cause has been identified and appropriately minimized, supportive counseling, behavioral therapy, or pharmacologic agents are next considered to bring these behavioral challenges under adequate control. Considerable caution is urged when one is prescribing medications to individuals who have TBI, particularly the elderly, given the frequency of TBI-related problems of impaired cognition, poor balance, and fatigue, because many medications worsen these problems. Additionally, benzodiazepines and traditional neuroleptics such as haloperidol have been shown to impair recovery following brain injury [62] and are best avoided following TBI, particularly during the acute phase. When medications are needed to control behavior, alternative agents are used; they often include beta-blockers and various anticonvulsants, which have fewer adverse cognitive and sedating effects than traditional neuroleptics and benzodiazepines. Treatment is typically initiated with the lowest possible dose and slowly titrated until the desired effect is achieved. After some time, consideration should be given to systematically tapering off psychotropic medications to determine whether they are still required, because TBI is a dynamic condition that often improves with treatment and over the course of time.

Specific emotional changes after traumatic brain injury

Following TBI, significant psychiatric challenges are observed that typically require focused interventions. The most common challenges are major depression and anxiety disorders.

Individuals who have TBI experience greater-than-expected rates of major depression, with depression being the most frequent co-occurring psychiatric disorder post-TBI [63–65]. Prevalences range between 30% and 77% [64,66,67], a finding that exceeds expected frequencies for community-based samples [67] or in populations of older adults [68,69]. Major depression may emerge at any time after TBI, with most episodes being time-limited [64,65,70]. Approximately 25% of individuals who experience a major depression remain chronically depressed [71]. Across studies, expected demographic factors (eg, age, marital status, education, socioeconomic status, diversity) and TBI-related factors (eg, duration after TBI) are unrelated to onset, resolution, or chronicity of depression [64,71,72]. However, several authors have found a relationship between female sex, a positive history of a pre-TBI psychiatric disorder [64,72], and more severe TBI [73] and the onset of post-TBI depression.

Older adults who have TBI are at increased risk for suicide, as are older depressed individuals in general [74]. For example, individuals who have had a reported loss of consciousness (and therefore a high probability of a prior TBI) have a fourfold increase in suicide attempts and greater psychopathology [75]. Increased risk for suicide has also been related to the length of time since injury and the degree of disruption in the individual's relationships and occupational functioning [76].

Finally, like their older peers who have major depressive disorders, a small proportion of older depressed adults who have TBI will present with psychotic features. Typically, the psychotic presentation reflects a nonbizarre paranoia, which on careful examination may be seen as a byproduct of decreased memory functioning secondary to the TBI. Secondary manic or hypomanic states have been reported in approximately 9% of individuals after TBI [77,78]. Mania has been associated with posttraumatic partial complex seizures and focal right hemisphere lesions [79]. The most problematic seizure disorders are those that are accompanied by depressive manifestations with suicidal thoughts or actual suicidal attempts [73,78].

Anxiety disorders are the second most common psychiatric diagnoses after TBI, with prevalences ranging from 2% to 15% for select disorders, findings that clearly exceed expected frequencies in either community-based samples [67] or older adults [69,70]. Minimal resolution of anxiety disorders after TBI is observed, with most disorders remaining chronic [64]. Although most demographic factors (eg, marital status, age, socioeconomic status) and TBI-related factors (eg, time since injury) appear to be unrelated to the onset of anxiety disorders after TBI, several authors have found relationships among sex, ethnic background [72], prior history of an anxiety disorder [64], and milder injuries [80–82].

The most frequent anxiety disorder following TBI is posttraumatic stress disorder (PTSD), with prevalences ranging from 19% to 33% as long as 8 years after TBI [64,72]. Other anxiety disorders commonly diagnosed after TBI include generalized anxiety disorder [65,72,83], panic disorder [64–66,72], and obsessive compulsive disorder [64]. Comorbidity of depression and anxiety after TBI is extremely common [64,66,84,85]. Comorbid psychiatric diagnoses after TBI create additional psychosocial stresses and have been shown to have a negative impact on functional [65] rehabilitation outcomes [86,87], family dysfunction [88], quality of life, and community integration [64]. Indeed, emotional disturbances have been viewed as more seriously handicapping than either the cognitive or the physical challenges of the TBI itself [89]. Thus, treatments offered in the form of pharmacologic interventions and psychotherapy are clearly indicated to minimize these secondary sequelae of the TBI.

Psychologic interventions in the elderly after traumatic brain injury

Treatment of psychiatric challenges after TBI typically encompasses both pharmacologic and nonpharmacologic (psychosocial) interventions, alone or in combination. The choice of clinical approach is dependent on many factors, including comorbid medical problems, age, and TBI-related challenges. Clinical decisions need to incorporate knowledge of the person's ability to comply with recommended interventions and a review of his or her current and prediagnosis medication history. Coexisting medical conditions may limit the choice of the pharmacology used to address the affective disorders, particularly in the elderly, who frequently have several comorbid conditions that may argue for use of a nonpharmacologic approach.

Pharmacologic interventions

When selecting medications for treatment of post-TBI mood disorders, the clinician must consider issues related to medication compliance, which are complicated by both the age of the individual and the presence of TBI.

For example, individuals may discontinue prescribed medications because of unpleasant side effects long before therapeutic levels of the medication have been attained. Memory declines may limit the individual's ability to follow the recommended medication regime. Noncompliance in the forms of overuse or abuse or, alternatively, underuse due to cost of the prescribed medication needs to be considered. Furthermore, consideration of dosage is important, because individuals who have TBI are more sensitive to the side effects of medications, especially psychotropic agents. Proposed general guidelines for medication use in TBI include prudent increases in medication doses, an emphasis on minimizing side effects ("start low, go slow"), an adequate therapeutic trial of the medication, often necessitating longer duration of treatment before evaluation of its efficacy, frequent reassessments to determine changes in treatment schedules, and monitoring of drug interactions. When clinical evidence suggests a partial response to medications, augmentation therapy is often suggested before one shifts to other pharmacologic agents [88].

Despite the known prevalence of depression after TBI [90], surprisingly little empiric research into efficacy of psychopharmacologic interventions for mood after TBI exists; most reports are limited to case studies and anecdotal experiences [91]. Selection of an antidepressant is usually guided by side effect profiles; one should opt to avoid medications that manifest high anticholinergic activity or lower seizure threshold or have high sedative effects [92]. Tricyclic antidepressants are generally avoided whenever possible, because they have significant anticholinergic effects that interfere with cognition and memory, have potentially lower seizure thresholds, and may cause orthostatic hypotension [93].

Selective serotonin reuptake inhibitors (SSRI) are currently the drugs of choice, because they have fewer adverse side effects, may be used to address both depressive and anxiety symptoms [91], and are extremely effective when depression is accompanied by vegetative or behavioral alterations [94]. Psychostimulants [95], select anxiolytic medications (eg, buspirone) [96], and mood stabilizers such as carbamazepine [97] are alternative considerations. Antidepressants appear to work best when augmented by individual or group psychotherapy to help the individual cope with permanent TBI-related changes in functioning. Some medications should be avoided following TBI, such as neuroleptics, benzodiazepines, and centrally acting antihypertensives, because they have been shown to inhibit recovery following brain injury [62].

Despite the lack of empiric research into the efficacy of anti-anxiety medications after TBI, usual interventions focus on the use of benzodiazepines, buspirone, or antidepressants, alone or in combination with psychotherapy and psychoeducation, to address anxiety. Although benzodiazepines are useful for treatment of anxiety in the general population, they are best avoided when treating individuals who have TBI because of their adverse effects on concentration, motor coordination, and memory [91] and their tendency to create drug dependency. SSRI have become the primary choice for treatment of a wide variety of anxiety disorders because of their low side effect profiles, minimal abuse potential, and effectiveness for a wide range of anxiety symptoms. Alternative approaches to treatment of anxiety include buspirone and anticonvulsants [91].

Psychotherapy approaches

Research on the efficacy of psychotherapeutic approaches in the treatment of post-TBI mood disorders is limited to case reports and one randomized trial comparing cognitive behavioral therapy (CBT) with supportive counseling [98]. CBT is the most frequently used psychotherapeutic approach to treating depression in individuals with other neurologic impairments [99,100]; it has been modified to address the specific cognitive challenges presented by individuals who have acquired brain injury [101–103]. Case studies have supported the use of CBT as an effective approach to TBI-related depression [104], anger management [105], and anxiety disorders [106]. CBT has been found to reduce subsequent development of PTSD in individuals who have mild TBI [98]. The CBT approach provides several advantages when applied to individuals who have TBI. It is a flexible approach that permits individualized interventions necessary to address specific cognitive and behavioral issues as they emerge during the course of recovery from brain injury, it incorporates the high level of structure necessary for an individual's maximum functioning secondary to acquired cognitive limitations, and it is factual in nature and deals with current and important situations for the individual. Typically, CBT is used in conjunction with antidepressant and anti-anxiety medications. Psychoeducation groups as well as individual supportive psychotherapy may be beneficial as well.

Summary

The growing population of older adults who have TBI will present numerous challenges to health care providers in our society over the next decades. Medical professionals, family members, and policy makers will need to address these unique challenges to ensure that proper care is provided and functional outcomes are maximized. Many older individuals are capable of making significant improvements and living quality lives following TBI. But they can only accomplish this with a proper diagnosis, appropriate and timely medical care, including intensive rehabilitation, and cognitive and emotional support in their communities.

References

[1] US Census Bureau. US interim projections by age, sex, race and Hispanic origin. March 18, 2004. Available at: http://www.census.gov/ipc/www/usinterimproj. Accessed July 30, 2005.
[2] Langlois JA, Kegler SR, Butler JA, et al. Traumatic brain injury–related hospital discharges: results from a 14-state surveillance system, 1997. MMWR CDC Surveill Summ 2003;52:1–20.
[3] Injury fact book 2001–2002. Atlanta (GA): Centers for Disease Control and Prevention, National Center for Injury Prevention and Control; 2001.
[4] Traumatic brain injury in the United States. Emergency room visits, hospitalizations and deaths. Atlanta (GA): Centers for Disease Control and Prevention; 2004.

[5]   Thurman DJ, Alverson CA, Dunn KA, et al. Traumatic brain injury in the United States: a
      public health perspective. J Head Trauma Rehabil 1999;14:602–15.
[6]   Krause JF, Arthur DL. Incidence and prevalence of, and costs associated with traumatic
      brain injury. In: Rosenthal M, Griffith ER, Bond MR, et al, editors. Rehabilitation of the
      adult and child with traumatic brain injury. 3rd edition. Philadelphia: F.A. Davis Co.; 1999.
      p. 3–18.
[7]   Centers for Disease Control and Prevention. Public health and aging: nonfatal fall-related
      traumatic brain injury among older adults—California 1996–1999. MMWR Morb Mortal Wkly
      Rep 2003;52:276–8.
[8]   Adekoya N, Thurman DJ, White DD, et al. Surveillance for traumatic brain injury deaths—
      United States, 1989–1998. MMWR Morb Mortal Wkly Rep 2002;51:1–14.
[9]   Tinetti ME, Doucette J, Claus E, et al. Risk factors for serious injury during falls by older
      persons in the community. J Am Geriatr Soc 1995;43:1214–21.
[10] Speechley M, Tinetti M. Falls and injuries in frail and vigorous community elderly persons.
      J Am Geriatr Soc 1991;39:46–52.
[11] Ray WA, Griffin MR, Downey W, et al. Long-term use of thiazide diuretics and risk of hip
      fracture. Lancet 1989;1:687–90.
[12] Thapa PB, Gidean P, Fought RL, et al. Psychotropic drugs and risk of recurrent falls in
      ambulatory nursing home residents. Am J Epidemiol 1995;142:202–11.
[13] Susman M, DiRusso SM, Sullivan T, et al. Traumatic brain injury in the elderly: increased
      mortality and worse functional outcome at discharge despite lower injury severity. J Trauma
      2002;53:219–23.
[14] Gubler KD, Davis R, Koepsell T, et al. Long-term survival of elderly trauma patients. Arch
      Surg 1997;132:1010–4.
[15] Servadei F, Murray GD, Teasdale GM, et al. Traumatic subarachnoid hemorrhage: demographic
      and clinical study of 750 patients from the European Brain Injury Consortium survey of head
      injuries. Neurosurgery 2002;50:261–7.
[16] Sato S, Suzuki J. Ultra structural observations of the capsule of chronic subdural hematoma in
      various clinical stages. J Neurosurg 1975;43:569–78.
[17] Ito H, Yamamoto S, Saito K, et al. Quantitative estimation of hemorrhage in chronic subdural
      hematoma using the ^{51}Cr erythrocyte labeling method. J Neurosurg 1987;66:862–4.
[18] Traynelis VC. Chronic subdural hematomas in the elderly. Clin Geriatr Med 1991;7:
      583–98.
[19] Feldman RG, Pincus JH, McEntee WJ. Cerebrovascular accident or subdural fluid collection?
      Arch Intern Med 1963;112:966–76.
[20] Rozzelle CJ, Wofford JL, Branch CL. Predictors of hospital mortality in older patients with
      subdural hematoma. J Am Geriatr Soc 1995;43:240–4.
[21] Gennarelli TA. The spectrum of traumatic axonal injury. Neuropathol Appl Neurobiol 1996;
      22:509–13.
[22] Gale SD, Johnson SC, Bigler ED, et al. Trauma-induced degenerative changes in brain injury:
      a morphometric analysis of three patients with pre-injury and post-injury MR scans. J Neuro-
      trauma 1995;12:151–8.
[23] Anderson CV, Wood DG, Bigler ED, et al. Lesion volume, injury severity, and thalamic
      integrity following head injury. J Neurotrauma 1996;13:59–65.
[24] The Brain Trauma Foundation. Guidelines for the management of severe head injury. New
      York: Brain Trauma Foundation; 1995.
[25] Cifu DX, Kreutzer JS, Marwitz JH, et al. Functional outcomes of older adults with trau-
      matic brain injury: a prospective, multicenter analysis. Arch Phys Med Rehabil 1996;77:
      883–8.
[26] Hoffman JM, Doctor JN, Chan L, et al. Potential impact of the new Medicare prospective
      payment system on reimbursement for traumatic brain injury inpatient rehabilitation. Arch Phys
      Med Rehabil 2003;84:1165–72.
[27] Mosenthal AC, Lavery RF, Addis M, et al. Isolated traumatic brain injury: age is an
      independent predictor of mortality and early outcome. J Trauma 2002;52:907–11.

[28] Kilaru S, Garb J, Emhoff T, et al. Long-term functional status and mortality of elderly patients with severe closed head injuries. J Trauma 1996;41:957–63.

[29] Hukkelhoven CW, Steyerberg EW, Rampen AJ, et al. Patient age and outcome following severe traumatic brain injury: an analysis of 5600 patients. J Neurosurg 2003;41:9966–73.

[30] Ritchie PD, Cameron PA, Ugoni A, et al. A study of the functional outcome and mortality in elderly patients with head injuries. J Clin Neurosci 2000;7:301–4.

[31] Mayer NH. Choosing upper limb muscles for focal intervention after traumatic brain injury. J Head Trauma Rehabil 2004;19:119–42.

[32] Fock J, Galen MP, Stillman BC, et al. Functional outcome following botulinum toxin A injection to reduce spastic equines in adults with traumatic brain injury. Brain Inj 2005;18: 57–63.

[33] Brashear A, McAfee AL, Kuhn ER, et al. Treatment with botulinum toxin type B for upper-limb spasticity. Arch Phys Med Rehabil 2003;84:103–7.

[34] Ellis GL. Subdural hematoma in the elderly. Emerg Med Clin North Am 1990;8:281–94.

[35] Cummings JL, Benson D. Dementia: a clinical approach. 2nd edition. Boston: Butterworth-Heinemann; 1992.

[36] Flanagan SR, Hibbard M, Gordon WA. The impact of age on traumatic brain injury. Phys Med Rehabil Clin N Am 2005;16:163–77.

[37] Goldstein FC, Levin HS, Oresley RM, et al. Neurobehavioral consequences of closed head injury in older adults. J Neurol Neurosurg Psychiatry 1994;57:961–6.

[38] Whyte JM, Plansky M, Fleming M, et al. Sustained arousal and attention after traumatic brain injury. Neuropsychologia 1995;33:797–813.

[39] Goodglass H. Disorders of naming following brain injury. Am Sci 1980;68:647–55.

[40] McDonald BC, Flashman LA, Saykin AJ. Executive dysfunction following traumatic brain injury: neural substrates and treatment strategies. NeuroRehabilitation 2002;17:333–44.

[41] Grady CL, Haxby JV, Horowitz B, et al. Longitudinal study of the early neuropsychological and cerebral metabolic changes in dementia of the Alzheimer's type. J Clin Exp Neuropsychol 1998;10:576–96.

[42] Welsh K, Butter N, Hughes J, et al. Detection of abnormal memory decline in mild cases of Alzheimer's disease using CERAD neuropsychological measures. Arch Neurol 1991;48: 278–81.

[43] Perry RJ, Hodges RJ. Attention and executive deficits in Alzheimer's disease. Brain 1999;122: 383–404.

[44] Hibbard MR, Uysal S, Sliwinski M, et al. Undiagnosed health issues in individuals with traumatic brain injury living in the community. J Head Trauma Rehabil 1998;13:47–57.

[45] Ashman T, Spielman LA, Hibbard MA, et al. Psychiatric challenges in the first 6 years after traumatic brain injury: cross-sequential analysis of Axis I disorders. Arch Phys Med Rehabil 2004;85(Suppl 2):S36–42.

[46] Alexopoulos GS. Affect disorders. In: Sadavoy L, Lazarus L, Jarvik L, et al, editors. Comprehensive review of geriatric psychiatry II. 2nd edition. Washington, DC: American Psychiatric Press; 1990. p. 563–92.

[47] Berger AK, Fratiglioni L, Forsell Y, et al. The occurrence of depressive symptoms in the preclinical phase of AD. Neurology 1999;53:1998–2002.

[48] McCurry SM, Gibbons LE, Logsdon RG, et al. Anxiety and nighttime behavioral disturbances. Awakenings in patients with Alzheimer's disease. J Gerontol Nurs 2004;30:12–20.

[49] Teri L, Ferretti LE, Gibbons LE, et al. Anxiety of Alzheimer's disease: prevalence and comorbidity. J Gerontol A Biol Sci Med Sci 1999;54:348–52.

[50] Corder EH, Saunders AM, Strittmatter WJ, et al. Gene dose and apolipoprotein E type 4 allele and the risk of Alzheimer's disease in late onset families. Science 1993;261:921–3.

[51] Twamley EW, Bondi MW. The differential diagnosis of dementia. In: Ricker J, editor. Differential diagnosis in adults' neuropsychological assessment. New York: Springer Publishing Co.; 2004. p. 276–326.

[52] Mayeux R, Saunders AM, Shea S, et al. Utility of the apolipoprotein E genotype in the

diagnosis of Alzheimer's disease. Alzheimer's Disease Centers Consortium of Apolipoprotein E. N Engl J Med 1998;338:506–11.

[53] Jellinger KA, Paulus W, Wrocklage C, et al. Traumatic brain injury as a risk factor for
Alzheimer's disease. Comparison of two retrospective autopsy cohorts with evaluation of ApoE
genotype. BMC Neurol 2001;1:3.

[54] Lye TC, Shored EA. Traumatic brain injury as risk factor for Alzheimer's disease: a review.
Neuropsychol Rev 2000;10:115–29.

[55] Plassman BL, Havlik RJ, Steddens DC, et al. Documented head injury in early adulthood and
risk of Alzheimer's disease and other dementias. Neurology 2000;55:1158–66.

[56] Guo Z, Cupples LS, Kurz A, et al. Head injury and risk of AD in the MIRAGE Study.
Neurology 2000;54:1316–23.

[57] Mayeux R, Ottman R, Maestre G, et al. Synergistic effects of traumatic head injury and
apolipoprotein-epsilon 4 in patients with Alzheimer's disease. Neurology 1995;45:555–7.

[58] Petersen RC, Smith G, Kokmen E, et al. Memory function in normal aging. Neurology
1992;42:396–401.

[59] Small SA, Stern Y, Tang M, et al. Selective declines in memory function among healthy elderly.
Neurology 1999;52:1392–6.

[60] Salthouse TA, Coon VE. Influence of task specific processing speed on age difference in
memory. J Gerontol 1993;48:245–55.

[61] Breed ST, Dahlman K, Gordon WA, et al. A comparison of cognitive functioning among
individuals with TBI, AD and no cognitive impairments. Brain Inj, in press.

[62] Goldstein LB. Common drugs may influence motor recovery after stroke. The Sygen in Acute
Stroke Study investigators. Neurology 1995;45:865–71.

[63] Hibbard MR, Uysal S, Kepler K, et al. Axis I psychopathology in individuals with TBI. Head
Trauma Rehabil 1998;13:24–39.

[64] Fann J, Katon W, Uomoto J, et al. Psychiatric disorders and functional disability in outpatient
treatment with traumatic brain injury. Am J Psychiatry 1995;151:1493–9.

[65] Van Reekum R, Bolago I, Finlayson M, et al. Psychiatric disorders after traumatic brain injury.
Brain Inj 1996;10:319–27.

[66] Varney N, Martzke J, Robert R. Major depression in patients with closed head injury.
Neuropsychology 1987;1:7–8.

[67] American Psychiatric Association. Diagnostic and statistical manual of mental disorders. 4th
edition. Washington, DC: American Psychiatric Press; 1994.

[68] Weissman MA, Bruce M, Leaf PJ, et al. Affective disorders. In: Robins LN, Regier LA, editors.
Psychiatric disorders in America: the Epidemiologic Catchment Area study. New York: Free
Press; 1991. p. 53–80.

[69] American Psychological Association. The psychological problems of older Americans.
Available at: http://www.apa.org/pi/aging/older/psychological.html. Accessed April 13, 2004.

[70] Hibbard MR, Ashman TA, Spielman LA, et al. Relationship between depression
and psychosocial functioning after traumatic brain injury. Arch Phys Med Rehabil 2004;
85(Suppl 2):S43–53.

[71] Ashman T, Spielman LA, Hibbard MR, et al. Psychiatric challenges in the first six years after
traumatic brain injury: cross-sequential analyses of axis I disorders. Arch Phys Med Rehabil
2004;85(Suppl 2):36–42.

[72] Fedoroff JP, Starkstein SE, Forrester AW, et al. Depression in patients with acute traumatic
brain injury. Am J Psychiatry 1992;149:918–23.

[73] Holsinger T, Steffens DC, Phillips C, et al. Head injury in early adulthood and the lifetime risk
of depression. Arch Gen Psychiatry 2002;59:17–24.

[74] National Institute of Mental Health. Older adults: depression and suicide facts. Bethesda (MD):
2003. NIH Publication #03–4593.

[75] Silver JM, Kramer R, Greenwood S, et al. The association between head injuries and
psychiatric disorders: findings from the New Haven NIMH Epidemiologic Catchment Area
study. Brain Inj 2001;15:935–45.

[76] Yudofsky SC, Hales RE, editors. The American Psychiatric Press textbook of neuropsychology. Washington, DC: American Psychiatric Press; 1992.

[77] Shukla S, Cook BL, Mukherjee S, et al. Mania following head trauma. Am J Psychiatry 1987;144:93–6.

[78] Robinson RG, Jorge R. Mood disorders. In: Silver JM, Yudofsky SC, Hales R, editors. Neuropsychiatry of traumatic brain injury. Washington, DC: American Psychiatric Press; 1994. p. 219–50.

[79] Starkstein SE, Mayberg HD, Berthier ML, et al. Mania after brain injury: neuroradiological and metabolic findings. Ann Neurol 1990;27:652–9.

[80] Ohry A, Rattok J, Solomon Z. Post-traumatic stress disorder in brain injury patients. Brain Inj 1996;10:687–95.

[81] Rattock J. Do patients with mild brain injuries have post traumatic stress disorder too? J Head Trauma Rehabil 1996;11:95–6.

[82] Silver JM, Rattok J, Anderson K. Post traumatic stress disorder and traumatic brain injury. Neurocase 1997;3:1–7.

[83] Jorge RE, Robinson RG, Starkstein SE, et al. Influence of major depression on 1-year outcome in patients with traumatic brain injury. Neurosurgery 1994;81:726–33.

[84] Deb S, Lyons I, Koutzoukis C, et al. Rate of psychiatric illness 1 year after traumatic brain injury. Am J Psychiatry 1999;156:774–8.

[85] Levin HS, Brown SA, Song JX, et al. Depression and post traumatic stress disorder at three months after mild to moderate traumatic brain injury. J Clin Exp Neuropsychol 2001;23:754–69.

[86] Brooks N, Campsie L, Symington C, et al. The effects of head injury on patients and relatives within seven years of injury. J Head Trauma Rehabil 1987;2:1–13.

[87] Thomsen IV. Late outcome of very severe blunt head trauma: a 10–15 year second follow up. J Neurol Neurosurg Psychiatry 1984;47:260–8.

[88] Silver JM, Yudofsky SC, Hales RE. Depression in traumatic brain. Neuropsych Behav Neurol 4:12–23.

[89] Lezak MD. Neuropsychological assessment. 2nd edition. New York: Oxford University Press; 1983.

[90] Rosenthal M, Christensen BK, Ross TP. Depression following traumatic brain injury. Arch Phys Med Rehabil 1998;79:90–103.

[91] Robinson RG, Jorge R. Mood disorders. In: Silver J, McAllister TW, Yudofsky SC, editors. Textbook of traumatic brain injury. Arlington (VA): American Psychiatric Publishing Co.; 2005. p. 201–12.

[92] Silver JM, Hales RE, Yudofsky SC. Psychopharmacology of depression in neurologic disorders. J Clin Psychiatry 1990;51:33–9.

[93] Wroblewski BA, McColgan K, Smith K, et al. The incidence of seizures during tricyclic antidepressant drug treatment in a brain injured population. J Clin Psychopharmacol 1990; 10:124–8.

[94] Kim E. Elderly. In: Silver J, McAllister TN, Yudofsky SC, editors. Textbook of traumatic brain injury. Arlington (VA): American Psychiatric Publishing Co.; 2005. p. 495–508.

[95] Zasler ND. Advances in neuropharmacological rehabilitation for brain dysfunction. Brain Inj 1992;6:1–14.

[96] Gaultieri CT. Pharmacotherapy and the neurobehavioral sequelae of traumatic brain injury. Brain Inj 1991;2:101–29.

[97] Kunik ME, Yudofsky SC, Silver JM, et al. Pharmacologic approach to management of agitation associated with dementia. J Clin Psychiatry 1994;55(Suppl):13–7.

[98] Bryant RA, Moulds M, Guthrie R, et al. Treating acute stress disorder following traumatic brain injury. Am J Psychiatry 2003;65:585–7.

[99] Birkett DP. The psychiatry of stroke. 1st edition. Washington, DC: American Psychiatric Press; 1996.

[100] Langenbahn DM, Sherr RL, Simon D, et al. Group psychotherapy. In: Langer KG, Lastsch L, Lewis L, editors. Psychotherapeutic interventions for adults with brain injury or stroke: a clinician's treatment resource. Madison (CT): Psychosocial Press; 1999. p. 167–89.

[101] Hibbard MR, Grober SE, Gordon WA, et al. Modification of cognitive psychotherapy for the treatment of post stroke depression. The Behavior Therapist 1990;1:15–7.

[102] Hibbard MR, Grober SE, Gordon WA, et al. Cognitive therapy and the treatment of post stroke depression. Topics in Geriatric Rehabilitation 1990;5:43–55.

[103] Hibbard MR, Grober SE, Stein PN, et al. Post stroke depression. In: Freeman A, Datillio FM, editors. Comprehensive casebook of cognitive therapy. New York: Plenum Press; 1992. p. 303–10.

[104] Payne HC. Traumatic brain injury, depressions and cannabis use—assessing their effects on cognitive performance. Brain Inj 2000;5:479–89.

[105] Medd J, Tate RL. Evaluation of an anger management therapy programme following acquired brain injury: a preliminary study. Neuropsychol Rehabil 2000;10:185–201.

[106] Hibbard MR, Gordon WA, Kothera L. Traumatic brain injury. In: Dattilio FM, Freeman A, editors. Cognitive-behavioral approaches to crisis interventions. 4th edition. New York: Guilford Press; 2000. p. 219–42.

ELSEVIER
SAUNDERS

Clin Geriatr Med 22 (2006) 469–489

CLINICS IN
GERIATRIC
MEDICINE

Rehabilitation of the Older Adult with Stroke

Monika V. Shah, DO[a,b,c,*]

[a]*Department of Physical Medicine and Rehabilitation, Baylor College of Medicine,
1333 Moursund Avenue, D-111, Houston, TX 77030, USA*
[b]*Traumatic Brain Injury and Stroke Program, The Institute for Rehabilitation and Research,
1333 Moursund Avenue, D-111, Houston, TX 77030, USA*
[c]*Long-Term Acute Care Brain Injury Program, Kindred Hospital, Baylor College of Medicine,
1333 Moursund Avenue, Houston, TX 77030, USA*

Stroke is an increasing public health concern throughout the world as the leading cause of long-term disability. There is estimated to be over 3.5 million survivors of stroke in the United States. It is responsible for 10% to 12% of all deaths in industrialized countries. Almost 90% of these deaths are among people aged over 65 years. It is well known that there exist differences related to epidemiology, pathophysiology, comorbidity, and functional outcome of patients with advanced age compared with the young. Factors that have been suggested to influence this disparity include age-related complications, availability of resources, lack of aggressive management, and possible diminished capacity for neuroplasticity. Despite these differences across age groups, there is compelling evidence that good outcomes can be achieved after comprehensive stroke rehabilitation [1–4]. The number of individuals aged >65 years is projected to increase from 39 million in 1995 to 69 million, or 20% of the total population, in 2030. The fastest growing age group will be the population aged >85 years, doubling its 1995 size by 2025 and increasing fivefold by 2050. This article reviews the current medical and rehabilitative aspects of stroke and the possible disparities related to advanced age.

* Department of Physical Medicine and Rehabilitation, Baylor College of Medicine, The Institute for Rehabilitation and Research, 1333 Moursund Avenue, D-111, Houston, TX 77030.
E-mail address: shahm@tirr.tmc.edu

0749-0690/06/$ – see front matter © 2006 Elsevier Inc. All rights reserved.
doi:10.1016/j.cger.2005.12.012   *geriatric.theclinics.com*

Stroke subtypes

Cerebrovascular disease is divided into ischemic or hemorrhagic lesions. Ischemic lesions comprise 80% of strokes and are caused by thrombotic (60%) or embolic (20%) mechanisms. Hemorrhagic strokes have an incidence of approximately 15% and are divided into intracerebral (10%) or subarachnoid (5%). Other causes (5%) of stroke include tumor, aneurysm, and arteriovenous malformation. The incidence of each stroke subtype and its etiology vary with age. Overall, cerebral infarction accounts for most strokes across all age groups. There is an increased incidence of hemorrhagic stroke with younger age when compared with the elderly primarily because of the differences in risk factors. Strokes are classified further by the brain's anatomic blood supply and related neurologic structures. They can be divided generally into anterior, middle, and posterior cerebral artery distributions (Table 1).

Stroke risk factors

The outcome of a patient with a treated stroke may never be as good as that of someone in whom a stroke is prevented [5]. The identification and modification of risk factors should begin as a primary prevention measure and continue after a stroke as a secondary prevention measure during the acute care and rehabilitation phase. There are specific and well-defined risk factors for stroke, both modifiable and unmodifiable, that are well-known to most clinicians. Advanced age, hypertension, atrial fibrillation, statin use, and alcohol consumption are discussed in terms of their impact on the elderly.

Age is the most important unmodifiable risk factor for all stroke types including ischemic stroke. For each successive 10 years after the age 55, the stroke rate more than doubles in both men and women [6,7]. Approximately 65% of all strokes occur in those who are over the age of 65. Data from Rochester, Minnesota, demonstrated that more than half of the strokes in this population

Table 1
Common stroke syndromes by territory

Vascular distribution	Clinical
ACA	Contralateral weakness (leg> arm) and hemianesthesia, contralateral cortical sensory loss, incontinence, abulia, apraxia, personality changes, frontal release signs, conjugate eye deviation toward lesion
MCA	Contralateral hemiplegia (arm and face> leg) and hemianesthesia, homonymous hemianopsia, conjugate eye deviation toward lesion, aphasia (d), aprosody (n), apraxia (d), hemineglect (n), visuoperceptual deficits (n), anosognosia
PCA	Contralateral visual field defects (hemianopsia) with macular sparing, language or memory deficits, alexia with or without agraphia (d)

Abbreviations: ACA, anterior cerebral artery; MCA, Middle cerebral artery; PCA, posterior cerebral artery; (d), dominant; (n), nondominant.

affected subjects aged >75 years and nearly one quarter affected subjects aged >85 years. Furthermore, elderly stroke patients are reported to have more severe strokes, higher case-fatality rates, and larger proportion discharged to long-term institutional care. In general, the frequency of stroke is higher in males than females until the age of 55. After the age of 55, the risk is nearly equal for both men and women. Because women tend to live longer than men, however, more women die of stroke each year.

Hypertension is considered the most important modifiable risk factor. The efficacy of antihypertensive treatment in preventing stroke is well established in all age groups. Using blood pressure of over 140/90 mm Hg to define hypertension, about 20% of the adult population has hypertension, whereas for people over the age of 65 years the prevalence is as high as 65% [8]. Since 1991, the results of three major trials (the British Medical Research Council trial of treatment in older adults, the Swedish Trial in Old Patients with Hypertension, and the Systolic Hypertension in the Elderly Program) have conclusively established the benefits of treating older patients (>60 years) with both diastolic and isolated systolic hypertension. International guidelines for the management of hypertension (including the Fifth Report of the Joint National Committee, the 1993 report of the World Health Organization and the International Society of Hypertension, and the second report of the British Hypertension Society Working Party) have all been modified to reflect the emerging evidence concerning the benefits of treating older patients. Cost-effectiveness data are similarly in accord with giving high priority to the treatment of older individuals with hypertension.

Atrial fibrillation is an important cardiac risk factor in the elderly and is estimated to cause almost half of all cardioembolic strokes. The prevalence of atrial fibrillation in people over 60 is approximately 5% and rises to almost 15% after the age of 75. Studies have shown that stroke patients with atrial fibrillation are significantly more likely to be dead, disabled, or handicapped at 3 months than those without atrial fibrillation [9]. There is an increased risk of subsequent stroke in the elderly patient with atrial fibrillation, yet many are not being treated. Although warfarin therapy with international normalized ratio between 2 and 3 dramatically reduces the risk of stroke, the risk of intracranial hemorrhage is increased in patients older than 75 years and in those anticoagulated with an international normalized ratio above 3. The decision to treat with warfarin therapy should be made by weighing the benefits against the risks for that individual.

There is compelling evidence that 3-hydroxy-3-methylglutaryl-CoA reductase inhibitors (statins) are strongly associated with lower risk of coronary disease. In the Prospective Study of Pravastatin in the Elderly at Risk trial, pravastatin was shown to reduce the risk of coronary events in elderly people with a history or risk of vascular disease [10]. Until recently, data regarding the specific relationship between hypercholesterolemia and stroke were less robust. According to data from the Heart Protection Study, there was an overall 25% reduction of first event rate for stroke. Among patients with pre-existing cerebrovascular disease there was no apparent reduction in the stroke rate, but there was a significant reduction in the rate of any major vascular event [11,12]. The association between plasma cholesterol levels and risk of stroke seems to diminish with in-creased age [13]. Statins have shown worsening of cognitive function in two randomized trials [14,15] and several case reports [16–18]. The Heart Protection Study and Prospective Study of Pravastatin in the Elderly at Risk trial, however, did not show favorable or deleterious effects on cognitive measures that were tested. There is still controversy over the finding that statins increased the frequency of new cancer diagnoses in elderly individuals [10], although recent experience in long-term trials allay concerns that there was a cause and effect relationship. Although there are clear benefits of statin therapy after a stroke, the potential side effects should be considered in the elderly.

There is a variable association between alcohol consumption and stroke. Alcohol has been reported to be a possible risk factor for thromboembolic stroke [19], and as a protective factor for stroke with light or moderate consumers [20,21]. Moderate consumption of alcohol (one to two drinks per day) may reduce cardiovascular disease including ischemic stroke; however, there seems to be a dose-response relationship between moderate consumption and the risk of intracerebral and subarachnoid hemorrhage. There is only limited evidence that moderate amount of drinking may have a protective effect among those older than 65 [22]. Alcohol should not be considered as a preventive agent for stroke. There are serious concerns of alcohol use in the elderly including alcohol-medication interactions, acceleration of age-related postural instability, and increase in falls [23]. It is recommended that the elderly abstain from alcohol use.

Other causes of stroke

The work-up for an older adult with stroke may be quite different from that of a young person. It is generally accepted that a hypercoagulable work-up in an elderly person with otherwise obvious stroke etiology, such as carotid stenosis, has a low yield. The differential diagnosis in young adults may include hematologic abnormalities and drug abuse, whereas advanced age may boast its own specific causes for stroke that warrant further investigation. The differential diagnosis of an elderly stroke patient may include such causes as hyperhomocysteinemia, amyloid angiopathy, and multi-infarct dementia.

Hyperhomocysteinemia is now established as a major risk factor for stroke [24]. It has been attributed to dietary deficiency of vitamin B_6, vitamin B_{12}, or folic acid, especially in older patients with poor nutritional intake. The interplay of folate, vitamin B_{12}, and vitamin B_6 helps control blood levels of homocysteine. Some individuals may have an inherited deficiency and develop premature atherosclerosis and often experience a stroke early in life. The use of antiepileptic drugs, such as phenytoin, has also been shown to increase the level of homocysteine in the blood [25]. Patients with stroke can have homocysteine levels 1.5 times those of age- and sex-matched controls [26]. Two large randomized multicenter trials, the Vitamin Intervention for Stroke Prevention and the Vitamins to Prevent Stroke studies, are designed to determine if, in addition to best medical and surgical management, high-dose folic acid, vitamin B_6, and vitamin B_{12} supplements reduce recurrent stroke or transient ischemic attack [27].

Cerebral amyloid angiopathy is caused by deposition of β-amyloid sheets in media and adventitia of small to mid-sized arteries of the cerebral cortex and the leptomeninges. Vessels become more rigid and fragile increasing the risk of rupture. Advanced age increases the incidence of cerebral amyloid angiopathy, which has been reported as 5% of those in the seventh decade of life, and up to 50% of those older than 90 years. Fifteen percent of all intracerebral hemorrhages in patients older than 60 years and about 50% of nontraumatic lobar intracerebral hemorrhages in those older than 70 years are attributable to cerebral amyloid angiopathy. Incidence remains elusive because definitive diagnosis is made only by histologic examination or postmortem brain biopsy. The most common symptoms are headache, occurring 60% to 70% at onset, followed by dementia, transient neurologic symptoms, or coma. The most common and devastating effect of cerebral amyloid angiopathy is lobar intracerebral hemorrhages, but it is associated with a lower mortality rate and a better functional outcome than hypertensive deep ganglionic bleeds. It is estimated that at least 40% of patients with intracerebral hemorrhages–related hemorrhage have some degree of dementia. Although patient management is unchanged from standard intracerebral hemorrhages, priority should be given to reversing anticoagulation. Blood thinners, such as warfarin, and antiplatelet agents, such as aspirin, should be avoided if possible. If these medications are required for other conditions, such as heart disease, the potential benefits must be carefully weighed against the increased risks.

Multi-infarct dementia, or vascular dementia, is the second most common cause of dementia in the elderly after Alzheimer's disease. The diagnosis requires (1) cognitive loss, often subcortical; (2) imaging studies demonstrating vascular brain lesions; and (3) exclusion of other causes of dementia, such as Alzheimer's disease [28]. It affects people between the ages of 60 and 75 with a slight predilection for men. Multi-infarct dementia is caused by small, multiple cerebral infarcts with the progression of cognitive impairment being insidious, stepwise, or both, usually affecting executive dysfunction, memory loss, or aphasia. A familial form of dementia associated with cerebrovascular disease is observed in a rare genetic condition, cerebral autosomal-dominant arteriopathy with subcortical infarcts and leukoencephalopathy. This condition is less common in the elderly because recurrent strokes usually begin before the age of 50.

Effective rehabilitation of the stroke patient with dementia is dependent on motivation and cognitive ability even more than on remaining motor or sensory function. Specifically, there should be a meaningful engagement with the therapist. Neuropsychologic evaluation commonly identifies impairment in executive dysfunction, memory, and language. Given its strong vascular component, the diagnosis of multi-infarct dementia is believed to be more preventable and offers a better likelihood for cognitive improvement compared with Alzheimer's disease [29]. Treatment often involves control of risk factors, such as hypertension, diabetes, smoking, hyperfibrinogenemia, hyperhomocysteinemia, orthostatic hypotension, and cardiac arrhythmias and pharmacologic management. Medications currently being used are similar to Alzheimer's disease. Anticholinergic medications, atypical antipsychotic agents, and antidepressants (eg, selective serotonin reuptake inhibitors) may be useful in some patients [28]. Pentoxifylline has been studied to slow the progression of dementia in patients who meet Diagnostic and Statistical Manual-III criteria for multi-infarct dementia and have clinical and neuroradiologic evidence of cerebrovascular disease [30]. Small open-label studies using rivastigmine, a second-generation acetylcholinesterase inhibitor, have shown improved attention, executive function, and apathy in vascular dementia [31]. Memantine is an N-methyl-D-aspartate receptor antagonist, approved in October 2003 by the US Food and Drug Administration for treatment of moderate to severe Alzheimer's disease. In Alzheimer's disease it has been shown to promote less cognitive deterioration with early benefit on mood and behavior with a low incidence of adverse effects [32]. All of these medications seem to be promising agents in vascular dementia, but their effects need to be established in double-blind, placebo-controlled clinical trials.

Medical issues during stroke rehabilitation

Medical management of the stroke patient goes beyond the acute care period. This is especially true with the recent trend toward earlier discharge from acute care to a rehabilitation facility. The goals during the rehabilitation phase of a stroke patient include (1) ensuring medical stability by implementing secondary stroke prevention measures and controlling risk factors, (2) preventing and treating complications that may increase morbidity and mortality, and (3) promoting neurologic and functional recovery. Ensuring medical stability of a patient demands a thorough review of clinical history, physical examination including a detailed neurologic assessment, laboratory studies, imaging results, and diagnostic testing. Specific treatments should be noted, including use of tissue plasminogen activator or interventional procedures and initiation or discontinuation of medications. Secondary stroke prevention measures, including risk factor modification, pharmacologic management, and surgical management (ie, carotid endarterectomy), should be implemented or confirmed.

Specialized stroke units are associated with better prognosis than general medical units [33]. Effective early management of acute stroke and transient ischemic attack reduces morbidity and mortality and can reduce use of scarce health and social services resources. Stroke-related mortality has decreased in recent years partly because of better risk factor management, the advent of tissue plasminogen activator, and improvement in acute medical management after stroke. Despite this overall reduction in mortality, stroke still remains an important cause of death worldwide. Approximately 20% of first-ever stroke patients die within 30 days. In the first few days, mortality is usually caused by the stroke itself from edema, herniation, or disruption of brainstem centers. Patients who have suffered a stroke remain at an increased risk of recurrent stroke at 30% to

40% within 5 years. An individualized strategy for secondary stroke prevention should be implemented within a maximum of 7 days of acute stroke or transient ischemic attack.

Pneumonia, cardiac disease, and pulmonary embolism are the most frequent causes of death during the first 30 days. Pneumonia may occur in approximately one third of patients, commonly caused by aspiration secondary to dysphagia. All stroke patients should undergo a bedside screening before initiation of oral intake followed by a full bedside swallow study if needed. Cardiac disease after stroke is manifested as myocardial infarction, arrhythmias, or heart failure. Full cardiac work-up should be completed during the acute care of a stroke patient. The incidence of pulmonary embolism after stroke is between 10% and 15%. Its peak is usually during the first week after stroke; initiation of prophylactic measures for deep vein thrombosis should be done as soon as possible. The total duration of prophylaxis is still unknown, because the risk of deep vein thrombosis continues well beyond the first week. Risk factors for deep vein thrombosis should be assessed during the rehabilitation phase and at the time of discharge. It is generally accepted that an ambulation distance of 50 ft per day significantly reduces the risk of deep vein thrombosis after stroke [34]. Contraindications to chemical prophylaxis may warrant mechanical (sequential compression device) or surgical (inferior vena cava filter) interventions.

Recovery after stroke

Early recovery after a stroke is caused by spontaneous mechanisms related to resolution of harmful local factors (ie, local edema, resorption of local toxins, improved local circulation, and resolution of arterial spasm). Motor recovery has been well-described and the most studied of all stroke impairments. The classic paper by Twitchell [35] in 1951 first described the pattern of motor recovery following stroke from a flaccid state to progressive increase in tone. The phases of recovery described by Twitchell [35] were later formalized into stages by Brunnstrom in 1970 [36]. The general pattern of recovery in a classic middle cerebral artery infarction is as follows: (1) proximal recovery occurs before distal; (2) the lower extremity recovers earliest and most completely; and (3) synergy patterns, stereotyped mass movements, occur before isolated, voluntary movements.

Neural plasticity is the potential of the central nervous system to reorganize its structure and function based on the idea that the brain is responsive, flexible, and dynamic. There is modification of neural networks that are use-dependent. After early, spontaneous recovery after stroke, several mechanisms are thought to occur. Bach-Y-Rita [37] described several theories on recovery and neuroplasticity, including collateral sprouting, unmasking, and diaschisis. Regeneration or collateral sprouting describes when a neighboring axon branches to assume the territory of a denervated region or injured axon. Unmasking of pathways is the activation of previously latent pathways when the dominant system fails. There may exist redundant pathways in which there is unmasking of the uninjured parallel pathway. The concept of diaschisis, coined by Constantin Von Monakow in 1914, describes how a site away from the primary injury may be affected when there is loss of neural input from the injured part of brain. Reversal of this process may contribute to neurologic and functional recovery after a stroke [38].

There is a clinical perception that these restorative processes are age-dependent. The question remains whether brain plasticity still exists and to what extent in the aging human brain because most studies have reported on young animals. Animal studies by Popa-Wagner and coworkers [39] report quantitative changes in the hippocampus and qualitative changes in the cortex with increased age. There seems to be a regenerative potential of the aged brain that is competent but attenuated after a stroke. Human studies further evaluate the ability of the aging motor cortex to reorganize. It is now well-known that cortical reorganization underlies functional recovery after a stroke and is elicited by motor training that uses practiced movements. The influence of age on this form of plasticity has been specifically studied by Sawaki and coworkers [40] who found a significant decrease in training-dependent plasticity as a function of age. Further studies are needed to delve into the mechanism and to quantify these changes in the aged brain.

Pharmacologic agents and recovery

An important goal during rehabilitation is to identify and minimize the use of pharmacologic agents that may impede recovery after stroke. Many drugs commonly used to treat new or chronic conditions have central nervous system side effects. Studies in laboratory animals indicate that certain centrally acting drugs (ie, clonidine, prazosin, neuroleptics, and other dopamine receptor antagonists; benzodiazepines; phenytoin; and phenobarbital) impair behavioral recovery after focal brain injury. Even single doses may have long-term harmful effects [41]. Consistent with previous reports, haloperidol retards motor recovery after sensory motor cortex injury in rats. The use of low doses of atypical antipsychotics

Table 2
Clinical practice guidelines for pharmacologic management of stroke patients during rehabilitation

1. Recommend against the use of neuroleptics, benzodiazepines, phenobarbital, and phenytoin during the stroke recovery period. The benefit of these drugs versus the risk of potential adverse effect should be considered.
2. Recommend against centrally acting α_2-adrenergic receptor agonists as antihypertensive medications, such as clonidine, and α_1-receptor antagonists, such as prazosin, as antihypertensive medications. There is a potential to impair recovery in stroke patients.
3. Because there is insufficient evidence on the optimal dosing and safety of neurostimulant agents, no clear recommendation can be made. A trial of neurotransmitter-releasing agents should be considered in patients to improve participation in stroke rehabilitation or to enhance motor recovery.

Adapted from Duncan PW, Zorowitz R, Bates B, et al. Management of adult stroke rehabilitation care: a clinical practice guideline. Stroke 2005;36:e100–43.

provides a safer alternative to haloperidol in the treatment of agitated stroke patients [42]. The Stroke Council of the American Heart Association endorses the clinical practice guidelines for the pharmacologic management of stroke rehabilitation (Table 2) [43].

The practice of neurorehabilitation is unique in that it provides an opportunity to enhance intensive rehabilitation with pharmacologic interventions that facilitate the recovery of damaged neurons and plastic responses in underused and unused brain tissue. Animal studies reveal that norepinephrine, amphetamine, and other α-adrenergic stimulating drugs can enhance motor performance after unilateral ablation of the sensory motor cortex. Although widely used, there are limited data to support the use of neurostimulants in stroke recovery. The most studied in clinical trials is dextroamphetamine, which has been shown both to expedite motor recovery and improve aphasia [44–46]. Other agents commonly used and studied in small controlled trials or case series to treat motor, language, and cognitive-behavioral syndromes include methylphenidate, amantadine, levodopa, selective serotonin reuptake inhibitors, and modafinil [47–53].

General rehabilitation principles in the stroke patient

Stroke rehabilitation begins as soon as the diagnosis of stroke is established. Rehabilitation during the acute phase should be to prevent recurrent stroke, avoid medical complications, mobilize the patient, encourage the resumption of self-care activities, and provide emotional support to the patient and family. During this phase, specific goals may include measures to prevent deep vein thrombosis or pressure sores, to minimize spasticity or contracture, to manage bowel and bladder issues, and to prevent respiratory complications. Therapy involves range-of-motion exercises and bed positioning with progressive increase in intensity as tolerated. A study of 145 patients with first-ever strokes showed better effectiveness on a functional outcome scale, the Barthel Index, with early rehabilitation treatment compared with delayed initiation of services [54]. Pooling the results of nine controlled trials revealed a small, but statistically significant intensity-effect relationship in the rehabilitation of stroke patients [55]. Subsequent studies support higher intensity of upper and lower limb training to improve activities of daily living, walking ability, and dexterity [56]. The general consensus is that greater intensity of rehabilitation produces slightly better outcomes [57]. It is still unknown whether there is a minimum threshold of intensity, below which there is no benefit.

Rehabilitation techniques

There are several rehabilitation models for treatment of central nervous system dysfunction. The basis for the appropriate model and its concomitant goals should be a combined effort of the patient, family, or caregiver, and the multidisciplinary rehabilitation team. The general approach to rehabilitation of a stroke patient may include one or more of the following methods: (1) compensatory strategies; (2) strengthening exercises; (3) facilitation and neurophysiologic techniques (Bobath); and (4) task-oriented approaches. Advanced age should not preclude any of these strategies, including upper- and lower-extremity task-oriented training.

Compensatory strategies

Compensation refers to the use of alternate strategies to complete a task. The initial functional training of a hemiplegic patient should emphasize compensatory strategies. For example, self-care is performed using the unaffected arm and mobility is achieved using a wheelchair. Some experts suggest that compensation is detrimental for the patient because it may lead to "learned nonuse." It is generally believed that there are some compensatory strategies that are necessary for function, whereas others that are detrimental should be avoided.

Strengthening exercises

A decline in general fitness often occurs in the disabled and in the elderly. In randomized trials, progressive resistance exercises performed three to four times weekly for a period of 6 to 12 weeks by patients with adequate motor control improved strength and functional activities [58]. Even in chronic stroke patients, trials show gains in walking ability with progressive aerobic exercises that are tailored to each patient's tolerance [59]. Lower-extremity muscle strength has been correlated with gait speed in stroke patients [60]. Lower-extremity strength has also been inversely correlated with a risk of falling in older post-stroke patients. An appropriate strengthening program can be implemented at a variable point in the rehabilitation process of a stroke patient.

Neurophysiologic and facilitation techniques

The neurodevelopmental training, or Bobath, approach focuses on the progression of movement through inhibition of primitive reflexes and facilitation of higher-level control. With neurodevelopmental training, the stroke patient is encouraged to use the affected side of their body to promote and relearn normal movement and to reduce muscle spasticity. Although widely used, no randomized controlled studies have shown this to be more effective than any other approach to stroke rehabilitation.

Task-oriented retraining

Emerging evidence suggests that new models of task-oriented exercise have the potential to improve motor function even years after stroke. There is evidence supporting the efficacy of task-specific training protocols emphasizing the use of the more affected limb [61]. Constraint-induced movement therapy and body-weight–supported treadmill training use this model of high intensity, task-specific training for the upper and lower extremity, respectively. Protocols for constraint-induced movement therapy are based on the theory of learned nonuse associated with the great effort required to perform tasks with the affected hand [62]. This approach involves intensive task-specific practice with the affected hand for 3 to 6 hours a day over a period of 2 to 6 weeks. The therapy progresses gradually from small approximations to full movement. The protocol may additionally restrain the unaffected hand to force greater use of the affected hand. There are specific inclusion criteria, which greatly limits the application of this training protocol [63]. The clinical benefit of this treatment may be present if initiated early or even 1 year poststroke.

Recovery of walking is a complex phenomenon. Even after significant neurologic improvement, walking requires considerable practice to improve motor control. Body-weight–supported treadmill training uses task-specific training to allow patients to take more steps at faster speeds than may otherwise be feasible. The effectiveness of this therapy is still inconclusive. A recent Cochrane review in 2003 on body-weight–supported treadmill training showed that it may improve walking speed among people with stroke who could walk independently at the start of treatment, but not those who were dependent walkers. There were no statistically significant adverse events, which is an important concern in the elderly who may have cardiac comorbidties [64]. Emerging evidence suggests that new models of task-oriented exercise, including the introduction of robotics, have the potential to improve motor function and cardiovascular health even years after stroke. Still, there is a need for well-designed large-scale studies to evaluate the effects further.

Stroke-related impairments

Dysphagia

Stroke-related dysphagia may cause complications, such as aspiration, dehydration, and nutritional deficiencies. In stroke patients, aspiration usually occurs from dysfunction of the pharyngeal phase of swallowing and is likely to occur without clinical manifestation, called "silent aspiration." Nearly one third of patients with dysphagia have aspiration, which in addition to impaired cough and gag reflex, becomes a major risk factor for pneumonia. Formal evaluation of swallow function and compensatory strategies should be implemented before the initiation of any oral intake. Video fluoroscopic swallow study can reveal delayed initiation of swallow with alteration in pharyngeal transit time.

Elderly patients are particularly susceptible to the effects of dehydration and malnutrition. Dehydration may be due to lowered response, impaired ability to concentrate urine, use of diuretics, or decreased intake due to fear of incontinence. Malnutrition is most commonly related to depression followed by use of medications that decrease appetite. Age-related reduction in laryngeal elevation also increases risk of aspiration.

Aphasia

Communication disorders are present in more than one third of patients, with aphasia being the most common. Aphasia is a disorder of language, typically associated with lesions of the left or dominant hemisphere. It is also recognized that some aspects of language, such as prosody of speech, may be affected if the nondominant side is affected. The Boston School of Aphasia is a commonly used classification system that assesses fluency, comprehension, repetition, and word-finding ability to make a diagnosis. In addition, the Western Aphasia Battery is used to evaluate the severity of the impairment. Generally, the prognosis for recovery is worse for the patient with delayed treatment or with advanced age. Regardless, a speech-language pathologist can provide interventions to maximize recovery and prevent inappropriate compensatory strategies. Another important goal is the education of family, caregivers, and staff on the facilitation of communication to meet the patient's needs. Although drug therapy is unlikely to revolutionize the treatment of aphasia, it may serve to supplement intense treatment or strategies to improve performance. Trials using bromocriptine, amphetamines, piracetam, and donepezil have been promising [46,65–67]. Additional studies are necessary, however, to assess the full potential of aphasia pharmacotherapy. Until then, the initial severity of aphasia timeliness of therapy intervention and age are the main factors influencing speech recovery.

Bowel and bladder

The incidence of bladder incontinence is 50% to 70% during the first month after stroke, but returns to the level of the general population by about 6 months. Supraspinal injury, as in stroke, causes an uninhibited or hyperreflexic bladder that is best treated with a timed voiding schedule. Postvoid residuals should be carefully monitored initially until safe bladder volume can be documented. Urinary retention is much less common, but may require intermittent catheterization initially. The frequency of urinary tract infections increases as a result of prolonged catheter use, alterations in bladder emptying, or reduced fluid intake. Elderly patients may have increased risk of bladder dysfunction due to premorbid bladder incontinence retention from medications, infections or prostatic problems in males. Bladder incontinence can increase skin breakdown, decrease socialization, increase rate of depression, and eventually increase chance of institutionalization. Medication should be used with caution unless previously indicated because of premorbid conditions.

Bowel incontinence occurs in up to one third of patients. Unlike bladder incontinence, bowel dysfunction usually resolves in the first few weeks after stroke. Even more common is bowel impaction. This is usually related to the relative inactivity; decreased nutrition, especially fiber; and diminished fluid intake. Appropriate dietary modifications, the use of regular bowel medications, and progressive increase in activity level can aid in managing bowel dysfunction.

Spasticity

Approximately 65% of individuals develop spasticity after a stroke [68]. In 1980, Lance [69] published this frequently cited definition: "Spasticity is a motor disorder characterized by a velocity-dependent increase in tonic stretch reflexes (muscle tone) with exaggerated tendon jerks, resulting from hyperexcitability of the stretch reflex, as one component of the upper motor neuron syndrome." Treatment should be based on realistic goals for the patient, which may include reducing pain, simplifying activities of daily living, improving hygiene, or improving function. It is notable that some patients do not require treatment because they may rely on their spasticity for improved function (ie, "walk on their tone").

Management of spasticity begins with two fundamental interventions: daily, prolonged stretching program; and avoidance or management of noxious stimuli (ie, ingrown toenail, distended bowel or bladder, pressure sore, or even tight clothing). It was once thought that a step-wise approach should be taken next, consisting of trial of oral medications, then local injections of phenol or botulinum toxin, to surgical options (rhizotomy, orthopedic surgery). The current management for spasticity of cerebral origin now minimizes the role of oral antispasticity agents because there is only mild reduction of spasticity with significant impairment of cognition. Even dantrolene, which is thought to act peripherally, may cause sedation and muscle weakness. The side effects of oral agents may be magnified in the elderly patient. Weight-bearing exercises and serial casting are commonly incorporated in the treatment program. Focal injections with phenol or botulinum toxin can be more effective when appropriately administered. Serial casting can and should be used adjunctively with other spasticity interventions. Intrathecal baclofen pumps are now more widely used for generalized spasticity [70]. Preliminary studies have shown intrathecal baclofen pumps to be effective in improving walking speed and functional mobility in ambulatory stroke patients when combined with physical therapy [71].

Hemiplegic shoulder pain

Hemiplegic shoulder pain is a frequent pain syndrome seen in poststroke patients with a prevalence of 34% to 84%, affecting both motor rehabilitation and psychologic well-being. It interferes with activities of daily living, balance, and ambulation and is associated with poorer outcome and increased length of stay in hospital [72]. Major risk factors for hemiplegic shoulder pain are advanced age, muscle tone changes after stroke, and sidedness of stroke. Age-related changes include decreased range of motion, degenerative changes of the acromioclavicular joint and glenoid labrum, and calcified tendons that may exacerbate the pain condition. Spastic hemiplegic shoulder is more commonly associated with pain compared with a flaccid shoulder because the humeral head is displaced anteriorly, posteriorly, or medially. Still, Tobis [73] in 1957 proposed the "main cause of shoulder pain in hemiplegia is flaccidity." The weight of the unsupported arm stretches the capsule and ligaments causing inferior subluxation. Right-sided lesions are thought to cause increased risk of trauma-related hemiplegic shoulder pain, especially if associated with visuospatial deficits or neglect. The differential diagnosis of hemiplegic shoulder pain may include adhesive capsulitis, rotator cuff tears, neuropathic damage, chronic regional pain syndrome, and musculoskeletal imbalances. Clinical history, palpation, and plain radiographs with arms unsupported are reliable tools in making the diagnosis.

Treatment of hemiplegic shoulder pain starts with proper positioning and handling. There is evidence that hemiplegic shoulder pain increases during the first few weeks following discharge from a hospital, usually because of less skilled transfers, less therapy, and less medications [74]. Early range-of-motion exercises can prevent immobility, spasticity, and contracture. Slings and supports, if used appropriately, can reduce subluxation and protect from trauma; however, they also reduce upper-extremity mobility and sensory feedback, encourage flexor tone, and impair gait and body image. Functional electrical stimulation has been shown to maintain muscle bulk and tone in flaccid shoulder and enhance functional recovery through cortical feedback. More recently, intramuscular neuromuscular electric stimulation has been shown to reduce poststroke shoulder pain with improvement lasting at least 6 months [75]. Oral analgesic medications are limited by their cognitive and sedative side effects, especially in the elderly. Local steroid injections can provide temporary relief, but atrophic effects of repeated injections further weaken the cuff. In chronic regional pain syndrome, sympathetic nerve block of the stellate ganglion may be effective if more conservative measures fail. Botulinum toxin injections have been used to relieve hemiplegic shoulder pain at rest and with range-of-motion in some patients.

Falls

Stroke has been associated with a higher fall risk in both the acute care and rehabilitation settings [76–78]. The incidence of falls has been reported as 14% in acute care [79], 24% during inpatient rehabilitation [78], and 39% in geriatric rehabilitation setting [80]. These numbers are quite dramatic because the number of hospital falls in stroke patients is a strong predictor of falls after discharge. Studies have shown increased age, male gender, visuospatial neglect, right hemisphere strokes, urinary incontinence, bilateral motor involvement, postural instability, impaired activities of daily living, impulsivity, and use of certain medications (ie, diuretics, antidepressants, or sedatives) to be positively associated with fall risk [80–83]. Because rehabilitation has become an increasingly significant part of stroke care and falls are one of the most common complications, there is a unique obligation to work on fall prevention strategies without lowering activity levels. Fall prevention measures begin with a fall assessment screening to identify patients at risk, implementing fall prevention strategies that minimize the use of restraints and sedating medications, and making ongoing reassessments at scheduled intervals. Despite these interventions, falls remain a significant complication after stroke.

Depression

Poststroke depression is a frequent complication after stroke that is associated with a negative impact on rehabilitation and functional recovery [84–87]. Over the years, literature has supported a relationship between stroke and depression with an incidence between 15% and 70%. According to a population-based study, the prevalence of major depression was 25% at hospital discharge, 30% at 3 months after stroke, 16% at 1 year, and 29% at 3 years with a mean age of 73 [88]. The Framingham study reported a 47% incidence of depression at 6 months poststroke with no difference between left- and right-sided lesions [89]. Other studies reported predisposition to depression after left anterior or right posterior infarcts [90]. The pathophysiology is not entirely elucidated and might involve several mechanisms including direct consequences of brain lesions, neuroendocrine mechanism, or even psychologic reaction to the stress or disability. Other causes include damage to left cerebral cortex, proximity of lesion to frontal pole, and premorbid history of a psychiatric disorder. Confounding factors may include medical comorbidities, impaired attention and initiation, or drugs that may depress mood (Table 3).

Treatment should be comprehensive to include patient and caregiver education, therapeutic exercises, psychotherapy, and pharmacologic agents. Counseling during rehabilitation may decrease the risk of depression, especially when directed toward concerns of being a burden on family or society. Several drugs have been shown to be effective in treating depression with a potential benefit of improving short-term motor recovery after stroke [91]. Currently, such drugs as methylphenidate, nortriptyline, citalopram, and fluoxetine are commonly used to treat poststroke depression [92,93].

Table 3
Medications commonly associated with worsening of depressive symptoms

Drug class	Medications
Analgesics	Codeine, propoxyphene
Antihypertensives	Clonidine, reserpine
Hormones	Estrogen, progesterone, prednisone, anabolic steroids
Cardiac medications	Digitalis, propanalol
Anticancer agents	Cycloserine, tamoxifen, vincristine
Parkinson's agents	Levodopa, bromocriptine
Anti-inflammatories	Indomethacin
Anxiolytics	Diazepam, triazolam

The search for depression should be systematic and early to ensure appropriate treatment. The elderly population may already be at high risk for depression because of associated chronic disease. Even more, advanced age is often accompanied by loss of key social support systems because of the death of a spouse or siblings, retirement, or relocation of residence at a time when it is most needed. Older adults with depression are more likely to commit suicide than are younger people with depression. Within 10 years after a stroke, the risk of death is 3.5 times higher in depressed patients than in those without depression [94].

Community and social reintegration

A comprehensive rehabilitation program should include appropriate community and social integration. A history of the patient's prior community activities and interests serves to guide the clinician in planning appropriate measures. The poststroke family support, financial status, and community resources should be evaluated to optimize successful return to the community. There are both physical and cognitive benefits associated with community participation. It has been shown that participation in physical activities can improve a patient's balance, decrease anxiety and depression, assist with pain management, and increase one's ability to maintain functional independence [95]. There is also a potential decreased risk of dementia with certain leisure activities [96].

The ability to drive is a vital aspect of maintaining functional independence in the community. Although many older adults voluntarily stop driving, there are still several elderly patients who wish to resume. The elderly are the fastest growing segment of the driving population. A person's crash risk per mile increases starting at age 55, exceeding that of a young, beginning driver by age 80 [97]. The effect of adding disability to these statistics is obvious. Counseling patients about their new disability and discussing alternative options may be appropriate. Driving assessment can be coordinated through a multidisciplinary driver's rehabilitation program, which may include an assessment of vision, attention, hearing, visuospatial skills, and motor function, followed by a behind-the-wheel assessment [98]. Opinions on driving fitness may be required by the physician; current licensing policies, liability, and reporting procedures for potentially ineligible drivers should be reviewed for each state [99].

Summary

Because only thrombolytics have been demonstrated to be effective in minimizing brain damage and maximizing functional outcome, intensive rehabilitation remains the most significant means by which stroke survivors may recover. Previously, the rehabilitation approach to the older stroke patient was supportive and focused on prevention of complications while spontaneous recovery occurs. Now, even these older stroke patients are undergoing relatively aggressive rehabilitation with good outcomes in morbidity, mortality, and function. In addition, the quality of life of these individuals is significantly improved. The recently published National Service Framework for Older People specifically highlights the importance of preventing age discrimination, encouraging respect and dignity, and promoting general health and well-being to ensure a well-coordinated approach to providing services that address conditions that are significant for older people. The Stroke Treatment and Ongoing Prevention Act is currently in the approval process with the 109th Congress, which will provide resources to improve stroke education, research, and patient care. In the meantime, it is important for clinicians to understand the current state of stroke rehabilitation so they can continue to provide quality care and improve outcomes.

Acknowledgments

The author acknowledges the assistance of Richard L. Harvey, MD, and the staff at the Rehabilitation Institute of Chicago for their support in preparation of this article.

References

[1] Di Carlo A, Lamassa M, Pracucci G, et al. Stroke in the very old: clinical presentation and determinants of 3-month functional outcome: a European perspective. European BIOMED Study of Stroke Care Group. Stroke 1999;30:2313–9.
[2] Ergeletzis D, Kevorkian CG, Rintala D. Rehabilitation of the older stroke patient: functional outcome and comparison with younger patients. Am J Phys Med Rehabil 2002;81:881–9.
[3] Lieberman D, Lieberman D. Rehabilitation following stroke in patients aged 85 and above. J Rehabil Res Dev 2005;42:47–54.
[4] Paolucci S, Antonucci G, Troisi E, et al. Aging and stroke rehabilitation. a case-comparison study. Cerebrovasc Dis 2003;15:98–105.
[5] Bronner LL, Kanter DS, Manson JE. Primary prevention of stroke. N Engl J Med 1995;333: 1392–400.
[6] Brown RD, Whisnant JP, Sicks JD, et al. Stroke incidence, prevalence, and survival: secular trends in Rochester, Minnesota, through 1989. Stroke 1996;27:373–80.
[7] Wolf PA, D'Agostino RB, O'Neal MA, et al. Secular trends in stroke incidence and mortality. The Framingham Study. Stroke 1992;23:1551–5.
[8] Goldstein LB, Adams R, Becker K, et al. Primary prevention of ischemic stroke: aA statement for healthcare professionals from the Stroke Council of the American Heart Association. Stroke 2001;32:280–99.
[9] Lamassa M, Di Carlo A, Pracucci G, et al. Characteristics, outcome, and care of stroke associated with atrial fibrillation in Europe: data from a multicenter multinational hospital-based registry (The European Community Stroke Project). Stroke 2001;32:392–8.
[10] Shepherd J, Blauw GJ, Murphy MB, et al. Pravastatin in elderly individuals at risk of vascular disease (PROSPER): a randomised controlled trial. Lancet 2002;360:1623–30.
[11] Collins R, Armitage J, Parish S, et al. Effects of cholesterol-lowering with simvastatin on stroke and other major vascular events in 20536 people with cerebrovascular disease or other high-risk conditions. Lancet 2004;363:757–67.
[12] Sacks FM, Pfeffer MA, Moye LA, et al. The effect of pravastatin on coronary events after

myocardial infarction in patients with average cholesterol levels. Cholesterol and Recurrent Events Trial investigators. N Engl J Med 1996;335:1001−9.

[13] Schatz IJ, Masaki K, Yano K, et al. Cholesterol and all-cause mortality in elderly people from the Honolulu Heart Program: a cohort study. Lancet 2001;358:351−5.

[14] Muldoon MF, Barger SD, Ryan CM, et al. Effects of lovastatin on cognitive function and psychological well-being. Am J Med 2000;108:538−46.

[15] Muldoon MF, Waldstein SR, Ryan CM, et al. Effects of six anti-hypertensive medications on cognitive performance. J Hypertens 2002;20:1643−52.

[16] King DS, Wilburn AJ, Wofford MR, et al. Cognitive impairment associated with atorvastatin and simvastatin. Pharmacotherapy 2003;23:1663−7.

[17] Orsi A, Sherman O, Woldeselassie Z. Simvastatin-associated memory loss. Pharmacotherapy 2001;21:767−9.

[18] Wagstaff LR, Mitton MW, Arvik BM, et al. Statin-associated memory loss: analysis of 60 case reports and review of the literature. Pharmacotherapy 2003;23:871−80.

[19] Ben-Shlomo Y, Markowe H, Shipley M, et al. Stroke risk from alcohol consumption using different control groups. Stroke 1992;23:1093−8.

[20] Camargo Jr CA, Hennekens CH, Gaziano JM, et al. Prospective study of moderate alcohol consumption and mortality in US male physicians. Arch Intern Med 1997;157:79−85.

[21] Stampfer MJ, Colditz GA, Willett WC, et al. A prospective study of moderate alcohol consumption and the risk of coronary disease and stroke in women. N Engl J Med 1988;319:267−73.

[22] Fried LP, Kronmal RA, Newman AB, et al. Risk factors for 5-year mortality in older adults: the Cardiovascular Health Study. JAMA 1998;279:585−92.

[23] Malmivaara A, Heliovaara M, Knekt P, et al. Risk factors for injurious falls leading to hospitalization or death in a cohort of 19,500 adults. Am J Epidemiol 1993;138:384−94.

[24] Green D. Thrombophilia and stroke. Top Stroke Rehabil 2003;10:21−33.

[25] Tamura T, Aiso K, Johnston KE, et al. Homocysteine, folate, vitamin B-12 and vitamin B-6 in patients receiving antiepileptic drug monotherapy. Epilepsy Res 2000;40:7−15.

[26] Coull BM, Malinow MR, Beamer N, et al. Elevated plasma homocyst(e)ine concentration as a possible independent risk factor for stroke. Stroke 1990;21:572−6.

[27] Spence JD, Howard VJ, Chambless LE, et al. Vitamin Intervention for Stroke Prevention (VISP) trial: rationale and design. Neuroepidemiology 2001;20:16−25.

[28] Roman GC. Vascular dementia revisited: diagnosis, pathogenesis, treatment, and prevention. Med Clin North Am 2002;86:477−99.

[29] Schut LJ. Dementia following stroke. Clin Geriatr Med 1988;4:767−84.

[30] Black RS, Barclay LL, Nolan KA, et al. Pentoxifylline in cerebrovascular dementia. J Am Geriatr Soc 1992;40:237−44.

[31] Roman GC. Rivastigmine for subcortical vascular dementia. Expert Rev Neurother 2005;5:309−13.

[32] Areosa Sastre A, McShane R, Sherriff F. Memantine for dementia. Cochrane Database Syst Rev 2004;4:CD003154.

[33] Indredavik B, Bakke F, Solberg R, et al. Benefit of a stroke unit: a randomized controlled trial. Stroke 1991;22:1026−31.

[34] Reding MJ, Potes E. Rehabilitation outcome following initial unilateral hemispheric stroke: life table analysis approach. Stroke 1988;19:1354−8.

[35] Twitchell TE. The restoration of motor function following hemiplegia in man. Brain 1951;74:443−80.

[36] Brunnstrom S. Movement therapy in hemiplegia: a neurophysiological approach. Philadelphia (PA): Harper and Row; 1970.

[37] Bach y Rita P. Central nervous system lesions: sprouting and unmasking in rehabilitation. Arch Phys Med Rehabil 1981;62:413−7.

[38] Seitz RJ, Azari NP, Knorr U, et al. The role of diaschisis in stroke recovery. Stroke 1999;30:1844−50.

[39] Popa-Wagner A, Schroder E, Schmoll H, et al. Upregulation of MAP1B and MAP2 in the rat brain after middle cerebral artery occlusion: effect of age. J Cereb Blood Flow Metab 1999;19: 425–34.

[40] Sawaki L, Yaseen Z, Kopylev L, et al. Age-dependent changes in the ability to encode a novel elementary motor memory. Ann Neurol 2003;53:521–4.

[41] Goldstein LB. Common drugs may influence motor recovery after stroke. The Sygen In Acute Stroke Study Investigators. Neurology 1995;45:865–71.

[42] Goldstein LB, Bullman S. Differential effects of haloperidol and clozapine on motor recovery after sensorimotor cortex injury in rats. Neurorehabil Neural Repair 2002;16:321–5.

[43] Duncan PW, Zorowitz R, Bates B, et al. Management of adult stroke rehabilitation care: a clinical practice guideline. Stroke 2005;36:e100–43.

[44] Crisostomo EA, Duncan PW, Propst M, et al. Evidence that amphetamine with physical therapy promotes recovery of motor function in stroke patients. Ann Neurol 1988;23:94–7.

[45] Sonde L, Nordstrom M, Nilsson CG, et al. A double-blind placebo-controlled study of the effects of amphetamine and physiotherapy after stroke. Cerebrovasc Dis 2001;12:253–7.

[46] Walker-Batson D, Curtis S, Natarajan R, et al. A double-blind, placebo-controlled study of the use of amphetamine in the treatment of aphasia. Stroke 2001;32:2093–8.

[47] Smith BW. Modafinil for treatment of cognitive side effects of antiepileptic drugs in a patient with seizures and stroke. Epilepsy Behav 2003;4:352–3.

[48] Grade C, Redford B, Chrostowski J, et al. Methylphenidate in early poststroke recovery: a double-blind, placebo-controlled study. Arch Phys Med Rehabil 1998;79:1047–50.

[49] Scheidtmann K, Fries W, Muller F, et al. Effect of levodopa in combination with physiotherapy on functional motor recovery after stroke: a prospective, randomised, double-blind study. Lancet 2001;358:787–90.

[50] Pariente J, Loubinoux I, Carel C, et al. Fluoxetine modulates motor performance and cerebral activation of patients recovering from stroke. Ann Neurol 2001;50:718–29.

[51] Pleger B, Schwenkreis P, Grunberg C, et al. Fluoxetine facilitates use-dependent excitability of human primary motor cortex. Clin Neurophysiol 2004;115:2157–63.

[52] Bassetti CL. Sleep and stroke. Semin Neurol 2005;25:19–32.

[53] Greener J, Enderby P, Whurr R. Pharmacological treatment for aphasia following stroke. Cochrane Database Syst Rev 2001;4:CD000424.

[54] Paolucci S, Antonucci G, Grasso MG, et al. Early versus delayed inpatient stroke rehabilitation: a matched comparison conducted in Italy. Arch Phys Med Rehabil 2000;81:695–700.

[55] Kwakkel G, Wagenaar RC, Koelman TW, et al. Effects of intensity of rehabilitation after stroke: a research synthesis. Stroke 1997;28:1550–6.

[56] Kwakkel G, Wagenaar RC, Twisk JW, et al. Intensity of leg and arm training after primary middle-cerebral-artery stroke: a randomised trial. Lancet 1999;354:191–6.

[57] Langhorne P, Wagenaar R, Partridge C. Physiotherapy after stroke: more is better? Physiother Res Int 1996;1:75–88.

[58] Patten C, Lexell J, Brown HE. Weakness and strength training in persons with poststroke hemiplegia: rationale, method, and efficacy. J Rehabil Res Dev 2004;41:293–312.

[59] Saunders DH, Greig CA, Young A, et al. Physical fitness training for stroke patients. Cochrane Database Syst Rev 2004;1:CD003316.

[60] Bohannon RW, Walsh S. Nature, reliability, and predictive value of muscle performance measures in patients with hemiparesis following stroke. Arch Phys Med Rehabil 1992;73:721–5.

[61] Page SJ. Intensity versus task-specificity after stroke: how important is intensity? Am J Phys Med Rehabil 2003;82:730–2.

[62] Wolf SL, Blanton S, Baer H, et al. Repetitive task practice: a critical review of constraint-induced movement therapy in stroke. Neurologist 2002;8:325–38.

[63] Grotta JC, Noser EA, Ro T, et al. Constraint-induced movement therapy. Stroke 2004;35(Suppl 1): 2699–701.

[64] Moseley AM, Stark A, Cameron ID, et al. Treadmill training and body weight support for walking after stroke. Cochrane Database Syst Rev 2003;3:CD002840.

[65] Albert ML, Bachman DL, Morgan A, et al. Pharmacotherapy for aphasia. Neurology 1988;38: 877–9.

[66] Enderby P, Broeckx J, Hospers W, et al. Effect of piracetam on recovery and rehabilitation after stroke: a double-blind, placebo-controlled study. Clin Neuropharmacol 1994;17:320–31.

[67] Berthier ML. Poststroke aphasia: epidemiology, pathophysiology and treatment. Drugs Aging 2005;22:163–82.

[68] McGuire JR, Harvey RL. The prevention and management of complications after stroke. Phys Med Rehabil Clin N Am 1999;10:857–74.

[69] Lance JW. Symposium synopsis. Chicago: Year Book Medical; 1980.

[70] Francisco GE, Hu MM, Boake C, et al. Efficacy of early use of intrathecal baclofen therapy for treating spastic hypertonia due to acquired brain injury. Brain Inj 2005;19:359–64.

[71] Francisco GE, Boake C. Improvement in walking speed in poststroke spastic hemiplegia after intrathecal baclofen therapy: a preliminary study. Arch Phys Med Rehabil 2003;84:1194–9.

[72] Roy CW, Sands MR, Hill LD, et al. The effect of shoulder pain on outcome of acute hemi-plegia. Clin Rehabil 1995;9:21–7.

[73] Tobis JS. Posthemiplegic shoulder pain. N Y State J Med 1957;57:1377–80.

[74] Wanklyn P, Forster A, Young J. Hemiplegic shoulder pain (HSP): natural history and investigation of associated features. Disabil Rehabil 1996;18:497–501.

[75] Yu DT, Chae J, Walker ME, et al. Intramuscular neuromuscular electric stimulation for post-stroke shoulder pain: a multicenter randomized clinical trial. Arch Phys Med Rehabil 2004;85: 695–704.

[76] Mayo NE, Korner-Bitensky N, Becker R, et al. Predicting falls among patients in a rehabilitation hospital. Am J Phys Med Rehabil 1989;68:139–46.

[77] Salgado R, Lord SR, Packer J, et al. Factors associated with falling in elderly hospital patients. Gerontology 1994;40:325–31.

[78] Vlahov D, Myers AH, al-Ibrahim MS. Epidemiology of falls among patients in a rehabilitation hospital. Arch Phys Med Rehabil 1990;71:8–12.

[79] Tutuarima JA, van der Meulen JH, de Haan RJ, et al. Risk factors for falls of hospitalized stroke patients. Stroke 1997;28:297–301.

[80] Nyberg L, Gustafson Y. Fall prediction index for patients in stroke rehabilitation. Stroke 1997; 28:716–21.

[81] Byers V, Arrington ME, Finstuen K. Predictive risk factors associated with stroke patient falls in acute care settings. J Neurosci Nurs 1990;22:147–54.

[82] Nyberg L, Gustafson Y. Patient falls in stroke rehabilitation: a challenge to rehabilitation strate-gies. Stroke 1995;26:838–42.

[83] Rapport LJ, Webster JS, Flemming KL, et al. Predictors of falls among right-hemisphere stroke patients in the rehabilitation setting. Arch Phys Med Rehabil 1993;74:621–6.

[84] Parikh RM, Lipsey JR, Robinson RG, et al. A two year longitudinal study of poststroke mood disorders: prognostic factors related to one and two year outcome. Int J Psychiatry Med 1988; 18:45–56.

[85] Robinson RG, Lipsey JR, Rao K, et al. Two-year longitudinal study of post-stroke mood dis-orders: comparison of acute-onset with delayed-onset depression. Am J Psychiatry 1986;143: 1238–44.

[86] Robinson RG, Starr LB, Kubos KL, et al. A two-year longitudinal study of post-stroke mood disorders: findings during the initial evaluation. Stroke 1983;14:736–41.

[87] Robinson RG, Starr LB, Lipsey JR, et al. A two-year longitudinal study of post-stroke mood disorders: dynamic changes in associated variables over the first six months of follow-up. Stroke 1984;15:510–7.

[88] Astrom M, Adolfsson R, Asplund K. Major depression in stroke patients: a 3-year longitudinal study. Stroke 1993;24:976–82.

[89] Kase CS, Wolf PA, Kelly-Hayes M, et al. Intellectual decline after stroke: the Framingham Study. Stroke 1998;29:805–12.

[90] Robinson RG, Kubos KL, Starr LB, et al. Mood disorders in stroke patients: importance of location of lesion. Brain 1984;107(Pt 1):81–93.

[91] Robinson RG, Schultz SK, Castillo C, et al. Nortriptyline versus fluoxetine in the treatment of depression and in short-term recovery after stroke: a placebo-controlled, double-blind study. Am J Psychiatry 2000;157:351–9.

[92] Lazarus LW, Moberg PJ, Langsley PR, et al. Methylphenidate and nortriptyline in the treatment of poststroke depression: a retrospective comparison. Arch Phys Med Rehabil 1994;75:403–6.

[93] Andersen G, Vestergaard K, Lauritzen L. Effective treatment of poststroke depression with the selective serotonin reuptake inhibitor citalopram. Stroke 1994;25:1099–104.

[94] Raj A. Depression in the elderly: tailoring medical therapy to their special needs. Postgrad Med 2004;115:26–8, 37–42.

[95] Bean JF, Vora A, Frontera WR. Benefits of exercise for community-dwelling older adults. Arch Phys Med Rehabil 2004;85(7 Suppl 3):S31 [quiz: S3–4].

[96] Verghese J, Lipton RB, Katz MJ, et al. Leisure activities and the risk of dementia in the elderly. N Engl J Med 2003;348:2508–16.

[97] Waller PF. Alcohol, aging, and driving. In: Gomberg ESL, Hegedus AM, Zucker RA, editors. Alcohol problems and aging. NIAAA Research Monograph No.33. Bethesda: NIAAA; 1998.

[98] Carr DB. The older adult driver. Am Fam Physician 2000;61:141–6, 8.

[99] Kelly R, Warke T, Steele I. Medical restrictions to driving: the awareness of patients and doctors. Postgrad Med J 1999;75:537–9.

ELSEVIER
SAUNDERS

Clin Geriatr Med 22 (2006) 491–497

CLINICS IN
GERIATRIC
MEDICINE

Index

Note: Page numbers of article titles are in **bold face** type.

0749-0690/06/$ – see front matter © 2006 Elsevier Inc. All rights reserved.
doi:10.1016/S0749-0690(06)00010-3

geriatric.theclinics.com

Changing Your Address?

Make sure your subscription changes too! When you notify us of your new address, you can help make our job easier by including an exact copy of your Clinics label number with your old address (see illustration below.) This number identifies you to our computer system and will speed the processing of your address change. Please be sure this label number accompanies your old address and your corrected address—you can send an old Clinics label with your number on it or just copy it exactly and send it to the address listed below.

We appreciate your help in our attempt to give you continuous coverage. Thank you.

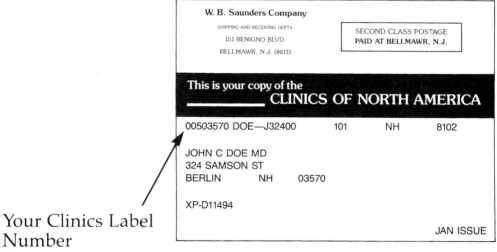

Your Clinics Label Number

Copy it exactly or send your label along with your address to:
W.B. Saunders Company, Customer Service
Orlando, FL 32887-4800
Call Toll Free 1-800-654-2452

Please allow four to six weeks for delivery of new subscriptions and for processing address changes.